An Evolutionary and Environmental Perspective of the Interaction of Nanomaterials with the Immune System-The Outcomes of the EU Project PANDORA

An Evolutionary and Environmental Perspective of the Interaction of Nanomaterials with the Immune System-The Outcomes of the EU Project PANDORA

Editor

Diana Boraschi

MDPI • Basel • Beijing • Wuhan • Barcelona • Belgrade • Manchester • Tokyo • Cluj • Tianjin

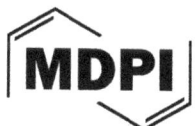

Editor
Diana Boraschi
National Research Council
Italy

Editorial Office
MDPI
St. Alban-Anlage 66
4052 Basel, Switzerland

This is a reprint of articles from the Special Issue published online in the open access journal *Nanomaterials* (ISSN 2079-4991) (available at: https://www.mdpi.com/journal/nanomaterials/special_issues/Immune_PANDORA).

For citation purposes, cite each article independently as indicated on the article page online and as indicated below:

LastName, A.A.; LastName, B.B.; LastName, C.C. Article Title. *Journal Name* **Year**, *Volume Number*, Page Range.

ISBN 978-3-0365-3947-8 (Hbk)
ISBN 978-3-0365-3948-5 (PDF)

Cover image courtesy of Diana Boraschi
SEM image of human monocytes in a collagen matrix; from Imaging Facility of Stazione Zoologica Anton Dohrn, Napoli, Italy.

© 2022 by the authors. Articles in this book are Open Access and distributed under the Creative Commons Attribution (CC BY) license, which allows users to download, copy and build upon published articles, as long as the author and publisher are properly credited, which ensures maximum dissemination and a wider impact of our publications.

The book as a whole is distributed by MDPI under the terms and conditions of the Creative Commons license CC BY-NC-ND.

Contents

About the Editor ix

Preface to "An Evolutionary and Environmental Perspective of the Interaction of
Nanomaterials with the Immune System-The Outcomes of the EU Project PANDORA" xi

Diana Boraschi
An Evolutionary and Environmental Perspective of the Interaction of Nanomaterials with the
Immune System
Reprinted from: *Nanomaterials* 2022, 12, 957, doi:10.3390/nano12060957 1

Lena M. Ernst, Eudald Casals, Paola Italiani, Diana Boraschi and Victor Puntes
The Interactions between Nanoparticles and the Innate Immune System from a
Nanotechnologist Perspective
Reprinted from: *Nanomaterials* 2021, 11, 2991, doi:10.3390/nano11112991 5

**Eleonora Ferrari, Francesco Barbero, Marti Busquets-Fité, Mirita Franz-Wachtel,
Heinz-R. Köhler, Victor Puntes and Birgit Kemmerling**
Growth-Promoting Gold Nanoparticles Decrease Stress Responses in Arabidopsis Seedlings
Reprinted from: *Nanomaterials* 2021, 11, 3161, doi:10.3390/nano11123161 25

**Natividad Isabel Navarro Pacheco, Radka Roubalova, Jaroslav Semerad, Alena Grasserova,
Oldrich Benada, Olga Kofronova, Tomas Cajthaml, Jiri Dvorak, Martin Bilej
and Petra Prochazkova**
In Vitro Interactions of TiO_2 Nanoparticles with Earthworm Coelomocytes:
Immunotoxicity Assessment
Reprinted from: *Nanomaterials* 2021, 11, 250, doi:10.3390/nano11010250 49

**Craig Mayall, Andraz Dolar, Anita Jemec Kokalj, Sara Novak, Jaka Razinger,
Francesco Barbero, Victor Puntes and Damjana Drobne**
Stressor-Dependant Changes in Immune Parameters in the Terrestrial Isopod Crustacean,
Porcellio scaber: A Focus on Nanomaterials
Reprinted from: *Nanomaterials* 2021, 11, 934, doi:10.3390/nano11040934 65

**Manon Auguste, Craig Mayall, Francesco Barbero, Matej Hočevar, Stefano Alberti,
Giacomo Grassi, Victor F. Puntes, Damjana Drobne and Laura Canesi**
Functional and Morphological Changes Induced in *Mytilus* Hemocytes
by Selected Nanoparticles
Reprinted from: *Nanomaterials* 2021, 11, 470, doi:10.3390/nano11020470 83

**Riccardo Catalano, Jérôme Labille, Daniela Gaglio, Andi Alijagic, Elisabetta Napodano,
Danielle Slomberg, Andrea Campos and Annalisa Pinsino**
Safety Evaluation of TiO_2 Nanoparticle-Based Sunscreen UV Filters on the Development and
the Immunological State of the Sea Urchin *Paracentrotus lividus*
Reprinted from: *Nanomaterials* 2020, 10, 2102, doi:10.3390/nano10112102 99

**Elmer Swart, Jiri Dvorak, Szabolcs Hernádi, Tim Goodall, Peter Kille, David Spurgeon,
Claus Svendsen and Petra Prochazkova**
The Effects of In Vivo Exposure to Copper Oxide Nanoparticles on the Gut Microbiome, Host
Immunity, and Susceptibility to a Bacterial Infection in Earthworms
Reprinted from: *Nanomaterials* 2020, 10, 1337, doi:10.3390/nano10071337 115

Rujiu Hu, Haojing Liu, Mimi Wang, Jing Li, Hua Lin, Mingyue Liang, Yupeng Gao and Mingming Yang
An OMV-Based Nanovaccine Confers Safety and Protection against Pathogenic *Escherichia coli* via Both Humoral and Predominantly Th1 Immune Responses in Poultry
Reprinted from: *Nanomaterials* **2020**, *10*, 2293, doi:10.3390/nano10112293 . . . . **137**

Mayra M. Ferrari Barbosa, Alex Issamu Kanno, Leonardo Paiva Farias, Mariusz Madej, Gergö Sipos, Silverio Sbrana, Luigina Romani, Diana Boraschi, Luciana C. C. Leite and Paola Italiani
Primary and Memory Response of Human Monocytes to Vaccines: Role of Nanoparticulate Antigens in Inducing Innate Memory
Reprinted from: *Nanomaterials* **2021**, *11*, 931, doi:10.3390/nano11040931 . . . . **157**

Benjamin J. Swartzwelter, Craig Mayall, Andi Alijagic, Francesco Barbero, Eleonora Ferrari, Szabolcs Hernadi, Sara Michelini, Natividad Isabel Navarro Pacheco, Alessandra Prinelli, Elmer Swart and Manon Auguste
Cross-Species Comparisons of Nanoparticle Interactions with Innate Immune Systems: A Methodological Review
Reprinted from: *Nanomaterials* **2021**, *11*, 1528, doi:10.3390/nano11061528 . . . . **173**

About the Editor

Diana Boraschi is an immunologist who built her experience in academic institutions and industrial settings in her home country (Italy) and abroad. She is Senior Associate Researcher at the Italian National Research Council and at the Stazione Zoologica Anton Dohrn in Napoli, Italy. She is currently serving as Director of the Center of Immunology and Biomaterials at the Shenzhen Institute of Advanced Technologies (SIAT) of the Chinese Academy of Sciences and as Distinguished Professor at the Department of Pharmacology SIAT in Shenzhen, China. She is the author of over 200 research articles in immunology (h-index 62, over 13500 citations). She is closely involved in higher education training activities in Europe, Asia, Africa, and South America, with a focus on poverty-related diseases. In 2017, she received an honorary PhD degree from the University of Salzburg (Austria). Her area of expertise is innate immunity and inflammation, with a particular focus on macrophages and cytokines of the IL-1 superfamily and the interaction of engineered nanomaterials with immunity in humans and environmental species.

Preface to "An Evolutionary and Environmental Perspective of the Interaction of Nanomaterials with the Immune System-The Outcomes of the EU Project PANDORA"

This book collects scientific contributions aiming to describe the mechanism common to all living species by which innate immunity interacts with nanomaterials. The overall goal is to harness such interactions for improving environmental and human safety and exploiting them for modulating immunity in vaccination strategies.

Most of the studies gathered here are the results of a successful collaboration effort across Europe, funded by the Horizon 2020 project PANDORA. The PANDORA scientists wish to dedicate this book to Valeria Matranga, a rigorous scientist and a good friend. Although Valeria left us at the very beginning of the PANDORA project, we have always kept in mind her approach to being a scientist.

Diana Boraschi
Editor

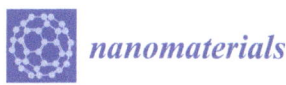

Editorial

An Evolutionary and Environmental Perspective of the Interaction of Nanomaterials with the Immune System

Diana Boraschi [1,2,3]

1. Institute of Biochemistry and Cell Biology (IBBC), National Research Council (CNR), 80131 Napoli, Italy; diana.boraschi@ibbc.cnr.it
2. Shenzhen Institute of Advanced Technology (SIAT), Chinese Academy of Sciences (CAS), Shenzhen 518055, China
3. Stazione Zoologica Anton Dohrn, 80121 Napoli, Italy

Assessing the modes of interaction between engineered nanomaterials and the immune system is a topic of particular interest for research in several fields, from a toxicological and safety perspective to potential nano-based immunomodulatory strategies for medical use. This Special Issue gathers results and new information—mostly collected within the EU Horizon 2020 project PANDORA (probing the safety of nano-objects by defining the immune responses of environmental organisms), which specifically focuses on nano-immune interaction across living organisms, from plants to human beings. The underlying concept is that several of the immune defensive mechanisms used for tackling exogenous agents (including nanomaterials) are conserved across evolution with little modification. Thus, we looked for common mechanisms of recognition and reaction, based on the high evolutionary conservation of innate immunity, the ancient and highly efficient defensive system shared by all living organisms [1]. We wanted to find answers to the following questions:

1. Do nanomaterials pose threats to the organisms' integrity or do the immune defensive mechanisms successfully deal with them?
2. Can we exploit our understanding of nano-immune interactions to devise nano-based tools to improve immune responses in vaccination?
3. Can we identify immune rections that are common across living organisms, and therefore we can use for a general nanosafety assessment of environmental and human health?

First question: **are nanomaterials seen by the immune system as a threat?** Yes, in some cases, in that the innate immune system, in particular phagocytes, can "see" the nanomaterials and begin action to eliminate the nanomaterials and maintain the organism's functionality. Most interestingly, we should also consider the inverse interaction, i.e., how nanomaterials "see" the immune system and are modified by their interaction with it [2]. Notably, upon interaction, we can even observe beneficial biological effects, as in the case of decreased stress responses and growth promotion in the model plant *Arabidopsis thaliana* [3]. In many other cases, it is possible to observe an immune reaction, with morphological and functional changes in innate immune cells; however, these changes are not long-lasting and do not hamper the organism's integrity. This means that a successful immune reaction has taken place, which has recognised the nanomaterials as a possible threat and has acted to eliminate them and re-establish normal tissue/organism functions [4–7]. A very important point that should be considered is that exposure to nanomaterials may affect immunity indirectly by interacting with immune-modulating entities. In particular, when nanomaterials are ingested, the interaction of nanomaterials with the resident microbiota must be considered, as microbiota are well known to shape intestinal and systemic immunity [8].

Second question: **can we use our knowledge of nano-immune interactions for designing "smart" nano-based vaccines?** The use of nanoparticles is a very promising

Citation: Boraschi, D. An Evolutionary and Environmental Perspective of the Interaction of Nanomaterials with the Immune System. *Nanomaterials* **2022**, *12*, 957. https://doi.org/10.3390/nano12060957

Received: 13 February 2022
Accepted: 7 March 2022
Published: 14 March 2022

Publisher's Note: MDPI stays neutral with regard to jurisdictional claims in published maps and institutional affiliations.

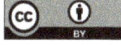

Copyright: © 2022 by the author. Licensee MDPI, Basel, Switzerland. This article is an open access article distributed under the terms and conditions of the Creative Commons Attribution (CC BY) license (https://creativecommons.org/licenses/by/4.0/).

approach to vaccination because the particles may double their scope by acting as a carrier for the vaccine antigens, being able to shuttle them preferentially to antigen-presenting cells while being active as an adjuvant, i.e., they are able to induce an innate/inflammatory response that is necessary for the optimal induction of a specific long-lasting immunity [9]. Two aspects have been considered here: the induction of a specific anti-infective protective immunity in poultry [10] and the possibility of modulating innate memory in human innate cells towards a more protective secondary response, thereby generating not only adaptive memory (resulting in enhanced secondary specific response) but also innate memory (i.e., a long-lasting amplification of the specific response) [11]. In both cases, nanoparticles derived from bacterial cells were used, and were able to act both as antigen carriers and adjuvant particles.

Third question: **can we design common assays that enable us to assess the cross-species effects of nanomaterials on immunity** (i.e., valid for both environmental species and human beings)? To this end, we have compared the most representative methods for evaluating immune reactivity across species in order to identify common conserved innate immune responses activated by interaction with nanomaterials. Excluding plants, whose extreme specialisation also impacts the type of immune defensive tools and responses, we have compiled a list of common assays, both in vivo and in vitro, that can be used to evaluate a response to nanomaterials (in terms, for instance, of safety) across animal species [12–14]. Notably, this implies that we can use some invertebrate models in vivo for predicting the effects of nanomaterials on human innate immunity [14].

To conclude, by examining immune response to nanomaterials across living organisms we have observed that immunity is, in general, able to cope with the nano-challenge and prevent detrimental effects to the organism. Both environmental species (marine and terrestrial invertebrates) and human beings display an array of common defensive mechanisms that are engaged in the interaction with nanomaterials, which allows us to identify model assays (in vivo and in vitro) which are predictive of nano-effects across species, making them useful for both environmental and human nano-safety testing. By evaluating nano-effects on the immune system, we can design nano-based vaccination strategies that exploit the immunomodulatory capacity of nanomaterials to achieve optimal long-term protective immunity.

Funding: This research was funded by the EU Commission H2020 project PANDORA (GA 671881) and by the Presidential International Fellowship Programme (PIFI) of CAS (2020VBA0028).

Acknowledgments: The author is grateful to all the PANDORA partners for their enthusiastic and active collaboration. Special thanks to Giuliana Donini for her relentless support of this project.

Conflicts of Interest: The author declares no conflict of interest.

References

1. Pinsino, A.; Bastús, N.G.; Busquets-Fité, M.; Canesi, L.; Cesaroni, P.; Drobne, D.; Duschl, A.; Ewart, M.-A.; Gispert, I.; Horejs-Höck, J.; et al. Probing the immunological responses to nanoparticles across environmental species: A perspective of the EU-funded PANDORA project. *Environ. Sci. Nano* **2020**, *7*, 3216–3232. [CrossRef]
2. Ernst, L.M.; Casals, E.; Italiani, P.; Boraschi, D.; Puntes, V. The interaction between nanoparticles and the innate immune system from a nanotechnologist perspective. *Nanomaterials* **2021**, *11*, 2991. [CrossRef] [PubMed]
3. Ferrari, E.; Barbero, F.; Busquet-Fité, M.; Franz-Wachtel, M.; Köhler, H.-R.; Puntes, V.; Kemmerling, B. Growth-promoting gold nanoparticles decrease stress responses in *Arabidopsis thaliana* seedlings. *Nanomaterials* **2021**, *11*, 3161. [CrossRef] [PubMed]
4. Navarro Pacheco, N.I.; Roubalova, R.; Semerad, J.; Grasserova, A.; Benada, O.; Kofronova, O.; Cajthmi, T.; Dvorak, J.; Bilej, M.; Prochazkova, P. In vitro interactions of TiO_2 nanoparticles with earthworm coelomocytes: Immunotoxicity assessment. *Nanomaterials* **2021**, *11*, 250. [CrossRef] [PubMed]
5. Mayall, C.; Dolar, A.; Kokalj, A.J.; Novak, S.; Razinger, J.; Barbero, F.; Puntes, V.; Drobne, D. Stressor-dependent changes in immune parameters in the terrestrial isopod crustacean *Porcellio scaber*: A focus on nanomaterials. *Nanomaterials* **2021**, *11*, 934. [CrossRef] [PubMed]
6. Auguste, M.; Mayall, C.; Barbero, F.; Hočevar, M.; Alberti, S.; Grassi, G.; Puntes, V.F.; Drobne, D.; Canesi, L. Functional and morphological changes induced in *Mytilus* hemocytes by selected nanoparticles. *Nanomaterials* **2021**, *11*, 470. [CrossRef] [PubMed]

7. Catalano, R.; Labille, J.; Gaglio, D.; Alijagic, A.; Napodano, E.; Slomberg, D.; Campos, A.; Pinsino, A. Safety evaluation of TiO_2 nanoparticle-based sunscreen UV filters on the development and the immunological state of the sea urchin *Paracentrotus lividus*. *Nanomaterials* **2020**, *10*, 2102. [CrossRef] [PubMed]
8. Swart, E.; Dvorak, J.; Hernádi, S.; Goodall, T.; Kille, P.; Spurgeon, D.; Svendsen, C.; Prochazkova, P. The effects of in vivo exposure to copper dioxide nanoparticles on the gut microbiome, host immunity and susceptibility to bacterial infection in earthworms. *Nanomaterials* **2020**, *10*, 1337. [CrossRef] [PubMed]
9. Boraschi, D.; Italiani, P. From antigen delivery to adjuvanticity: The broad application of nanoparticles in vaccinology. *Vaccines* **2015**, *3*, 930–939. [CrossRef] [PubMed]
10. Hu, R.; Liu, H.; Wang, M.; Li, J.; Liang, M.; Gao, Y.; Yang, M. An OMV-based nanovaccine confers safety and protection against pathogenic *Escherichia coli* via both humoral anmd predominantly Th1 immune responses in poultry. *Nanomaterials* **2020**, *10*, 2293. [CrossRef] [PubMed]
11. Barbosa, M.M.F.; Kanno, A.I.; Farias, L.P.; Madej, M.; Sipos, G.; Sbrana, S.; Romani, L.; Boraschi, D.; Leite, L.C.C.; Italiani, P. Primary and memory response of human monocytes to vaccines: Role of nanoparticulate antigens in inducing innate memory. *Nanomaterials* **2021**, *11*, 931. [CrossRef] [PubMed]
12. Swartzwelter, B.J.; Mayall, C.; Alijagic, A.; Barbero, F.; Ferrari, E.; Hernádi, S.; Michelini, S.; Navarro Pacheco, N.I.; Prinelli, A.; Swart, E.; et al. Cross-species comparisons of nanoparticle interactions with innate immune systems: A methodological review. *Nanomaterials* **2021**, *11*, 1528. [CrossRef] [PubMed]
13. Boraschi, D.; Li, D.; Li, Y.; Italiani, P. In vitro and in vivo models to assess the immune-related effects of nanomaterials. *Int. J. Environ. Res. Public Health* **2021**, *18*, 11769. [CrossRef] [PubMed]
14. Auguste, M.; Melillo, D.; Corteggio, A.; Marino, R.; Canesi, L.; Pinsino, A.; Italiani, P.; Boraschi, D. Methodological approaches to assess innate immunity and innate memory in marine invertebrates and humans. *Front. Toxicol.* **2022**, *4*, 842469. [CrossRef]

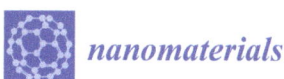

Review

The Interactions between Nanoparticles and the Innate Immune System from a Nanotechnologist Perspective

Lena M. Ernst [1], Eudald Casals [2], Paola Italiani [3], Diana Boraschi [3,4,5] and Victor Puntes [1,6,7,*]

1. Vall d'Hebron Research Institute (VHIR), 08035 Barcelona, Spain; lena.montana@vhir.org
2. School of Biotechnology and Health Sciences, Wuyi University, Jiangmen 529020, China; wyuchemecm@126.com
3. Institute of Protein Biochemistry and Cell Biology (IBBC), National Research Council (CNR), 80131 Napoli, Italy; paola.italiani@ibbc.cnr.it (P.I.); diana.boraschi@ibbc.cnr.it (D.B.)
4. Shenzhen Institute of Advanced Technology (SIAT), Chinese Academy of Sciences (CAS), Shenzhen 518055, China
5. Stazione Zoologica Anton Dohrn, 80121 Napoli, Italy
6. Institut Català de Nanociència i Nanotecnologia (ICN2), CSIC and The Barcelona Institute of Science and Technology (BIST), Campus UAB, 08193 Barcelona, Spain
7. Institució Catalana de Recerca I Estudis Avançats (ICREA), 08010 Barcelona, Spain
* Correspondence: victor.puntes@vhir.org

Abstract: The immune system contributes to maintaining the body's functional integrity through its two main functions: recognizing and destroying foreign external agents (invading microorganisms) and identifying and eliminating senescent cells and damaged or abnormal endogenous entities (such as cellular debris or misfolded/degraded proteins). Accordingly, the immune system can detect molecular and cellular structures with a spatial resolution of a few nm, which allows for detecting molecular patterns expressed in a great variety of pathogens, including viral and bacterial proteins and bacterial nucleic acid sequences. Such patterns are also expressed in abnormal cells. In this context, it is expected that nanostructured materials in the size range of proteins, protein aggregates, and viruses with different molecular coatings can engage in a sophisticated interaction with the immune system. Nanoparticles can be recognized or passed undetected by the immune system. Once detected, they can be tolerated or induce defensive (inflammatory) or anti-inflammatory responses. This paper describes the different modes of interaction between nanoparticles, especially inorganic nanoparticles, and the immune system, especially the innate immune system. This perspective should help to propose a set of selection rules for nanosafety-by-design and medical nanoparticle design.

Keywords: nanoparticles; immune system; innate immunity; inflammation; tolerance

1. Introduction

The immune system of higher vertebrates encompasses a collection of different specialized cells and specialized soluble molecules distributed throughout the body, being present in all organs and tissues, circulating in blood and lymph (to reach every corner of the body in case of need), and concentrated in some lymphoid organs (lymph nodes, spleen, bone marrow, where hematopoiesis takes place in adult life). These cells have been classified into two functional branches, namely innate and the adaptive immunity, which have different roles, complementing each other very efficiently in complex organisms such as mammals (simpler organisms such as invertebrates only display a perfectly efficient innate immunity). The innate immune system's role is to scan the body to remove apoptotic bodies, cell debris, and protein aggregates; recognize and eliminate pathogens or abnormal cells; and keep commensals outside tissues. Additionally, it promotes the repair of damaged tissue and is involved in the control of embryogenesis and delivery. We can say that the innate immune system is the actual immune system, active throughout evolution with conserved and very efficient defensive mechanisms. The other system, adaptive immunity, developed much

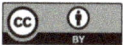

later as a complement of innate immunity, providing slower but more specific protective responses, good for long-living and mobile organisms that do not stably reside in the same environment [1]. The adaptive immune responses are tools for the innate immune system with subordinated or programmed functions—tools because they develop without making any decision [2]. It is the innate immune system that detects, categorizes, and triggers the immune response and, in the case of additional needs, calls for adaptive immunity to come in when the innate activation has reached a certain threshold level indicative of excessive danger and the need for more specific defensive tools.

These complex defensive actions that body tissues perform in response to harmful stimuli, such as pathogens or damaged cells, are described as inflammation. Inflammation requires an excess biological workout and therefore it is closely related to metabolism. Immunometabolism has become increasingly popular since the publication of Mathis and Shoelson's perspective in 2011 [3]. This is crucial in the context of interactions with nanoparticles (NPs), since they have been observed to have the capacity to increase or decrease reactive oxygen species (ROS), which directly correlates with the onset or remission of inflammation [4]. ROS are free radical molecules resulting from natural metabolism, which, when excessive and unregulated, may contribute to cell damage and aggravate human pathologies such as cancer [5], neurodegeneration, and stroke, among others [6].

Following the great oxidation event some 2.3 billion years ago, oxidation has been the leading force of metabolism. A delicate equilibrium between heat generation (enthalpy) and biological organization (entropy) was established, which allowed natural systems to decrease their free energy in a particular controlled fashion [7]. Deregulation of a living system, for instance, in the case of a disease, increases enthalpy generation at the expense of entropy. The system over-burns, which in biological terms is described as inflammation (literally *setting in flames*). Inflammation is correlated with a particular metabolic pathway, anaerobic glycolysis, providing higher energy power output, in which cells defend themselves from aggression. Furthermore, aerobic glycolysis, with a broken Krebs cycle, provides important metabolic intermediates and ROS [8]. Inflammation provokes the unbalance between endogenous production of free radicals and antioxidant defenses, resulting in oxidative stress [9]. While this metabolic defense mechanism is an ability of all eukaryotic cells, it is reasonable to imagine that, through evolution, some cells adapted the unbalanced energy equation to becoming professional defensive cells forming a whole discontinued system distributed across the body and responsible for the maintenance, defense, and repair of our biological tissues. In normal conditions, these cells have a patrolling role based on scanning and surveying tissues to eliminate senescent or damaged cells and become aggressive when encountering some possible dangers, capable of initiating, developing, and controlling inflammation.

The innate cell response is different, depending on the type of stimulus or combination of stimuli, the stimulus intensity (quantitative and temporal), the location of the innate cells (the tissue and its specialization), and the microenvironmental conditions. All these cues trigger a defined activation profile in innate cells, which is different based on the combination of microenvironmental conditions that have triggered it. Engineered NPs may share several characteristics of microbial agents, such as size and ordered molecular surface patterns, presenting "eat-me" or "eat-me-not" surface signals that favor or prevent macrophages from engulfing them. Thus, they are expected to develop complex and intense interactions with immunity. Bachmann et al. [10] showed that the immune system readily recognized antigen repetitive organization on the surface of viral particles.

In contrast, poor antigen organization does not induce an immune response. The same holds for complement (in particular C1q, an ancient version of immunoglobulins) [11], which recognizes ordered antigenic structures as those present on microorganisms but do not react to disordered patterns as those present in mammalian cell surfaces. The same has been observed with NP coatings [12]. These interactions mainly concern innate immunity, as responsible for detecting and categorizing foreign matter inside the body.

In order to navigate the described interactions between NPs and the immune system, it is recommendable to remember the different type of immune cells and their different functions (Figure 1). A major role in the innate immune system is played by macrophages, which in mammals develop some specialized functions depending on the tissue where they reside and are named accordingly: Langerhans cells in the skin, Kupffer cells in the liver, osteoclasts in the bone, microglia in the brain. Other innate immune cells are the innate lymphoid cells (ILCs), such as natural killer cells. ILCs contribute to patrolling tissues (abundant in the barrier tissues such as mucosal surfaces), identifying and killing/eliminating abnormal cells and microorganisms, and contributing to tissue development and homeostasis. Contrary to macrophages, they cannot phagocytose, but they are endowed with cytotoxic tools that literally kill the target. Similarly, mast cells are highly efficient defensive cells, abundant in all barrier tissues, endowed with an array of pre-formed proteolytic enzymes and other bioactive substances, which they release upon challenge and can detoxify snake and bee venoms, release factors that initiate/enhance a tissue-localized protective inflammatory reaction against parasites, and contribute to tissue repair and remodeling. Other important innate cells are neutrophils (short-lived, very abundant in the blood, highly phagocytic and inflammatory, strong producers of reactive oxygen species (ROS) in response to microbes), basophils (functionally similar to mast cells but residing in the blood), and eosinophils (with partially overlapping functions with mast cells and basophils, involved in response to multicellular parasites). Moreover, cells of adaptive immunity include T and B lymphocytes, which develop membrane receptors or antibodies able to recognize different pathogenic molecules/antigens specifically. In between, there are dendritic cells, which share with macrophages the capacity of taking up, processing, and presenting pathogen-derived antigens to adaptive immune cells, thereby enabling T and B cells to develop their antigen-specific membrane receptors and antibodies.

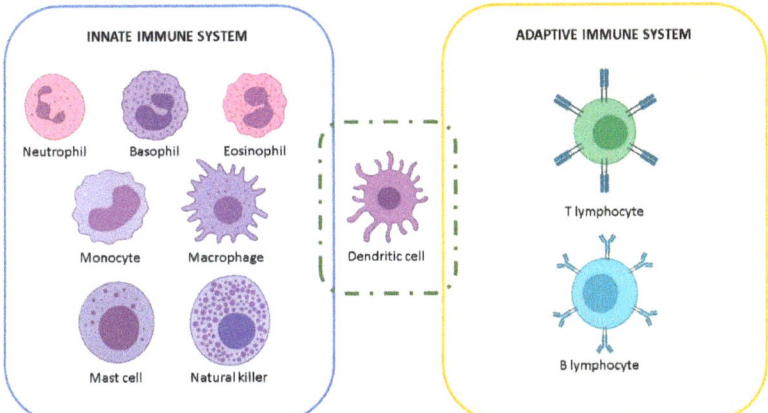

Figure 1. Representative classification of the most common mammalian immune cells.

The majority of the works on NP and immune system interactions [13] have focused on circulating blood monocytes (macrophage precursors) and tissue-resident macrophages [14]. Blood monocytes come from the bone marrow, while tissue macrophages can be a mixture of self-replicating cells that have populated the tissue during embryogenesis (developed from precursors in the yolk sac or fetal liver) and cells developed from blood monocytes that enter the tissue for replenishing the resident macrophage pool [15]. Macrophages present higher phagocytic activity than monocytes and can be easily identified based on size (monocytes are smaller than macrophages) and some biochemical markers (e.g., esterases) and surface molecules (e.g., CD14, CD16, CD68, CD11b, MAC-1) that are differentially expressed between the two cell types. The functional profile of monocytes and macrophages is exceptionally plastic, as the role of these cells is that of rapidly reacting to different microenvironmental signals by adopting an appropriate activation profile, which will contribute to danger elimination and, eventually, instructing the subsequent adaptive immune responses.

2. The NP-Immune System Interactions

It is essential to realize that inorganic matter is commonly nanostructured and that NPs and nanostructures have naturally occurred on the planet's surface since its origin before life emerged. This suggests that the immune system of living organisms has developed in an environment rich in such structures and substances, and therefore it should know how to deal with them. However, since the advent of nanotechnology, we are building more artificial nanostructures and artificial combinations of nanostructures and molecules, which may result in stronger interactions with the immune system, beneficial or detrimental. They depend on the nature of the employed material and its evolution in the environment before encountering the immune cell. The observed interactions between NPs and the immune system can be classified as in Figure 2. It is essential to understand that the interaction of NPs and the immune system can be multifactorial; size, shape, and surface state (including composition, structure, charge. and hydrophilicity) are primary factors, together with the presence of bioactive moieties in the sample, or the promotion of chemical reactions resulting in immune activation. These factors are closely related to the NP evolution in different media, which may result into aggregation, dissolution, or associate with bystander (bio)molecules. All these factors should be taken into account to develop safe NPs and functional NPs.

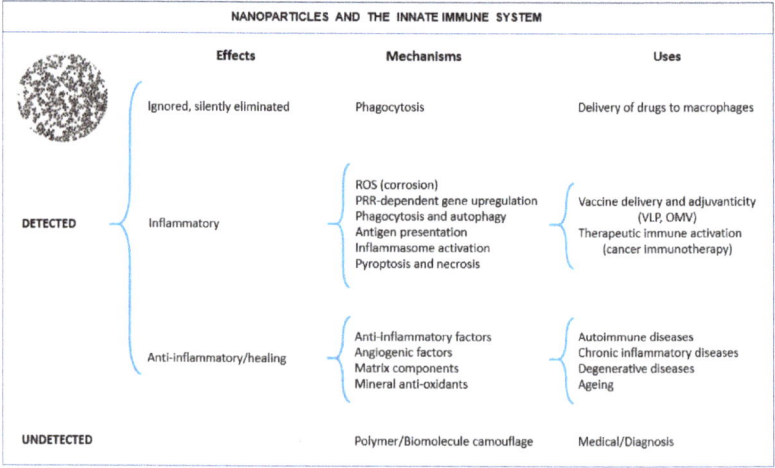

Figure 2. NP-immune system interactions. NPs can be undetected or detected by cells of the immune system, depending on different parameters such as their size, surface charge, and hydrophobicity/hydrophilicity of the surface coating. If detected, NPs can be either tolerated (either ignored or eliminated in a silent fashion, i.e., without inducing an inflammatory reaction) or generate an inflammatory response allowing for resolution of inflammation and tissue regeneration or an anti-inflammatory. With a proper NP design, these responses can be harnessed for developing different immunomodulating activities for medical exploitation (e.g., self-adjuvanted vaccines based on virus-like particles (VLPs), or outer membrane vesicles (OMVs), etc.).

2.1. When NPs Are Not Detected by the Immune System

The first scenario is when the NPs can escape from immune system detection. Indeed, the progress in the construction of synthetic nanostructures as delivery vehicles, contrast agents, or medical devices has allowed for the development of NPs able to escape the immune system and reach their target without inducing an undesirable inflammatory reaction. In order to escape from pattern recognition receptors inserted in the cell membrane of immune cells, or opsonization by complement molecules or antibodies (which mark foreign/dead cells for recycling, thereby enhancing phagocytosis), the use of polymers to camouflage the NP surface has been thoroughly developed. In pharmacology, polyethylene glycol (PEG) and polyvinylpyrrolidone (PVP) have been the most used polymers to stealthily NPs from the immune system [13,16,17], historically developed together with the liposomal formulation of antineoplastic drugs, such as in the case of Doxil® and, more recently, mRNA vaccine platforms [16]. Studies showed that these polymer functionalized NPs may appear invisible (stealth) to the immune system [17,18] by mimicking non-dangerous biological structures. As a consequence, the PEG coating increased the half-life of organic and inorganic NPs in the bloodstream from minutes to hours [19,20], similar to previous observations with PEGylated proteins [21]. Similarly, oligosaccharide- and peptide-derived NP coatings seem to afford escape from the immune system and allow for longer circulation times. Nevertheless, these coatings can reduce/delay opsonization and phagocytosis, but they do not completely prevent it. Thus, for example, the development of anti-PEG antibodies has been reported in several patients, which led to faster clearance of subsequent doses of PEG-coated formulations [22–24]. To circumvent these problems, researchers have explored the possibility of coating NPs with natural substances that can more finely deceive the immune system, for instance, by coating NPs with albumin or serum mixtures. As far as proteins are not denatured, and the resulting object is not too big, NPs seem to pass undetected [25].

The different coatings employed to escape immune system detection are listed in Table 1.

Table 1. Coatings employed to avoid immune detection.

Surface Coating	Nanoparticle Core	References
Albumin (rat, mouse, or human)	CeO$_2$ NPs as an anti-inflammatory mineral substance	[26–29]
	Abraxane as an albumin-based nanoparticle for chemotherapeutic delivery	[30]
Polyethylene glycol (PEG)	Au NPs for tumor targeting	[19]
	SiO$_2$ NPs for evasion of phagocytic clearance	[20]
	Polystyrene NPs for evasion of phagocytic clearance	[31]
Retinol	Polyethylenimine (PEI) NPs for drug delivery	[25]
CD47	Polystyrene NPs for evasion from phagocytic clearance	[31,32]
Erythrocyte membrane fragments	Poly(lactic-co-glycolic acid) (PLGA) NPs for drug delivery	[33]

Another way of camouflaging NPs from immune elimination is using coatings with proteins that are downregulatory immune signals. This is the case of the CD47 protein, a marker of "self" and "eat-me-not" that is expressed on all cell membranes [34]. In the work of Rodriguez et al. [32], the attachment of "self" peptides computationally designed from human CD47 protein onto polystyrene NPs achieved a delayed macrophage-mediated clearance of NPs in mice. In addition, this increased the circulation time of the NPs and enhanced the drug delivery to lung adenocarcinoma xenografts. Likewise, Hu et al. [33] coated PLGA NPs with a red blood cell (RBC)-membrane shell. These RBC-based polymeric NPs also showed a longer circulation half-life and sustained in vivo drug release compared with that achieved by using PEG-coated NPs. The coating with specific "self" molecules can also be used for the opposite reason, i.e., to induce an immune system activation by coating NPs with endogenous danger-associated molecular patterns. As an example, Aldossari et al. [35] coated AgNPs with high-density lipoprotein (HDL), which is recognized by scavenger receptors (SR-B1) expressed by macrophages. Once administered to mice, HDL-coated AgNPs provoked the recruitment of inflammatory cells, whereas SR-B1-deficient mice showed reduced cell recruitment. This strategy allowed the antimicrobial activity of AgNPs to be enhanced by targeting delivery. This indicates how important the NP coating is to escape the immune system, where a large body of knowledge has been developed to allow NPs to serve as drug delivery vehicles.

2.2. When NPs Are Detected by the Immune System and Tolerated

When the immune system detects NPs, they can be tolerated or induce an activation. Being tolerated means that NPs are silently removed, without inducing inflammation, as if they were protein aggregates, apoptotic cells, or cellular debris. This can be controlled mainly by modulating NP size, surface charge, and hydrophobicity/hydrophilicity of their surface [13,16,17,32,33], where small sizes, hydrophilicity, and negative surface charges often result in tolerable NPs [36]. In general, one can say that NPs below 4–6 nm can pass undetected and undergo rapid renal clearance after i.v. administration [37]. As the NP diameter increases, NPs become the target of the different immune cells. NPs of virus-like size (a few tens to a few hundreds of nm) can be endocytosed without triggering inflammation [12]. Larger objects, of micrometric size, like bacteria, are phagocytosed, while for sizes larger than 10–20 microns, objects are encapsulated [38].

This has critical consequences for the biodistribution of NPs inside the body. NPs are transported and accumulated in different organs depending on the administration route, their physicochemical properties, and their detection by the immune system. Accordingly, after intravenous (i.v.) injection, common NPs are often filtered in the liver by hepatocytes [17,18] or eventually Kupffer cells (the liver macrophages) depending on if they are detected or pass undetected by the immune system [31]. The first studies of biodistribution of colloidal particles (a few hundred nm) were reported in the 1970s in the *Journal of the Reticuloendothelial Society* (now *Journal of Leukocyte Biology*). Singer et al. [39] and Adlersberg et al. [40], by treating mice with i.v. and i.p. colloidal Au, found that after one hour, 90% of the administered dose was accumulated in the liver and 10% in the rest of the body (mainly kidneys). Subsequent histological studies with similar colloidal gold particles i.p. administered found them in the liver and lymph nodes primarily localized inside macrophages [41]. These results were later confirmed by numerous studies of the pharmacokinetic and biodistribution of different NPs. Sadauskas et al. [42], using AuNPs of different sizes (below 40 nm), showed that Kupffer cells were central in accumulating NPs once they entered the body. Similar results were also obtained with metal oxides, quantum dots, carbon nanostructures, etc. [43]. Yokel et al. [44] administered citrate capped nanoceria (5, 15, 30, and 55 nm) at 50 and 100 mg/kg bw i.v. into Sprague-Dawley rats and measured Ce content over time (1 h, 20 h, and 30 days). Remarkably, in all these works and many others, no inflammation or systemic injury was observed, except at larger doses (>100 mg/kg bw). Accordingly, we have observed by mass spectroscopy that after i.v. administration of albumin-conjugated nanoceria (CeO_2) at low doses (0.1 mg/kg bw), twice a week during two weeks, in control and fibrotic Wistar rats, that most of the Ce is in the liver (84% of the administered dose after one hour and 75% eight weeks after administration) [26].

This non-inflammatory capture of NPs can be exploited for harnessing these phagocytic immune cells to transport NPs towards the target area, be it a wound, an infection, or a tumor. For such delivery, circulating monocytes have been proposed as a sort of Trojan Horse or Cellular Shuttle, since they naturally migrate from the blood to the sites of damage and disease. Hence, they can be loaded with NPs to be transported through the body [45,46]. Thus, Choi et al. [47] explored the use of monocytes containing AuNPs for transport into tumor regions for subsequent photothermal therapy. This study showed the phagocytosis of AuNPs by both monocytes and macrophages and their recruitment into the tumor. Oude-Engberink et al. [48] showed the accumulation of monocytes laden with iron oxide NPs (30 nm) in the affected cerebral sites in a rat model of experimental neuroinflammation. More recently, Moore et al. [49], using a microfluidic in vitro model, showed increased activity of monocytes/macrophages to transport NP across a confluent endothelial cell layer, advancing in the design of cellular shuttles loaded with NPs. This tolerated elimination of NPs may limit the dispersibility of NPs inside the body. However, the immune system is by itself an important therapeutic target where nanocarriers can efficiently transport drugs assisting immunotherapy.

2.3. When NPs Are Detected by the Immune System and Not Tolerated

Many reports show that NPs may induce harmful immune responses and toxicity. NPs can induce an inflammatory immune activation because of aggregation or dissolution or because they accidentally carry immune-activating moieties (such as endotoxin, detergents, allergens, or cationic molecules). These biological effects are rather independent of the composition, size, or shape of the individual NP, described as extrinsic factors of NP toxicity [4]. Similarly, the organization of molecular epitopes in a non-conventional form (upon adhesion of the NP surface) may generate new antigens or allergens. The activation of the immune system induced by NPs can be classified as follows:

2.3.1. NP-Induced Oxidative Stress

The more universal inflammatory reaction to NPs corresponds to the most non-specific and rapid defense mechanism of macrophages, the overproduction of reactive oxygen species (ROS), which results in oxidative stress, responsible of lipid oxidation and DNA damage and, eventually, structural alterations, DNA mutations, and cell death. ROS refers to biogenic free radical molecules resulting from natural metabolism characterized by being highly oxidant. These free radicals are involved in different critical physiological processes, such as gene expression, signal transduction, growth regulation, and, significantly, inflammation, where high ROS concentrations are needed to sustain the energetic demands of a proinflammatory immune response [50].

Accordingly, independently of composition, large aggregates of TiO_2 [51], Al_2O_3 [52], and Fe_2O_3 [53] NPs showed a similar capacity to increase oxidative stress. Moreover, the corrosion process of metallic NPs itself produces a high concentration of free radicals, which may trigger an inflammatory immune response [54–56]. These processes are often neglected in NPs made up of bulk non-biodegradable materials. However, biodegradation of Ag, Fe_3O_4, and CdSe/ZnS NPs due to enzymatic or hydrolytic activities in lysosomes [57,58] have been described. Even the physiological disintegration of AuNPs through oxidative etching by cysteine and chlorine has been described [59–61]. Similarly, carbon nanotubes (CNTs) have been observed to dissolve in vivo through enzymatic catalysis [62]. Subsequently, an increased number of reports has established relationships between observed inflammatory effects after NP exposure and NP disintegration [63–66]. Related to that, it is worth mentioning the works of Burello et al. [67] and Zhang et al. [55]. They developed theoretical and experimental models to predict the oxidative stress potential of oxide NPs by looking at their bandgap energy and their ability to perturb the intracellular redox state. Note that NP dissolution may become a source of toxic cations. For instance, in the early 2000s, the studies of Derfus et al. [68] and Kirchner et al. [69] showed that the released Cd ions were responsible for the intracellular oxidation and toxicity caused by CdSe NPs. Similar effects were found later when comparing the toxicity of Ni NP and ions as a function of time [70].

2.3.2. When Phagocytosis Is Not Sufficient

When the immune system detects a foreign object, phagocytosis is the first mechanism for elimination that comes into play. However, when the object is too big (usually larger than 10–20 µm), rather than engulfing it, the immune cells start spreading on it to form a layer of cells that secludes the object from the rest of the tissue and initiate a chemical defense against the material that, if not non-biodegradable, is permanently kept secluded into a fibrous capsule or granuloma.

Historically, chronic inflammation has been observed in the case of penetration of non-biodegradable (persistent) large size (micrometric) particles in the lungs, as the well-known cases of particle-induced granulomatosis such as silicosis and asbestosis [71]. This is because when a phagocytic cell fails to digest these particles, phagolysosomal rupture, the release of lysosomal enzymes and particles, and subsequent activation of the inflammasome and other cytoplasmic sensing mechanisms may happen, thereby triggering inflammation. This may lead, as the material persists, to chronic inflammation, permanent oxidative stress, tissue damage, and alterations that favor tumorigenesis in the long term. Brandwood et al. [72] found that murine macrophages phagocytosed inert carbon fiber-reinforced carbon particles up to 20 microns in diameter, but larger particles were not engulfed and became surrounded by aggregations of macrophages. This reaction may have pathological aspects; fibromas and granulomas are non-functional neo-tissues, similar to scars, that may hamper the organ functions and be active, i.e., growing, for a long time. In some instances, the reaction can be overtly pathological, as in the case of long fibrous materials. Accordingly, when Poland et al. [73] instilled high doses of multiwalled carbon nanotubes between the membranes lining the lungs and abdominal organs in mice, they found that long straight nanotubes caused inflammation and lesions in membrane cells similar to those leading to cancer, just like asbestos fibers [74]. Similarly, Ag nanospheres did not elicit any immune response or toxicity, while Ag nanowires can elicit a high inflammatory response, directly correlated to nanowire length, in murine macrophages [75]. The same effects were observed by Ji et al. [76] in THP-1 cells when comparing nanoceria nanorods and high aspect ratio nanoceria nanowires at high doses and aggregation states. This suggests that the needle-like shape of NPs is prone to provoke inflammation. It has been observed that macrophages engulfing needle-shaped crystals and fibers end up getting pierced by the needle-like structures and, consequently, start inflammation [77]. Parental NPs usually are never grown to these sizes, but uncontrolled aggregation can transform objects of tens of nm to tens of μm.

2.3.3. NPs, Intendedly or Accidentally, Can Display Antigens, Allergens, or Toxins

The unintended or accidental absorption of biomolecules onto the NP surface may be a cause of concern. NPs may associate with specific bio-molecules, toxic by-standers, or pollutants, and present them to the immune system in an ordered pattern, thereby mimicking microorganisms and triggering the innate immune reaction of the host.

It is important to note that NPs have a strong tendency to adsorb many different molecules (hetero-aggregation) at their surface due to their high surface energy. Consequently, they are usually surrounded by a molecular coating, either provided intentionally (NP functionalization) and/or spontaneously by molecules present in the environment, forming the NP biocorona. These coatings also take part in the NP morphology and functions. The consequences of this are diverse; NPs can be good molecular aggregators and substrates for molecules to be presented to the immune system.

Among essential immunoactive biomolecules present in the environment, bacterial endotoxin is one of the most common and abundant. Endotoxins (also known as lipopolysaccharides (LPSs)) are large molecules present in the outer membrane of Gram-negative bacteria, able to elicit strong innate/inflammatory immune responses. Endotoxin is a ubiquitous environmental contaminant and can be present in all chemicals and glassware used in laboratories, even after sterilization (depyrogenation is needed to get rid of it). The presence of endotoxin, if not recognized, can be responsible for many of the in vitro and in vivo effects attributed to NPs [78]. Our study [79] showed that the endotoxin present on AuNPs turned those NPs from inactive to highly inflammatory and able to induce secretion of IL-1β in human primary monocytes. This could be an underlying factor in inflammatory responses and toxic effects associated with other metallic NPs and carbon nanomaterials [80,81]. Hence, special attention is needed to avoid endotoxin contamination when preparing NPs, which includes working in endotoxin-free conditions and glassware depyrogenation [82].

In other cases, the toxic ingredient may come from the formulation or derived chemicals employed during NPs preparation. If the synthesis process does not involve proper purification steps, the use of such NP samples may entail deleterious responses due to excess surfactants or unreacted precursors. This is the case of PEI molecules, a common NP stabilizer to enhance NP endocytosis, but with safety concerns due to the attachment to the negatively charged cell membranes that modify permeability and compromise viability [83]. Indeed, it is well-established that positively charged macromolecules can cause higher toxicity and immune activation than their neutral or negatively charged counterparts, as in the case of monolayer-coated silicon nanoparticles [84]. Similar is the case of amphipathic molecules such as cetyltrimethyl ammonium bromide (CTAB), employed in preparing Au nanorods [85], which act as a detergent to lyse cell membranes. Another example is in the work of Dowding et al. [86]. These authors prepared different nanoceria NPs using the identical precursor (cerium nitrate hexahydrate) through a similar wet chemical process but using other bases: NH_4OH, which yields negatively charged nanoceria, or hexamethylenetetramine (HMTA), which yields positively charged nanoceria at neutral pH. Results showed that HMTA-nanoceria NPs were readily taken into endothelial cells and reduced cell viability at a 10-fold lower concentration than the other NPs, which showed no toxicity.

Another type of immunoactive molecule that NPs can adsorb is allergens. This is unlikely to happen in the case of NPs since the concentration of allergens in the environment is very low, and the NP surface would be passivated before encountering them. However, it must be taken into account. Note that it has been reported that car combustion emission microparticles, when coated by pollen grains, enhance allergenic responses [87]. Radauer et al. [88] observed the formation of a stable allergen coating around NPs when exposed to different types of allergens (Der p1 and Bet v1), enhancing allergic responses against them. A recent review about the potential of NPs to trigger allergies via adsorption of allergens can be found in reference [89]. Here, it is essential to remark that allergy, understood as an anomalous immune response towards substances that are generally tolerated, has never been observed for engineered nanomaterials per se.

Regarding immune effects induced by biomolecules adsorbed on the NP surface, another possible source of inflammation comes from the potential modification of the structure of proteins upon adsorption at the NP surface [90]. Lynch et al. [91] pointed out how partial protein misfolding at the NP surface may result in the exposure of protein fractions usually buried in the core of the native structure. These cryptic epitopes may be recognized by immune cells and trigger inappropriate defensive reactions. Accordingly, in the work of Falagan [92], such modifications of the adsorbed proteins structure have been indicated as responsible for the long-term toxicity observed after a single low-dose exposure of AuNPs.

2.3.4. NPs Presenting Vaccine Antigens and Working as Vaccine Adjuvants

Regarding the intentional use of NPs for vaccination, conjugation of antigens to NPs can help both attain a more efficient presentation of poorly immunogenic soluble antigens and provide an adjuvant effect targeted to innate immunity (the NP as a foreign agent) [12]. An interesting example is the development of AuNP-based virus-like particles (VLPs), where the NP replaces the virus core, which scaffolds the proteic capsid structure [93]. Typically, capsid proteins need the highly negatively charged dense core of DNA/RNA to self-assemble properly. This core can be replaced by dense and highly negatively charged AuNPs. Nikura et al. [93] demonstrated that the size and shape of AuNP-VLPs allowed for shaping of the in vitro and in vivo immune response in terms of the production of antibodies against West Nile virus. This implies that by modulating the NP size and shape, and consequently the arrangement of viral proteins on the NP surface, it could be possible to obtain highly effective and efficient vaccines. NPs can also be employed as vaccine adjuvants by exploiting their capacity to target and modulate the activity of innate immune cells. For a long time, vaccines were prepared by precipitation of antigens within some matrix, initially bread crumbs (in the XIX century), and currently alum powder, where the antigens are absorbed, forming aggregates that vary in size from 1 to 20 µm, acting as an antigen depot [94]. In this way, slow release of antigens is achieved, prolonging antigen presence, improving its processing and presentation. Other NP aggregates have been used as adjuvants. Skarastina et al. [95] used silica NPs (10–20 nm) as adjuvants for the hepatitis B vaccine in a mouse model. The monodisperse silica NPs formed heterogeneous aggregates larger than 1 µm after formulation, resulting in the same IgG2a/IgG1 ratios as in the case of immunization with alum as an adjuvant. Other nanostructure used as vaccine adjuvants are nano-sized emulsions (sometimes called lipidic NPs). This is the case of the oil-in-water MF59 emulsion, which is used as an adjuvant, mainly for influenza vaccines (Flaud®, Novartis) and has been licensed in more than 20 countries. The MF59 adjuvant allows for significant cross-reactivity against viral strains and reduces antigen concentration to 50–200-fold lower doses [96].

The induction of inflammatory responses with non-pathogenic triggers has also been proposed as a preventive approach against exposure to unknown pathogens. Behind this concept, preventive activation of the innate immunity, there is the capacity of innate immune cells to develop a different response to a challenge as a consequence of previous contact with a different threat, a capacity known as innate memory [97,98]. All innate immune cells are able to develop a long lasting memory, despite their short lifespan in circulation. The reason lies mainly on the fact that the precursors in the bone marrow can be primed by a trigger and generate circulating immune cells with a different capacity to react against threats, as currently shown in monocytes/macrophages. Thus, after having previously experienced an inflammatory activation, the innate immune system becomes more efficient in preventing the rooting of newly incoming pathogens. For instance, this has been observed in the case of the administration of bacille calmette-guerin (BCG), the vaccine for tuberculosis, which increases resistance to other diseases [99]. The generation of innate memory thus represents an alternative, or better a complement, to the highly specific adaptive memory induced by vaccines. The strategy of innate memory induction leads to outcomes (enhanced protection) that have advantages (wider range of protection) and disadvantages (more unpredictable and less controllable side effects). Despite the controversy regarding safety, NPs can be used as adjuvants for the non-specific amplification of immune responses, and, even more, they can be excellent tools for generating or modulating innate memory [100]. In this regard, administration of AuNPs alone was observed to have little/no impact on the subsequent capacity of human monocytes to mount an innate/inflammatory response to a microbial challenge (LPS) [101]. However, the co-administration of AuNPs, or Fe_3O_4NPs, with memory-inducing microbial agents (e.g., LPS, BCG, muramyl dipeptide (MDP), Helicobacter pylori) led to a modulation of the innate memory response induced by the microbial agents depending on the priming stimulus and the NP type, shape, and size [102]. The implication is that vaccination with antigens and NPs could bring about a protective specific immunity based on adaptive immune memory and a non-specific innate memory induced by the antigen-NP combination.

The proinflammatory activation effects are listed in Table 2. In all these aspects, the uncontrolled proinflammatory activation of the immune system is, in principle, a common source of NP toxicity. In contrast, controlled activation can be employed for vaccination and other modes of defense against pathogens.

Table 2. Inflammatory activation induced by NPs.

NPs That Cause Inflammation		
Category	Surfactant	References
Inflammation induced by by-standers	Cetyltrimethyl ammonium bromide (CTAB)	[85]
	Hexamethylenetetramine (HMT)	[103]
Inflammation induced by pollutants	Bacterial endotoxin (LPS)	[78,79]
	Allergens	[88,89]
Category	Mechanism	References
	Non biocompatible size/shape	[72–76]
Inflammation induced by the core	Excess of aggregation/agglomeration	[51–53,96,102,104]
	Chemical transformations and corrosion	[54–70,102]
Category	Surfactant	References
Inflammation induced by the coating (bioactive molecules, VLPs…)	Virus like particles (VLP)	[93]
	Antigen/ordered peptides/proteins coatings	[91,92,100,105]
	Cationic polymers	[83]

2.4. When NPs Act as Enzymes and in This Way Can Modulate Immune Reactions

Rare-earth oxide NPs have been found to be biocompatible antioxidants able to buffer excess ROS in physiological conditions, showing powerful anti-inflammatory effects. Mineral antioxidants may offer superior activity to currently available substances due to their enhanced bioavailability and stability, longer tissue residence time, and resistance to biological degradation [106]. These features can be exploited in many diseases based on excessive immune/inflammatory activation, such as autoimmune diseases, chronic inflammation, organ rejection, asthma and other allergic diseases, neurodegenerative pathologies (Alzheimer's disease, Parkinson's disease), and aging [106]. They have been described as engineered inorganic materials with enzyme-like activities, especially cerium oxide NPs, nanoceria [106,107]. Nanoceria has been reported to display superoxide dismutase (SOD)-like activity (conversion of superoxide anion into hydrogen peroxide and finally oxygen) [108], catalase-like activity (conversion of hydrogen peroxide into oxygen and water) [109,110], peroxidase-like activity (conversion of hydrogen peroxide into hydroxyl radicals) [111], as well as NO scavenging ability [103]. Consequently, nanoceria has been shown to safely down-regulate oxidative stress by scavenging the excess of ROS in diseases such as retinal degeneration [112,113], neurological disorders (including Alzheimer's disease, Parkinson's disease, and ALS) [114–116], ischemia [117], cardiopathies [118], diabetes [119], gastrointestinal inflammation [120], liver diseases [26–28], and cancer [121,122], as well as in regenerative medicine [123] and tissue engineering [124], with better performance than other antioxidant substances in both efficacy and efficiency. Interestingly, nanoceria become active at high ROS concentrations. Otherwise, at homeostatic ROS levels, the NPs become inactive. This is because several free radicals have to be simultaneously absorbed onto the NP surface in order to be recombined into non-radical adducts, a condition that only happens for high ROS concentrations. In other words, the ROS scavenging capacities of nanoceria are ROS concentration dependent. With time, these NPs dissolve into innocuous ions, which are excreted via the urinary route [19]. The solid NPs have been observed to be excreted through the hepatobiliary route [26,125].

This aspect is significantly different from the previous ones, where activation of the immune system results in inflammatory responses. In this case, the enzyme-like catalytic activity of rare earth NPs results in anti-inflammatory activity. The different observed responses are listed in Table 3.

Table 3. Immune responses to NP exposure.

Category	Nanoparticle Core	Surface Coating	References
NPs that pass unnoticed	Au NPs	Polyethylene glycol (PEG)	[19]
	SiO_2 NPs	Polyethylene glycol (PEG)	[20]
	Polyethylenimine (PEI) NPs	Retinol	[25]
	Polystyrene NPs	CD47 or PEG	[31,32]
		Bovine serum albumin (BSA)	[46]
	Polymeric NPs	Erythrocyte membrane fragments	[33]
	Abraxane	Human serum albumin (HSA)	[30]
NPs that are tolerated	Au NPs	Sodium citrate	[42,92]
		Disordered peptidic coatings	[47]
	CeO_2 NPs	Rat serum albumin (RSA)	[44]
	Polystyrene NPs	Poly-L-lysine	[46]
	Fe_3O_4 NPs	Dextrane	[48]
	SiO_2 NPs	3-Aminopropyltriethoxysilane (APTES)	[49]

Table 3. Cont.

Category	Nanoparticle Core	Surface Coating	References
Immunoactive NPs with inflammatory activity	Au NPs	Peptides/proteins	[55,58,93,105]
		Bacterial endotoxin (LPS)	[78]
		Cetyltrimethyl ammonium bromide (CTAB)	[85]
		Allergens	[88]
		Poly(acrylic acid) (PAA)	[92]
		Polyethylene glycol (PEG)	[92]
	Ag NPs	High-density lipoprotein (HDL)	[35]
		Sodium citrate	[58,65,74]
	Alumina NPs	Fetal bovine serum (FBS)	[52]
	CeO$_2$ NPs	Hexamethylenetetramine (HMT)	[86]
		Polyethylenimine (PEI)-polyethylene glycol (PEG)	[122]
	Gadolinium endohedral metallofullerenols	Polyhydroxy	[80]
	Silica NPs	Hepatitis B virus core protein	[104]
Immunoactive NPs with anti-inflammatory activity	CeO$_2$ NPs	Murine serum albumin	[26–29]
		Polyethylene glycol (PEG)	[117]
		Gelatin	[124]

3. NP Evolution and Transformations in the Exposure Media

The interaction between NPs and the immune system strongly depends on the conditions in which such interaction occurs (route of exposure, co-exposure with other agents) and on the characteristics of both NPs and the host immune system. Here we have presented the variety of immune responses to NPs and how these responses can help us design immuno-active and immune-benign NPs, which could either avoid immune recognition and activation in order to persist in the body long enough for completing their theranostic tasks or directly interact with immune cells for triggering inflammatory or anti-inflammatory responses as desired for therapeutic purposes. Indeed, the scientific community is still struggling with the apparent contradiction of similar materials being toxic and non-toxic (even beneficial) at the same time. This paradox can be attributed to undescribed effects of NP modifications during their dispersion in the working media, such as aggregation and corrosion. The main modifications NPs may suffer during their dispersion in different media are shown in Figure 3. Basically, NPs can be coated with molecules (e.g., hydrophilic polymers) to both pass undetected by the immune system and avoid aggregation (1). They can also be coated with soluble antigenic molecules to induce a response against them (2). In the opposite direction, when dispersed in physiological media, NPs can aggregate (3) and adsorb other molecules present in the medium (e.g., protein corona) (4) or both (5). In addition, depending on the core composition, NPs can be used as ROS scavengers, thereby down-regulating inflammatory responses (6), or they can dissolve and act as an ion reservoir that may increase the level of oxidative stress and generate an inflammatory response (7).

NPs have different ways to minimize their high surface energy, basically aggregation and corrosion. These are common phenomena in nature, widely studied by geochemistry, where a NP is an intermediate state between a micrometric particle and the dissolved ions. Thus, NPs may aggregate or associate with coating molecules in different media. They may also disintegrate through corrosion (defined as the chemical degradation of a solid material) and dissolution.

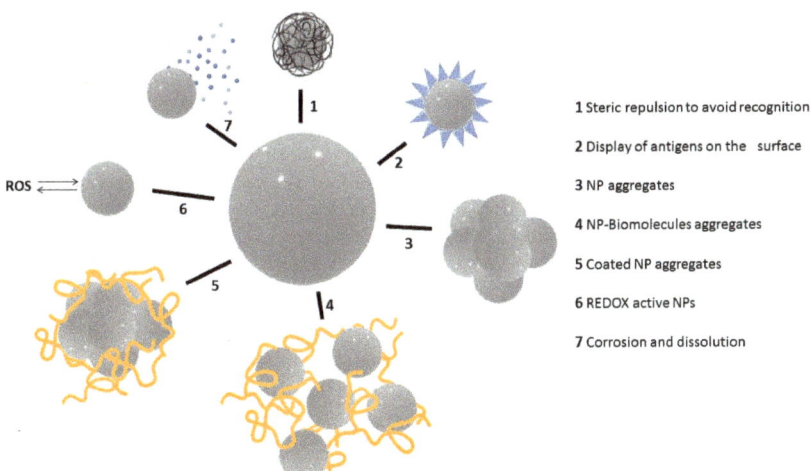

Figure 3. Intended or spontaneous NP modifications and their impact on immune responses.

Aggregation deserves particular attention. NPs are colloidally stable by repulsive electrostatic or steric forces or a combination of both. Aggregability depends on intrinsic NP parameters such as morphology, surface coating, and charge, and extrinsic parameters such as electrolyte concentration, pH, presence of organic matter, etc. Aggregation is common in physiological environments where NPs aggregate to submicrometric or micrometric sizes when not properly stabilized. To avoid it, one has to provide repulsive forces to the NP surface, either by electrostatic (high surface charge) or steric (entropic) means, usually provided by large soluble molecules associated with the NP surface; otherwise, they will aggregate and their unique physicochemical properties that arise at the nanoscale (quantum confinement, superparamagnetism, extreme catalytic activity, etc.) progressively lost. Note that aggregation entails modifications in terms of specific surface area, concentration, mobility, and dosing. Protein adsorption, the formation of a protein corona, is a particular aggregation phenomenon between NPs and proteins present in the dispersion media. It is a dynamic process in which, initially, proteins adsorb and desorb at the surface, followed by a set of re-organizational arrangements, which make this absorption more stable and finally irreversible [126,127]. This depends on NP size, surface state, type of protein, and protein-NP incubation media and conditions, where sophisticated functional patterns can be obtained [128]. The most straightforward strategy to cope with this issue is to passivate the NP surface in a controlled manner, e.g., by albuminization, PEGylation, or addition of PVP. These strategies usually decrease aggregation, even in high salt media, and the adsorption of microenvironmental biomolecules on the NP surface.

In addition to aggregation, chemical transformations, corrosion, and dissolution can also be a cause of immune activation via the alteration for the cellular redoxome, and the delivery of toxic cations. In this regard, the nanochemist or nanoengineer needs to control the redox potential (and the oxidative/reductive environment) where the NP will be stored, employed, and disposed of. In this regard, using NPs at their higher valence state is recommendable when possible [14] (passivating the surface with a continuous layer of oxide is sometimes an alternative). The chemical transformation and dissolution of NPs, which can cause immune activation or toxicity, is fundamental to determine NP fate and reduce its presence and persistence in the environment.

4. Concluding Remarks

After considering the different interactions NPs may have with the immune system, one can draw indications on how NPs have to be designed to control these interactions and consequent responses. Indeed, while many NP functions can be attributed to their core structure, the surface coating defines much of their bioactivity. By controlling the nano-bio interface, NPs can be designed to be safe and innocuous or active and have therapeutic benefits. From the NP point of view, and for the nanochemist and the nanoengineer, the NP immunological properties can be summarized as depicted in Figure 4. The composition of the NP core determines its chemical potential and catalytic activity, while the surface coating largely determines its bioactivity. NPs can aggregate, either with other NPs or with macromolecules present in the physiological media (e.g., biocorona), or they can dissolve, being redox-active and acting as an ion reservoir, consequently increasing the levels of oxidative stress.

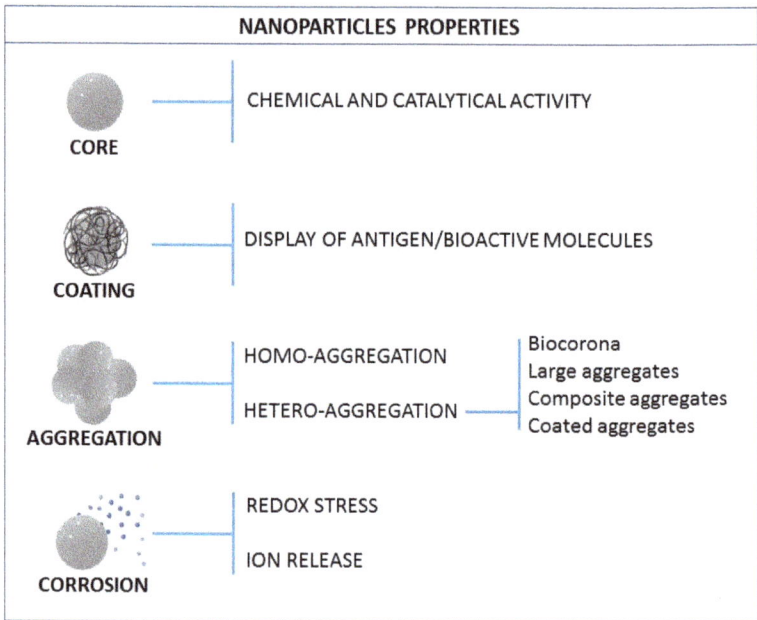

Figure 4. The NP properties that can impact the immune system.

In order to address the NP immune interactions, one has first to deal with the instability of the NP surface, and it should be passivated before introduction into biological systems. Otherwise, they may spontaneously aggregate, resulting in objects of increased size and decreased dose. Polymeric coatings have traditionally been the most commonly employed materials for such purposes. However, this surface engineering is sometimes costly and involves multi-step synthesis approaches, sometimes in the organic phase. One simple and effective solution could be to promote NP solubility in physiological media by pre-albuminization during the preparation process [118,119,128], a similar approach employed by Abraxane®, one of the first approved nanomedicines [30]. In addition to providing colloidal stability and avoiding opsonization, NP coatings can be designed to directly interact with the immune system, such as CD47 [32] for avoiding complement activation, LPS for inducing innate/inflammatory activation [79], or viral proteins for vaccination [95]. Finally, NPs that belong to the family of natural antioxidants, such as nanoceria that catalytically scavenge free radicals (ROS in the context of inflammation), provide powerful immunomodulatory effects.

Thus, by mainly playing with surface characteristics, it is possible to adjust the NP physicochemical characteristics (aggregation, surface display of given biomolecules, chemical stability) and consequently their modes of interaction with the immune system.

Author Contributions: V.P., L.M.E., E.C., P.I. and D.B. wrote the manuscript. L.M.E. also prepared the figures and managed references together with E.C. All authors have read and agreed to the published version of the manuscript.

Funding: This research was funded by the EU Commission H2020 project PANDORA (GA 671881; to D.B., P.I. and V.P.). Additional funds were provided by the EU Commission H2020 project ENDO-NANO (GA 812661; to P.I. and D.B.), the Italian MIUR InterOmics Flagship projects MEMORAT and MAME (to D.B. and P.I.), the Italian MIUR/PRIN-20173ZECCM (to P.I.), the CAS President's International Fellowship Programme (PIFI; award 2020VBA0028; to D.B.), Spanish Ministerio de Ciencia, Innovación y Universidades (MCIU) (RTI2018-099965-B-I00, AEI/FEDER, UE), and Generalitat de Catalunya (2017-SGR-1431) (V.P.).

Conflicts of Interest: The authors declare no conflict of interest. The funders had no role in the design of the study; in the collection, analyses, or interpretation of data; in the writing of the manuscript; or in the decision to publish.

References

1. Flajnik, M.F.; Kasahara, M. Origin and evolution of the adaptive immune system: Genetic events and selective pressures. *Nat. Rev. Genet.* **2010**, *11*, 47–59. [CrossRef]
2. Iwasaki, A.; Medzhitov, R. Control of adaptive immunity by the innate immune system. *Nat. Immunol.* **2015**, *16*, 343–353. [CrossRef]
3. Mathis, D.; Shoelson, S.E. Immunometabolism: An emerging frontier. *Nat. Rev. Immunol.* **2011**, *11*, 81. [CrossRef]
4. Casals, E.; Gusta, M.F.; Piella, J.; Casals, G.; Jiménez, W.; Puntes, V. Intrinsic and Extrinsic Properties Affecting Innate Immune Responses to Nanoparticles: The Case of Cerium Oxide. *Front. Immunol.* **2017**, *8*, 970. [CrossRef]
5. Reczek, C.R.; Chandel, N.S. The Two Faces of Reactive Oxygen Species in Cancer. *Annu. Rev. Cancer Biol.* **2017**, *1*, 79–98. [CrossRef]
6. Chen, Q.; Wang, Q.; Zhu, J.; Xiao, Q.; Zhang, L. Reactive oxygen species: Key regulators in vascular health and diseases. *Br. J. Pharmacol.* **2018**, *175*, 1279–1292. [CrossRef]
7. Ritort, F. The Noisy and Marvelous Molecular World of Biology. *Inventions* **2019**, *4*, 24. [CrossRef]
8. O'Neill, L.A. A broken krebs cycle in macrophages. *Immunity* **2015**, *42*, 393–394. [CrossRef]
9. Pizzino, G.; Irrera, N.; Cucinotta, M.; Pallio, G.; Mannino, F.; Arcoraci, V.; Squadrito, F.; Altavilla, D.; Bitto, A. Oxidative Stress: Harms and Benefits for Human Health. *Oxid. Med. Cell. Longev.* **2017**, *2017*, 8416763. [CrossRef]
10. Bachmann, M.F.; Rohrer, U.H.; Kündig, T.M.; Bürki, K.; Hengartner, H.; Zinkernagel, R.M. The influence of antigen organization on B cell responsiveness. *Science* **1993**, *262*, 1448–1451. [CrossRef]
11. Bachmann, M.F.; Jennings, G.T. Vaccine delivery: A matter of size, geometry, kinetics and molecular patterns. *Nat. Rev. Immunol.* **2010**, *10*, 787–796. [CrossRef]
12. Bastús, N.G.; Sánchez-Tilló, E.; Pujals, S.; Farrera, C.; López, C.; Giralt, E.; Celada, A.; Lloberas, J.; Puntes, V. Homogeneous Conjugation of Peptides onto Gold Nanoparticles Enhances Macrophage Response. *ACS Nano* **2009**, *3*, 1335–1344. [CrossRef]
13. Moghimi, S.M.; Szebeni, J. Stealth liposomes and long circulating nanoparticles: Critical issues in pharmacokinetics, opsonization and protein-binding properties. *Prog. Lipid Res.* **2003**, *42*, 463–478. [CrossRef]
14. Hume, D.A. The mononuclear phagocyte system. *Curr. Opin. Immunol.* **2006**, *18*, 49–53. [CrossRef]
15. Gordon, S.; Plüddemann, A. The Mononuclear Phagocytic System. Generation of Diversity. *Front. Immunol.* **2019**, *10*, 1893. [CrossRef]
16. Peracchia, M.T.; Harnisch, S.; Pinto-Alphandary, H.; Gulik, A.; Dedieu, J.C.; Desmaële, D.; d'Angelo, J.; Müller, R.H.; Couvreur, P. Visualization of in vitro protein-rejecting properties of PEGylated stealth polycyanoacrylate nanoparticles. *Biomaterials* **1999**, *20*, 1269–1275. [CrossRef]
17. Gref, R.; Lück, M.; Quellec, P.; Marchand, M.; Dellacherie, E.; Harnisch, S.; Blunk, T.; Müller, R.H. 'Stealth' corona-core nanoparticles surface modified by polyethylene glycol (PEG): Influences of the corona (PEG chain length and surface density) and of the core composition on phagocytic uptake and plasma protein adsorption. *Colloids Surf. B Biointerfaces* **2000**, *18*, 301–313. [CrossRef]
18. Hou, X.; Zaks, T.; Langer, R.; Dong, Y. Lipid nanoparticles for mRNA delivery. *Nat. Rev. Mater.* **2021**, *10*, 1–17.
19. Veronese, F.M.; Pasut, G. PEGylation, successful approach to drug delivery. *Drug Discov. Today* **2005**, *10*, 1451–1458. [CrossRef]
20. Harris, J.M.; Chess, R.B. Effect of pegylation on pharmaceuticals. *Nat. Rev. Drug Discov.* **2003**, *2*, 214–221. [CrossRef]
21. Perrault, S.D.; Walkey, C.; Jennings, T.; Fischer, H.C.; Chan, W.C.W. Mediating Tumor Targeting Efficiency of Nanoparticles Through Design. *Nano Lett.* **2009**, *9*, 1909–1915. [CrossRef]
22. He, Q.; Zhang, J.; Shi, J.; Zhu, Z.; Zhang, L.; Bu, W.; Guo, L.; Chen, Y. The effect of PEGylation of mesoporous silica nanoparticles on nonspecific binding of serum proteins and cellular responses. *Biomaterials* **2010**, *31*, 1085–1092. [CrossRef]
23. Abuchowski, A.; McCoy, J.R.; Palczuk, N.C.; van Es, T.; Davis, F.F. Effect of covalent attachment of polyethylene glycol on immunogenicity and circulating life of bovine liver catalase. *J. Biol. Chem.* **1977**, *252*, 3582–3586. [CrossRef]

24. Richter, A.W.; Akerblom, E. Antibodies against polyethylene glycol produced in animals by immunization with monomethoxy polyethylene glycol modified proteins. *Int. Arch. Allergy Appl. Immunol.* **1983**, *70*, 124–131. [CrossRef]
25. Cheng, T.-L.; Wu, P.-Y.; Wu, M.-F.; Chern, J.-W.; Roffler, S.R. Accelerated Clearance of Polyethylene Glycol-Modified Proteins by Anti-Polyethylene Glycol IgM. *Bioconjug. Chem.* **1999**, *10*, 520–528. [CrossRef]
26. Verhoef, J.J.F.; Carpenter, J.F.; Anchordoquy, T.J.; Schellekens, H. Potential induction of anti-PEG antibodies and complement activation toward PEGylated therapeutics. *Drug Discov. Today* **2014**, *19*, 1945–1952. [CrossRef]
27. Zhang, Z.; Wang, C.; Zha, Y.; Hu, W.; Gao, Z.; Zang, Y.; Chen, J.; Zhang, J.; Dong, L. Corona-Directed Nucleic Acid Delivery into Hepatic Stellate Cells for Liver Fibrosis Therapy. *ACS Nano* **2015**, *9*, 2405–2419. [CrossRef]
28. Oldenborg, P.-A.; Zheleznyak, A.; Fang, Y.-F.; Lagenaur, C.F.; Gresham, H.D.; Lindberg, F.P. Role of CD47, as a Marker of Self on Red Blood Cells. *Science* **2000**, *288*, 2051–2054. [CrossRef]
29. Rodriguez, P.L.; Harada, T.; Christian, D.A.; Pantano, D.A.; Tsai, R.K.; Discher, D.E. Minimal "Self" peptides that inhibit phagocytic clearance and enhance delivery of nanoparticles. *Science* **2013**, *339*, 971–975. [CrossRef]
30. Hu, C.-M.J.; Zhang, L.; Aryal, S.; Cheung, C.; Fang, R.H.; Zhang, L. Erythrocyte membrane-camouflaged polymeric nanoparticles as a biomimetic delivery platform. *Proc. Natl. Acad. Sci. USA* **2011**, *108*, 10980–10985. [CrossRef]
31. Aldossari, A.A.; Shannahan, J.H.; Podila, R.; Brown, J.M. Scavenger receptor B_1 facilitates macrophage uptake of silver nanoparticles and cellular activation. *J. Nanoparticle Res.* **2015**, *17*, 313. [CrossRef]
32. Seong, S.Y.; Matzinger, P. Hydrophobicity: An ancient damage-associated molecular pattern that initiates innate immune responses. *Nat. Rev. Immunol.* **2004**, *4*, 469–478. [CrossRef]
33. Bastús, N.G.; Casals, E.; Vázquez-Campos, S.; Puntes, V. Reactivity of engineered inorganic nanoparticles and carbon nanostructures in biological media. *Nanotoxicology* **2008**, *2*, 99–112. [CrossRef]
34. Choi, H.S.; Liu, W.; Misra, P.; Tanaka, E.; Zimmer, J.P.; Itty Ipe, B.; Bawendi, M.G.; Frangioni, J.V. Renal clearance of quantum dots. *Nat. Biotechnol.* **2007**, *25*, 1165–1170. [CrossRef]
35. Sperling, R.A.; Casals, E.; Comenge, J.; Bastús, N.G.; Puntes, V.F. Inorganic engineered nanoparticles and their impact on the immune response. *Curr. Drug Metab.* **2009**, *10*, 895–904. [CrossRef]
36. Qie, Y.; Yuan, H.; von Roemeling, C.A.; Chen, Y.; Liu, X.; Shih, K.D.; Knight, J.A.; Tun, H.W.; Wharen, R.E.; Jiang, W.; et al. Surface modification of nanoparticles enables selective evasion of phagocytic clearance by distinct macrophage phenotypes. *Sci. Rep.* **2016**, *6*, 26269. [CrossRef]
37. Singer, J.M.; Adlersberg, L.; Sadek, M. Long-term observation of intravenously injected colloidal gold in mice. *J. Reticuloendothel. Soc.* **1972**, *12*, 658–671.
38. Adlersberg, L.; Singer, J.M. The fate of intraperitoneally injected colloidal gold particles in mice. *J. Reticuloendothel. Soc.* **1973**, *13*, 325–342.
39. Williams, R.J.; Bradley, N.J. Distribution of intraperitoneal gold colloid (198-Au). *Acta Med. Austriaca* **1989**, *16*, 50–54.
40. Sadauskas, E.; Wallin, H.; Stoltenberg, M.; Vogel, U.; Doering, P.; Larsen, A.; Danscher, G. Kupffer cells are central in the removal of nanoparticles from the organism. *Part. Fibre Toxicol.* **2007**, *4*, 10. [CrossRef]
41. Casals, E.; Vázquez-Campos, S.; Bastús, N.G.; Puntes, V. Distribution and potential toxicity of engineered inorganic nanoparticles and carbon nanostructures in biological systems. *TrAC Trends Anal. Chem.* **2008**, *27*, 672–683. [CrossRef]
42. Yokel, R.A.; Tseng, M.T.; Dan, M.; Unrine, J.M.; Graham, U.M.; Wu, P.; Grulke, E.A. Biodistribution and biopersistence of ceria engineered nanomaterials: Size dependence. *Nanomed. Nanotechnol. Biol. Med.* **2013**, *9*, 398–407. [CrossRef]
43. Oro, D.; Yudina, T.; Fernandez-Varo, G.; Casals, E.; Reichenbach, V.; Casals, G.; de la Presa, B.; Sandalinas, S.; Carvajal, S.; Puntes, V.; et al. Cerium oxide nanoparticles reduce steatosis, portal hypertension and display anti-inflammatory properties in rats with liver fibrosis. *J. Hepatol.* **2016**, *64*, 691–698. [CrossRef]
44. Mehta, K.; Lopez-Berestein, G.; Hersh, E.M.; Juliano, R.L. Uptake of liposomes and liposome-encapsulated muramyl dipeptide by human peripheral blood monocytes. *J. Reticuloendothel. Soc.* **1982**, *32*, 155–164.
45. Thiele, L.; Rothen-Rutishauser, B.; Jilek, S.; Wunderli-Allenspach, H.; Merkle, H.P.; Walter, E. Evaluation of particle uptake in human blood monocyte-derived cells in vitro. Does phagocytosis activity of dendritic cells measure up with macrophages? *J. Control. Release* **2001**, *76*, 59–71. [CrossRef]
46. Choi, M.-R.; Stanton-Maxey, K.J.; Stanley, J.K.; Levin, C.S.; Bardhan, R.; Akin, D.; Badve, S.; Sturgis, J.; Robinson, J.P.; Bashir, R.; et al. A Cellular Trojan Horse for Delivery of Therapeutic Nanoparticles into Tumors. *Nano Lett.* **2007**, *7*, 3759–3765. [CrossRef]
47. Oude Engberink, R.D.; Blezer, E.L.; Hoff, E.I.; van der Pol, S.M.; van der Toorn, A.; Dijkhuizen, R.M.; de Vries, H.E. MRI of monocyte infiltration in an animal model of neuroinflammation using SPIO-labeled monocytes or free USPIO. *J. Cereb. Blood Flow Metab.* **2008**, *28*, 841–851. [CrossRef]
48. Moore, T.L.; Hauser, D.; Gruber, T.; Rothen-Rutishauser, B.; Lattuada, M.; Petri-Fink, A.; Lyck, R. Cellular Shuttles: Monocytes/Macrophages Exhibit Transendothelial Transport of Nanoparticles under Physiological Flow. *ACS Appl. Mater. Interfaces* **2017**, *9*, 18501–18511. [CrossRef]
49. Viola, A.; Munari, F.; Sanchez-Rodriguez, R.; Scolaro, T.; Castegna, A. The Metabolic Signature of Macrophage Responses. *Front. Immunol.* **2019**, *10*, 1462. [CrossRef]
50. Noel, A.; Maghni, K.; Cloutier, Y.; Dion, C.; Wilkinson, K.J.; Halle, S.; Tardif, R.; Truchon, G. Effects of inhaled nano-TiO_2 aerosols showing two distinct agglomeration states on rat lungs. *Toxicol. Lett.* **2012**, *214*, 109–119. [CrossRef]

51. Yoon, D.; Woo, D.; Kim, J.; Kim, M.; Kim, T.; Hwang, E.; Baik, S. Agglomeration, sedimentation, and cellular toxicity of alumina nanoparticles in cell culture medium. *J. Nanoparticle Res.* **2011**, *13*, 2543–2551. [CrossRef]
52. Zhu, X.; Tian, S.; Cai, Z. Toxicity Assessment of Iron Oxide Nanoparticles in Zebrafish (Danio rerio) Early Life Stages. *PLoS ONE* **2012**, *7*, 9. [CrossRef] [PubMed]
53. Liu, J.; Sonshine, D.A.; Shervani, S.; Hurt, R.H. Controlled Release of Biologically Active Silver from Nanosilver Surfaces. *ACS Nano* **2010**, *4*, 6903–6913. [CrossRef]
54. Zhang, H.; Ji, Z.; Xia, T.; Meng, H.; Low-Kam, C.; Liu, R.; Pokhrel, S.; Lin, S.; Wang, X.; Liao, Y.-P.; et al. Use of Metal Oxide Nanoparticle Band Gap to Develop a Predictive Paradigm for Oxidative Stress and Acute Pulmonary Inflammation. *ACS Nano* **2012**, *6*, 4349–4368. [CrossRef]
55. Semerád, J.; Filip, J.; Ševců, A.; Brumovský, M.; Nguyen, N.H.A.; Mikšíček, J.; Lederer, T.; Filipová, A.; Boháčková, J.; Cajthaml, T. Environmental fate of sulfidated nZVI particles: The interplay of nanoparticle corrosion and toxicity during aging. *Environ. Sci. Nano* **2020**, *7*, 1794–1806. [CrossRef]
56. Sabella, S.; Carney, R.P.; Brunetti, V.; Malvindi, M.A.; Al-Juffali, N.; Vecchio, G.; Janes, S.M.; Bakr, O.M.; Cingolani, R.; Stellacci, F.; et al. A general mechanism for intracellular toxicity of metal-containing nanoparticles. *Nanoscale* **2014**, *6*, 7052–7061. [CrossRef]
57. Jiang, X.; Miclăuş, T.; Wang, L.; Foldbjerg, R.; Sutherland, D.S.; Autrup, H.; Chen, C.; Beer, C. Fast intracellular dissolution and persistent cellular uptake of silver nanoparticles in CHO-K1, cells: Implication for cytotoxicity. *Nanotoxicology* **2015**, *9*, 181–189. [CrossRef]
58. Wiley, B.; Herricks, T.; Sun, Y.; Xia, Y. Polyol Synthesis of Silver Nanoparticles: Use of Chloride and Oxygen to Promote the Formation of Single-Crystal, Truncated Cubes and Tetrahedrons. *Nano Lett.* **2004**, *4*, 1733–1739. [CrossRef]
59. Kim, K.-H.; Kim, J.-U.; Cha, S.-H.; Lee, J.-C. Reversible Formation and Dissolution of Gold Nanoparticles through Turning On and Off Sequences of UV Light. *J. Am. Chem. Soc.* **2009**, *131*, 7482–7483. [CrossRef]
60. Xia, Y.; Xiong, Y.; Lim, B.; Skrabalak, S.E. Shape-controlled synthesis of metal nanocrystals: Simple chemistry meets complex physics? *Angew. Chem. Int. Ed. Engl.* **2009**, *48*, 60–103. [CrossRef] [PubMed]
61. Allen, B.L.; Kichambare, P.D.; Gou, P.; Vlasova, I.I.; Kapralov, A.A.; Konduru, N.; Kagan, V.E.; Star, A. Biodegradation of Single-Walled Carbon Nanotubes through Enzymatic Catalysis. *Nano Lett.* **2008**, *8*, 3899–3903. [CrossRef] [PubMed]
62. Franklin, N.M.; Rogers, N.J.; Apte, S.C.; Batley, G.E.; Gadd, G.E.; Casey, P.S. Comparative toxicity of nanoparticulate ZnO, bulk ZnO, and $ZnCl_2$, to a freshwater microalga (Pseudokirchneriella subcapitata): The importance of particle solubility. *Environ. Sci. Technol.* **2007**, *41*, 8484–8490. [CrossRef]
63. Auffan, M.; Rose, J.; Wiesner, M.R.; Bottero, J.Y. Chemical stability of metallic nanoparticles: A parameter controlling their potential cellular toxicity in vitro. *Environ. Pollut.* **2009**, *157*, 1127–1133. [CrossRef] [PubMed]
64. De Matteis, V.; Malvindi, M.A.; Galeone, A.; Brunetti, V.; De Luca, E.; Kote, S.; Kshirsagar, P.; Sabella, S.; Bardi, G.; Pompa, P.P. Negligible particle-specific toxicity mechanism of silver nanoparticles: The role of Ag+ ion release in the cytosol. *Nanomed. Nanotechnol. Biol. Med.* **2015**, *11*, 731–739. [CrossRef]
65. Wang, D.; Lin, Z.; Wang, T.; Yao, Z.; Qin, M.; Zheng, S.; Lu, W. Where does the toxicity of metal oxide nanoparticles come from: The nanoparticles, the ions, or a combination of both? *J. Hazard. Mater.* **2016**, *308*, 328–334. [CrossRef]
66. Burello, E.; Worth, A.P. A theoretical framework for predicting the oxidative stress potential of oxide nanoparticles. *Nanotoxicology* **2011**, *5*, 228–235. [CrossRef]
67. Derfus, A.M.; Chan, W.C.W.; Bhatia, S.N. Probing the Cytotoxicity of Semiconductor Quantum Dots. *Nano Lett.* **2004**, *4*, 11–18. [CrossRef]
68. Kirchner, C.; Liedl, T.; Kudera, S.; Pellegrino, T.; Muñoz Javier, A.; Gaub, H.E.; Stölzle, S.; Fertig, N.; Parak, W.J. Cytotoxicity of Colloidal CdSe and CdSe/ZnS Nanoparticles. *Nano Lett.* **2005**, *5*, 331–338. [CrossRef]
69. Zhou, C.; Vitiello, V.; Casals, E.; Puntes, V.F.; Iamunno, F.; Pellegrini, D.; Changwen, W.; Benvenuto, G.; Buttino, I. Toxicity of nickel in the marine calanoid copepod Acartia tonsa: Nickel chloride versus nanoparticles. *Aquat. Toxicol.* **2016**, *170*, 1–12. [CrossRef] [PubMed]
70. Heffner, D.K. The cause of sarcoidosis: The Centurial enigma solved. *Ann. Diagn. Pathol.* **2007**, *11*, 142–152. [CrossRef]
71. Brandwood, A.; Noble, K.R.; Schindhelm, K. Phagocytosis of carbon particles by macrophages in vitro. *Biomaterials* **1992**, *13*, 646–648. [CrossRef]
72. Poland, C.A.; Duffin, R.; Kinloch, I.; Maynard, A.; Wallace, W.A.H.; Seaton, A.; Stone, V.; Brown, S.; MacNee, W.; Donaldson, K. Carbon nanotubes introduced into the abdominal cavity of mice show asbestos-like pathogenicity in a pilot study. *Nat. Nanotechnol.* **2008**, *3*, 423. [CrossRef] [PubMed]
73. Stoehr, L.C.; Gonzalez, E.; Stampfl, A.; Casals, E.; Duschl, A.; Puntes, V.; Oostingh, G.J. Shape matters: Effects of silver nanospheres and wires on human alveolar epithelial cells. *Part. Fibre Toxicol.* **2011**, *8*, 36. [CrossRef] [PubMed]
74. Toybou, D.; Celle, C.; Aude-Garcia, C.; Rabilloud, T.; Simonato, J.-P. A toxicology-informed, safer by design approach for the fabrication of transparent electrodes based on silver nanowires. *Environ. Sci. Nano* **2019**, *6*, 684–694. [CrossRef]
75. Ji, Z.; Wang, X.; Zhang, H.; Lin, S.; Meng, H.; Sun, B.; George, S.; Xia, T.; Nel, A.E.; Zink, J.I. Designed Synthesis of CeO_2 Nanorods and Nanowires for Studying Toxicological Effects of High Aspect Ratio Nanomaterials. *ACS Nano* **2012**, *6*, 5366–5380. [CrossRef] [PubMed]
76. Fadeel, B. Hide and Seek: Nanomaterial Interactions with the Immune System. *Front. Immunol.* **2019**, *10*, 133. [CrossRef]

77. Li, Y.; Shi, Z.; Radauer-Preiml, I.; Andosch, A.; Casals, E.; Luetz-Meindl, U.; Cobaleda, M.; Lin, Z.; Jaberi-Douraki, M.; Italiani, P.; et al. Bacterial endotoxin (lipopolysaccharide) binds to the surface of gold nanoparticles, interferes with biocorona formation and induces human monocyte inflammatory activation. *Nanotoxicology* **2017**, *11*, 1157–1175. [CrossRef]
78. Li, Y.; Italiani, P.; Casals, E.; Valkenborg, D.; Mertens, I.; Baggerman, G.; Nelissen, I.; Puntes, V.F.; Boraschi, D. Assessing the Immunosafety of Engineered Nanoparticles with a Novel in Vitro Model Based on Human Primary Monocytes. *ACS Appl. Mater. Interfaces* **2016**, *8*, 28437–28447. [CrossRef]
79. Chen, Z.; Liu, Y.; Sun, B.; Li, H.; Dong, J.; Zhang, L.; Wang, L.; Wang, P.; Zhao, Y.; Chen, C. Polyhydroxylated metallofullerenols stimulate IL-1β secretion of macrophage through TLRs/MyD88/NF-κB pathway and NLRP$_3$ inflammasome activation. *Small* **2014**, *10*, 2362–2372. [CrossRef]
80. Chen, G.Y.; Yang, H.J.; Lu, C.H.; Chao, Y.C.; Hwang, S.M.; Chen, C.L.; Lo, K.W.; Sung, L.Y.; Luo, W.Y.; Tuan, H.Y.; et al. Simultaneous induction of autophagy and toll-like receptor signaling pathways by graphene oxide. *Biomaterials* **2012**, *33*, 6559–6569. [CrossRef]
81. Li, Y.; Italiani, P.; Casals, E.; Tran, N.; Puntes, V.F.; Boraschi, D. Optimising the use of commercial LAL assays for the analysis of endotoxin contamination in metal colloids and metal oxide nanoparticles. *Nanotoxicology* **2015**, *9*, 462–473. [CrossRef] [PubMed]
82. Kafil, V.; Omidi, Y. Cytotoxic impacts of linear and branched polyethylenimine nanostructures in a431 cells. *Bioimpacts* **2011**, *1*, 23–30.
83. Bhattacharjee, S.; de Haan, L.H.; Evers, N.M.; Jiang, X.; Marcelis, A.T.; Zuilhof, H.; Rietjens, I.M.; Alink, G.M. Role of surface charge and oxidative stress in cytotoxicity of organic monolayer-coated silicon nanoparticles towards macrophage NR8383 cells. *Part. Fibre Toxicol.* **2010**, *7*, 25. [CrossRef] [PubMed]
84. Alkilany, A.M.; Nagaria, P.K.; Hexel, C.R.; Shaw, T.J.; Murphy, C.J.; Wyatt, M.D. Cellular uptake and cytotoxicity of gold nanorods: Molecular origin of cytotoxicity and surface effects. *Small* **2009**, *5*, 701–708. [CrossRef] [PubMed]
85. Dowding, J.M.; Das, S.; Kumar, A.; Dosani, T.; McCormack, R.; Gupta, A.; Sayle, T.X.; Sayle, D.C.; von Kalm, L.; Seal, S.; et al. Cellular interaction and toxicity depend on physicochemical properties and surface modification of redox-active nanomaterials. *ACS Nano* **2013**, *7*, 4855–4868. [CrossRef]
86. Fujieda, S.; Diaz-Sanchez, D.; Saxon, A. Combined nasal challenge with diesel exhaust particles and allergen induces In vivo IgE isotype switching. *Am. J. Respir. Cell Mol. Biol.* **1998**, *19*, 507–512. [CrossRef]
87. Radauer-Preiml, I.; Andosch, A.; Hawranek, T.; Luetz-Meindl, U.; Wiederstein, M.; Horejs-Hoeck, J.; Himly, M.; Boyles, M.; Duschl, A. Nanoparticle-allergen interactions mediate human allergic responses: Protein corona characterization and cellular responses. *Part. Fibre Toxicol.* **2016**, *13*, 3. [CrossRef]
88. Martin, H.; Bettina, G.; Marlene, S.; Mark, G.; Albert, D. Immune Frailty and Nanomaterials: The Case of Allergies. *Curr. Bionanotechnol.* **2016**, *2*, 20–28.
89. Goy-López, S.; Juárez, J.; Alatorre-Meda, M.; Casals, E.; Puntes, V.F.; Taboada, P.; Mosquera, V. Physicochemical Characteristics of Protein–NP Bioconjugates: The Role of Particle Curvature and Solution Conditions on Human Serum Albumin Conformation and Fibrillogenesis Inhibition. *Langmuir* **2012**, *28*, 9113–9126. [CrossRef] [PubMed]
90. Lynch, I.; Dawson, K.A.; Linse, S. Detecting cryptic epitopes created by nanoparticles. *Sci. STKE* **2006**, *2006*, pe14. [CrossRef]
91. Falagan-Lotsch, P.; Grzincic, E.M.; Murphy, C.J. One low-dose exposure of gold nanoparticles induces long-term changes in human cells. *Proc. Natl. Acad. Sci. USA* **2016**, *113*, 13318–13323. [CrossRef]
92. Niikura, K.; Matsunaga, T.; Suzuki, T.; Kobayashi, S.; Yamaguchi, H.; Orba, Y.; Kawaguchi, A.; Hasegawa, H.; Kajino, K.; Ninomiya, T.; et al. Gold nanoparticles as a vaccine platform: Influence of size and shape on immunological responses in vitro and in vivo. *ACS Nano* **2013**, *7*, 3926–3938. [CrossRef]
93. Pulendran, B.; Arunachalam, P.S.; O'Hagan, D.T. Emerging concepts in the science of vaccine adjuvants. *Nat. Rev. Drug Discov.* **2021**, *20*, 454–475. [CrossRef] [PubMed]
94. Skrastina, D.; Petrovskis, I.; Lieknina, I.; Bogans, J.; Renhofa, R.; Ose, V.; Dishlers, A.; Dekhtyar, Y.; Pumpens, P. Silica nanoparticles as the adjuvant for the immunisation of mice using hepatitis B core virus-like particles. *PLoS ONE* **2014**, *9*, e114006. [CrossRef]
95. O'Hagan, D.T. MF59 is a safe and potent vaccine adjuvant that enhances protection against influenza virus infection. *Expert Rev. Vaccines* **2007**, *6*, 699–710. [CrossRef]
96. Boraschi, D.; Italiani, P. Innate Immune Memory: Time for Adopting a Correct Terminology. *Front. Immunol.* **2018**, *9*, 799. [CrossRef]
97. Mitroulis, I.; Ruppova, K.; Wang, B.; Chen, L.S.; Grzybek, M.; Grinenko, T.; Eugster, A.; Troullinaki, M.; Palladini, A.; Kourtzelis, I.; et al. Modulation of Myelopoiesis Progenitors Is an Integral Component of Trained Immunity. *Cell* **2018**, *172*, 147–161. [CrossRef]
98. Uthayakumar, D.; Paris, S.; Chapat, L.; Freyburger, L.; Poulet, H.; De Luca, K. Non-specific Effects of Vaccines Illustrated Through the BCG Example: From Observations to Demonstrations. *Front. Immunol.* **2018**, *9*, 2869. [CrossRef] [PubMed]
99. Barbosa, M.M.F.; Kanno, A.I.; Farias, L.P.; Madej, M.; Sipos, G.; Sbrana, S.; Romani, L.; Boraschi, D.; Leite, L.C.C.; Italiani, P. Primary and Memory Response of Human Monocytes to Vaccines: Role of Nanoparticulate Antigens in Inducing Innate Memory. *Nanomaterials* **2021**, *11*, 931. [CrossRef] [PubMed]
100. Della Camera, G.; Madej, M.; Ferretti, A.M.; La Spina, R.; Li, Y.; Corteggio, A.; Heinzl, T.; Swartzwelter, B.J.; Sipos, G.; Gioria, S.; et al. Personalised Profiling of Innate Immune Memory Induced by Nano-Imaging Particles in Human Monocytes. *Front. Immunol.* **2021**, *12*, 692165. [CrossRef] [PubMed]

101. Casals, E.; Zeng, M.; Parra-Robert, M.; Fernández-Varo, G.; Morales-Ruiz, M.; Jiménez, W.; Puntes, V.; Casals, G. Cerium Oxide Nanoparticles: Advances in Biodistribution, Toxicity, and Preclinical Exploration. *Small* **2020**, *16*, 1907322. [CrossRef]
102. Xu, C.; Qu, X. Cerium oxide nanoparticle: A remarkably versatile rare earth nanomaterial for biological applications. *Npg Asia Mater.* **2014**, *6*, e90. [CrossRef]
103. Korsvik, C.; Patil, S.; Seal, S.; Self, W. Superoxide dismutase mimetic properties exhibited by vacancy engineered ceria nanoparticles. *Chem. Commun.* **2007**, *10*, 1056–1058. [CrossRef] [PubMed]
104. Pirmohamed, T.; Dowding, J.; Singh, S.; Wasserman, B.; Heckert, E.; Karakoti, A.; King, J.; Seal, S.; Self, W. Nanoceria exhibit redox state-dependent catalase mimetic activity. *Chem. Commun.* **2010**, *46*, 2736–2738. [CrossRef] [PubMed]
105. Cafun, J.D.; Kvashnina, K.O.; Casals, E.; Puntes, V.F.; Glatzel, P. Absence of Ce^{3+} sites in chemically active colloidal ceria nanoparticles. *ACS Nano* **2013**, *7*, 10726–10732. [CrossRef] [PubMed]
106. Heckert, E.G.; Seal, S.; Self, W.T. Fenton-Like Reaction Catalyzed by the Rare Earth Inner Transition Metal Cerium. *Environ. Sci. Technol.* **2008**, *42*, 5014–5019. [CrossRef]
107. Dowding, J.; Dosani, T.; Kumar, A.; Seal, S.; Self, W. Cerium oxide nanoparticles scavenge nitric oxide radical ((NO)-N-center dot). *Chem. Commun.* **2012**, *48*, 4896–4898. [CrossRef]
108. Chen, J.P.; Patil, S.; Seal, S.; McGinnis, J.F. Rare earth nanoparticles prevent retinal degeneration induced by intracellular peroxides. *Nat. Nanotechnol.* **2006**, *1*, 142–150. [CrossRef]
109. Cai, X.; Sezate, S.A.; Seal, S.; McGinnis, J.F. Sustained protection against photoreceptor degeneration in tubby mice by intravitreal injection of nanoceria. *Biomaterials* **2012**, *33*, 8771–8781. [CrossRef]
110. Schubert, D.; Dargusch, R.; Raitano, J.; Chan, S.W. Cerium and yttrium oxide nanoparticles are neuroprotective. *Biochem. Biophys. Res. Commun.* **2006**, *342*, 86–91. [CrossRef]
111. D'Angelo, B.; Santucci, S.; Benedetti, E.; Di Loreto, S.; Phani, R.; Falone, S.; Amicarelli, F.; Cerù, M.P.; Cimini, A. Cerium Oxide Nanoparticles Trigger Neuronal Survival in a Human Alzheimer Disease Model By Modulating BDNF Pathway. *Curr. Nanosci.* **2009**, *5*, 167–176. [CrossRef]
112. Kalashnikova, I.; Mazar, J.; Neal, C.J.; Rosado, A.L.; Das, S.; Westmoreland, T.J.; Seal, S. Nanoparticle delivery of curcumin induces cellular hypoxia and ROS-mediated apoptosis via modulation of Bcl-2/Bax in human neuroblastoma. *Nanoscale* **2017**, *9*, 10375–10387. [CrossRef] [PubMed]
113. Kim, C.K.; Kim, T.; Choi, I.Y.; Soh, M.; Kim, D.; Kim, Y.J.; Jang, H.; Yang, H.S.; Kim, J.Y.; Park, H.K.; et al. Ceria nanoparticles that can protect against ischemic stroke. *Angew. Chem. Int. Ed. Engl.* **2012**, *51*, 11039–11043. [CrossRef] [PubMed]
114. Niu, J.L.; Azfer, A.; Rogers, L.M.; Wang, X.H.; Kolattukudy, P.E. Cardioprotective effects of cerium oxide nanoparticles in a transgenic murine model of cardiomyopathy. *Cardiovasc. Res.* **2007**, *73*, 549–559. [CrossRef]
115. Khurana, A.; Tekula, S.; Godugu, C. Nanoceria suppresses multiple low doses of streptozotocin-induced Type 1, diabetes by inhibition of Nrf2/NF-κB pathway and reduction of apoptosis. *Nanomedicine* **2018**, *13*, 1905–1922. [CrossRef] [PubMed]
116. Colon, J.; Hsieh, N.; Ferguson, A.; Kupelian, P.; Seal, S.; Jenkins, D.W.; Baker, C.H. Cerium oxide nanoparticles protect gastrointestinal epithelium from radiation-induced damage by reduction of reactive oxygen species and upregulation of superoxide dismutase 2. *Nanomedicine* **2010**, *6*, 698–705. [CrossRef]
117. Parra-Robert, M.; Casals, E.; Massana, N.; Zeng, M.; Perramón, M.; Fernández-Varo, G.; Morales-Ruiz, M.; Puntes, V.; Jiménez, W.; Casals, G. Beyond the Scavenging of Reactive Oxygen Species (ROS): Direct Effect of Cerium Oxide Nanoparticles in Reducing Fatty Acids Content in an In Vitro Model of Hepatocellular Steatosis. *Biomolecules* **2019**, *9*, 425. [CrossRef] [PubMed]
118. Fernández-Varo, G.; Perramón, M.; Carvajal, S.; Oró, D.; Casals, E.; Boix, L.; Oller, L.; Macías-Muñoz, L.; Marfà, S.; Casals, G.; et al. Bespoken Nanoceria: An Effective Treatment in Experimental Hepatocellular Carcinoma. *Hepatology* **2020**, *72*, 1267–1282. [CrossRef]
119. Tarnuzzer, R.W.; Colon, J.; Patil, S.; Seal, S. Vacancy engineered ceria nanostructures for protection from radiation-induced cellular damage. *Nano Lett.* **2005**, *5*, 2573–2577. [CrossRef]
120. Li, H.; Liu, C.; Zeng, Y.-P.; Hao, Y.-H.; Huang, J.-W.; Yang, Z.-Y.; Li, R. Nanoceria-Mediated Drug Delivery for Targeted Photodynamic Therapy on Drug-Resistant Breast Cancer. *ACS Appl. Mater. Interfaces* **2016**, *8*, 31510–31523. [CrossRef] [PubMed]
121. Das, S.; Chigurupati, S.; Dowding, J.; Munusamy, P.; Baer, D.R.; McGinnis, J.F.; Mattson, M.P.; Self, W.; Seal, S. Therapeutic potential of nanoceria in regenerative medicine. *MRS Bull.* **2014**, *39*, 976–983. [CrossRef]
122. Marino, A.; Tonda-Turo, C.; De Pasquale, D.; Ruini, F.; Genchi, G.; Nitti, S.; Cappello, V.; Gemmi, M.; Mattoli, V.; Ciardelli, G.; et al. Gelatin/nanoceria nanocomposite fibers as antioxidant scaffolds for neuronal regeneration. *Biochim. Biophys. Acta-Gen. Subj.* **2017**, *1861*, 386–395. [CrossRef] [PubMed]
123. Muhammad, F.; Wang, A.; Qi, W.; Zhang, S.; Zhu, G. Intracellular Antioxidants Dissolve Man-Made Antioxidant Nanoparticles: Using Redox Vulnerability of Nanoceria to Develop a Responsive Drug Delivery System. *Appl. Mater. Interfaces* **2014**, *6*, 19424–19433. [CrossRef] [PubMed]
124. Casals, E.; Pfaller, T.; Duschl, A.; Oostingh, G.J.; Puntes, V. Time evolution of the nanoparticle protein corona. *ACS Nano* **2010**, *4*, 3623–3632. [CrossRef] [PubMed]
125. Casals, E.; Pfaller, T.; Duschl, A.; Oostingh, G.J.; Puntes, V. Hardening of the Nanoparticle Protein Corona in Metal (Au, Ag) and Oxide (Fe_3O_4, CoO and CeO_2) Nanoparticles. *Small* **2011**. [CrossRef] [PubMed]

126. Astorga-Gamaza, A.; Vitali, M.; Borrajo, M.L.; Suárez-López, R.; Jaime, C.; Bastus, N.; Serra-Peinado, C.; Luque-Ballesteros, L.; Blanch-Lombarte, O.; Prado, J.G.; et al. Antibody cooperative adsorption onto AuNPs and its exploitation to force natural killer cells to kill HIV-infected T cells. *Nano Today* **2021**, *36*, 101056. [CrossRef]
127. Ribera, J.; Rodríguez-Vita, J.; Cordoba, B.; Portolés, I.; Casals, G.; Casals, E.; Jiménez, W.; Puntes, V.; Morales-Ruiz, M. Functionalized cerium oxide nanoparticles mitigate the oxidative stress and pro-inflammatory activity associated to the portal vein endothelium of cirrhotic rats. *PLoS ONE* **2019**, *14*, e0218716. [CrossRef]
128. O'Shaughnessy, J.A.; Tjulandin, S.; Davidson, N. ABI-007 (ABRAXANE™), a Nanoparticle Albumin-Bound (nab) Paclitaxel Demonstrates Superior Efficacy vs Taxol in MBC: A Phase III Trial. In Proceedings of the 26th Annual San Antonio Breast Cancer Symposium, San Antonio, TX, USA, 3–6 December 2003. Abstract 44.

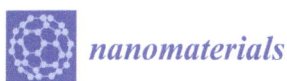

Article

Growth-Promoting Gold Nanoparticles Decrease Stress Responses in Arabidopsis Seedlings

Eleonora Ferrari [1], Francesco Barbero [2,3], Marti Busquets-Fité [4], Mirita Franz-Wachtel [5], Heinz-R. Köhler [6], Victor Puntes [2,7,8] and Birgit Kemmerling [1,*]

1 ZMBP, University of Tübingen, 72076 Tübingen, Germany; eleonora.ferrari@uni-tuebingen.de
2 Catalan Institute of Nanoscience and Nanotechnology (ICN2), CSIC and BIST, Campus UAB, Bellaterra, 08193 Barcelona, Spain; fra.barbero@gmail.com (F.B.); victor.puntes@icn.cat (V.P.)
3 Universitat Autònoma de Barcelona (UAB), Bellaterra, 08193 Barcelona, Spain
4 Applied Nanoparticles, S.L., 08018 Barcelona, Spain; marti.busquets@appliednanoparticles.eu
5 Proteome Center, University of Tübingen, 72076 Tübingen, Germany; mirita.franz-wachtel@uni-tuebingen.de
6 Animal Physiological Ecology, University of Tübingen, 72076 Tübingen, Germany; heinz-r.koehler@uni-tuebingen.de
7 Institució Catalana de Recerca i Estudis Avançats (ICREA), 08010 Barcelona, Spain
8 Vall d'Hebron Institut de Recerca (VHIR), 08032 Barcelona, Spain
* Correspondence: birgit.kemmerling@zmbp.uni-tuebingen.de

Abstract: The global economic success of man-made nanoscale materials has led to a higher production rate and diversification of emission sources in the environment. For these reasons, novel nanosafety approaches to assess the environmental impact of engineered nanomaterials are required. While studying the potential toxicity of metal nanoparticles (NPs), we realized that gold nanoparticles (AuNPs) have a growth-promoting rather than a stress-inducing effect. In this study we established stable short- and long-term exposition systems for testing plant responses to NPs. Exposure of plants to moderate concentrations of AuNPs resulted in enhanced growth of the plants with longer primary roots, more and longer lateral roots and increased rosette diameter, and reduced oxidative stress responses elicited by the immune-stimulatory PAMP flg22. Our data did not reveal any detrimental effects of AuNPs on plants but clearly showed positive effects on growth, presumably by their protective influence on oxidative stress responses. Differential transcriptomics and proteomics analyses revealed that oxidative stress responses are downregulated whereas growth-promoting genes/proteins are upregulated. These omics datasets after AuNP exposure can now be exploited to study the underlying molecular mechanisms of AuNP-induced growth-promotion.

Keywords: engineered nanomaterial (ENM); nanoparticle (NP); gold nanoparticle (AuNP); plant; *Arabidopsis thaliana*; plant growth; stress response; transcriptomics; proteomics

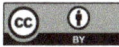

1. Introduction

Engineered nanomaterials (ENMs) are distributed into the environment in drastically increasing amounts, yet knowledge on the resulting effects of ENMs on the environment is limited [1,2]. Although naturally occurring nanomaterials have always existed, in the last decade the emission rate of anthropogenic nanoparticles (NPs), intentionally or unintentionally released, has been continuously rising [3,4]. For these reasons, novel nanosafety approaches to assess the environmental impact of ENMs are required [5].

Gold ENMs are used worldwide in various fields, including medicine, biology, chemistry, physics, electronics, and cosmetics [6–8]. The unique optical and electrochemical properties of AuNPs [9], as well as their accessibility for various surface functionalizations [10], have been exploited in many applications ranging from diagnostics and cancer therapy [11] to industrial catalysis [12] and water purification [13]. Furthermore, the latest developments in nanotechnology have opened up new opportunities in the food safety industry [14,15] and agronomy [16]. Several studies have shown that biosynthesized AuNPs have larvicidal and nematicidal effects in crop cultivation without adversely affecting their growth and development [17,18], implicating the application of more agro-ecological practices in the future.

The increasing production, use, and disposal of ENMs has translated into a higher and uncontrolled release of such materials in the environment [19]. As a result of the unique size-dependent physicochemical properties of NMs, such as higher reactivity than their respective bulk materials, concerns about potential adverse effects have arisen [20,21]. In order to assess the risk of ENMs on biosystems, a comprehensive characterization of the material is required, as their physicochemical properties and behavior after release into the environment depend on their chemical composition, size, shape, and surface [22,23]. Stable colloidal ENMs can be obtained by steric or electrostatic surface functionalization with coating materials [24,25]. Despite the stabilizing function of such surface modifications, it must be taken into account that the chemistry of coatings can change under natural conditions, affecting the properties of ENMs and their biocompatibility [26,27].

To study the risk of ENMs, ecological effects should be studied under natural conditions, but model systems also need to be optimized for stable, non-toxic assay conditions and adequate characterization of ENMs. As ENMs can change their properties in different environments, characterization is necessary for the starting material as well as under experimental conditions.

Positive, negative, and no effects of ENMs on human health, animals, and plants have been described. In vitro toxicity studies of AuNPs did not find detectable changes in the concentration of inflammatory markers in either humans or animals [28–31]. On the other hand, AuNPs were associated with dose-dependent imbalances of oxidative stress levels in vitro [32,33], with higher doses of particles responsible for initial oxidative cell damage [34,35]. Many studies have reported that the effects of AuNPs on living organisms are strictly related not only to their concentration, but especially to their size and the physicochemical properties of the coatings [36,37]. Environmental AuNP concentration predicted by screening models are 0.14 µg L^{-1} in natural waters and 5.99 µg kg^{-1} in soils [38]. Under lab conditions, for these concentrations no measurable physiological effect on plants have been reported [39]. To evaluate whether AuNPs have any effect on plants, higher concentrations are tested to assess the maximum potential risk that could be caused by AuNP accumulation. The effects of AuNPs on plants were reviewed by Siddiqi and Husen [40]. Overall, despite a few contradictory studies, AuNPs have been found to have detrimental effects at high concentrations ($\geq$100 mg/L) [41], with particles with a diameter below 5 nm showing increasing toxicity [42–44]. By contrast, lower concentrations of AuNPs can enhance seed germination and chlorophyll content, and improve growth and productivity in several crops and model plants under laboratory conditions [45–47]. Enhanced and reduced toxic effects and stress responses, such as reactive oxygen species (ROS) production and activation of immune responses, have both been reported in plants after AuNP treatment [40,47–50]. Furthermore, growth-promoting effects are common for nanofertilizers such as ZnNPs, for example, but were also observed for inert AuNPs [18,47]. AuNPs are widely inert and the special physicochemical properties of NPs can be studied without physiological side effects of the bulk material [51]. The mechanism underlying AuNP-induced growth-promotion is not yet understood. Understanding how NPs influence plant growth could be useful for improving crop yield in the future [52].

AuNP uptake is controversially discussed in the community, with studies showing uptake and even transport within the plant and others ruling it out [53–56]. The pore size of cell walls has been determined to be approximately 3–6 nm, a size that precludes the uptake of larger molecules, but some properties of NPs, such as surface charge, may induce morphological changes in the cell wall, thereby affecting pore size and uptake rate [57,58]. Though many plants have been tested for their ability to take up various kinds of ENMs, our knowledge is still limited and many aspects remain elusive. The mechanisms underlying the physiological effects caused by AuNPs in or outside the plant cells will be interesting to elucidate in the future.

Transcriptomics and proteomics studies after exposure to multi-walled carbon nanotubes (MWCNT), titanium dioxide (TiO_2), cerium dioxide (CeO_2), and silver (Ag) NPs have been reported in Arabidopsis plants [59–62]. Furthermore, Simon et al. [63] performed a transcriptome sequencing study on the eukaryotic green alga *Chlamydomonas reinhardtii* after treatment with Ag, TiO_2, zinc oxide (ZnO) NPs, and quantum dots (QDs). Conversely, the transcriptome and proteome changes in plants exposed to AuNPs have not yet been adequately studied.

Here, we show that well-characterized AuNPs stabilized with sodium citrate and tannic acid (SCTA) are stable, sterilizable, and functional in promoting the growth of Arabidopsis seedlings and do not show any negative effects at moderate concentration levels. Stress responses are downregulated after AuNP exposure at the ROS burst level and also on the transcriptome and proteome level. We studied transcriptome and proteome changes after AuNP-SCTA treatment, and those omics data revealed candidate genes/proteins that could explain the growth-promoting effect of AuNPs on a molecular level.

2. Materials and Methods

2.1. AuNP Synthesis

Aqueous dispersions of citrate-stabilized AuNPs were synthesized following two kinetically controlled seeded growth approaches as reported by Bastús et al. [64] and Piella et al. [65]. Tetrachloroauric (III) acid trihydrate (99.9% purity), sodium citrate tribasic dihydrate (99%), and tannic acid were purchased from Sigma-Aldrich (Madrid, Spain). Briefly, 150 mL of sodium citrate (SC) aqueous solution (2.2 mM) were brought to a boil in a three-neck flask under reflux; subsequently, 1 mL of 25 mM chloroauric acid ($HAuCl_4$) was injected into the citrate solution. After few minutes the solution became reddish, indicative of AuNP formation (~10 nm, seeds). Afterwards, different sequential steps of growth, consisting of sample dilution plus further addition of gold precursor, led to the desired AuNP size. In the second method, the main difference was the addition of traces of tannic acid (TA) (200 µM) as a co-reducer and an increase in the starting pH to produce highly monodispersed and stable AuNPs. Several batches of the AuNPs were synthesized with and without the addition of TA. All batches presented very similar features and produced similar results in the assays described. The AuNPs were synthesized by the Catalan Institute of Nanoscience and Nanotechnology and purchased from Applied Nanoparticles SL.

The AuNP dispersions were concentrated by Amicon® Ultra Centrifugal Filters (100 kDa) (Merck, Darmstadt, Germany).

2.2. AuNP Characterization

2.2.1. Size Determination by Electron Microscopy

The diameter of the synthesized AuNPs was measured by analysis of images obtained by scanning electron microscopy (SEM) with FEI Magellan XHR SEM (FEI, Hillsboro, OR, USA) in transmission mode (STEM) operated at 20 kV. Samples were prepared by drop-casting 3 µL of the NP dispersion onto a carbon-coated copper TEM grid and left to dry under mild vacuum. To prevent aggregation of the NPs during the drying procedure, they were previously conjugated with 55 kDa polyvinylpyrrolidone (PVP) (Sigma-Aldrich, Madrid, Spain). More than 500 particles from different regions of the grid were measured.

2.2.2. UV-Vis Spectroscopy

The UV-Vis absorption spectra of AuNPs are due to the collective oscillation of their metallic surface electrons, called localized surface plasmon resonance (LSPR). The LSPR profile and maximum position strictly depend on the material, shape, and size of the NPs, as well as the refractive index of the solvent and the vicinity of the NP surfaces. The LSPR profile is highly sensitive to NP aggregation. At inter-particle distances that are less than their diameter, the NP near-field electromagnetic coupling applies, leading to significant UV-Vis spectra changes that translate to a LSPR red-shift and/or to the occurrence of a second peak at a higher wavelength. For large aggregates, an increase in the baseline can be observed [66–68].

UV-Vis spectra were acquired with a Shimadzu UV-2400 spectrophotometer (SSI, Kyoto, Japan). One mL of sample was placed in a plastic cuvette and analyses were performed at time zero or over time in the 300–800 nm range at room temperature. In the case of solidified media, samples were poured into the cuvette prior to jellification. MilliQ water or $\frac{1}{2}$ Murashige and Skoog (MS) agar (Duchefa, Haarlem, The Netherlands) were taken as reference for the different samples.

2.2.3. Size and Zeta Potential Measurements

Laser doppler velocimetry and dynamic light scattering were used to determine the Z potential and the hydrodynamic diameter of the AuNPs, respectively, employing a Malvern Zetasizer Nano ZS instrument (light source wavelength at 638.2 nm; detector at a fixed scattering angle of 173°) (Malvern Panalytical Ltd., Malvern, UK). Measurements were performed at 25 °C. Diameters were reported as Z-average and polydispersity index (PDI) calculated by cumulative analysis.

2.2.4. Au Quantification

Samples were digested with aqua regia (1:3 HNO_3 (70%):HCl (37%)) for 24 h and then diluted with MilliQ water to be further analyzed by induced coupled plasma-mass spectroscopy (ICP-MS) using an ICP-MS NexION 300 from Perkin Elmer (Shelton, CT, USA).

2.3. AuNP Sterilization

AuNP suspensions were sterilized by filter sterilization with cellulose mixed ester (CME) and polyethersulfone (PES) filters (Carl Roth, Karlsruhe, Germany), both with a pore size of 0.2 µm, according to the manufacturer's protocol. UV-Vis spectra of AuNPs before and after filtration were acquired as previously mentioned.

2.4. Plant Growth Conditions and Plant NP Exposition

2.4.1. Seed Sterilization

Arabidopsis thaliana ecotype Columbia 0 (Col-0) seeds were surface sterilized by chlorine gas treatment in a desiccator containing 50 mL of 12% sodium hypochlorite and 2 mL of 37% HCl for 4 h. The chemicals were purchased from Merck (Darmstadt, Germany). The seeds were dried in a laminar air flow sterile bench for 30 min. The seeds were grown on agar-solidified medium or in hydroponic cultures.

2.4.2. Plant Growth Conditions

All plants were grown in long day conditions with 16 h light, 8 h dark, 22 °C, 110 µmol $m^{-2} s^{-1}$ light, and 60% relative humidity.

2.4.3. NP Exposure in Agar-Solidified Medium

Sterilized seeds were sown on agar plates containing $\frac{1}{2}$ MS plant medium and stratified at 4 °C for 2 days in the dark. Afterwards, plates were incubated for 7 days under controlled long day conditions. Plates were placed vertically to allow root growth along the agar surface. The reducing and stabilizing agents sodium citrate and tannic acid (SCTA) or AuNP-SCTA were mixed with the medium at the indicated concentrations before jellification. Physicochemical characterization of AuNP-SCTA dispersed in $\frac{1}{2}$ MS agar showed high colloidal stability up to 3 weeks, allowing for 1 week exposure experiments.

2.4.4. NP Exposure in Hydroponic Culture

Sterilized seeds were sown on a thin layer of $\frac{1}{2}$ MS agar medium and stratified at 4 °C for 2 days in the dark. Subsequently, the seeds were germinated and grown for 2 weeks under controlled long day conditions. The seedling roots grew through the agar into liquid $\frac{1}{2}$ MS plant medium. After 2 weeks, SCTA or AuNP-SCTA were mixed in the indicated concentration with the $\frac{1}{2}$ MS medium and were incubated for 6 h. Since UV-Vis spectroscopic analyses of AuNP-SCTA dispersed in $\frac{1}{2}$ MS revealed no changes in the shape of the spectrum at 6 h, whereas a typical aggregation profile was shown after 9 h, this interval was chosen for short-term experiments.

2.5. Physiological Effects

Arabidopsis thaliana seedlings were grown in agar-solidified medium, as described previously, with SCTA or AuNP-SCTA to a final concentration of 10 mg/L. Photographs of 7 day-old seedlings were taken. Growth parameters, i.e., rosette diameter, primary root length, and lateral root length, were measured using the software ImageJ. The lateral root number was determined by counting the number of lateral roots per seedling with 20 seedlings being analyzed for each individual parameter (n = 20).

2.6. Statistical Analysis

Statistical significance between groups was evaluated using one-way ANOVA combined with Tukey's honest significant difference (HSD) test. FOX assay data were tested with a two-way nested ANOVA followed by Dunnett's post-hoc test; data were normally distributed (Shapiro–Wilk test) and showed homogeneity of variances (Levene's test). Significant differences are indicated with different letters ($p < 0.01$). Statistical evaluations were performed using JMP (version 15.0.0, Heidelberg, Germany) software.

2.7. Detection of Immune-Related Responses

2.7.1. Oxidative Burst

Production of reactive oxygen species (ROS) was measured in a luminol-based assay using a microplate luminometer (CentroPRO LB 962; Berthold Technologies, Bad Wildbad, Germany) as described by Albert et al. [69]. The elicitor flg22 (final concentration 100 nM) was used in the assay as positive control. The horseradish peroxidase, in the presence of ROS, catalyzed the oxidation of luminol to 3-aminophthalate with emission of light at 428 nm. The monitored oxidative burst was measured as emitted light and recorded as relative light units (RLU). The ROS burst was monitored for 30 min for 3 plants per treatment and three leaf pieces per plant (n = 9).

2.7.2. FOX Assay

The level of lipid hydroperoxides (LOOHs) was assessed with the modified colorimetric ferrous oxidation xylenol orange (FOX) assay as described by Hermes-Lima et al. [70] and adjusted by Schmieg et al. [71]. Leaves of 5 week-old *A. thaliana* plants were cut into square pieces (about 2 mm^2) and left to equilibrate overnight in milliQ water. Then the leaf pieces were elicited for 30 min with flg22 (100 nM) or the tested compounds and immediately stored at -80 °C. Three plants and three leaf pieces per plant (n = 9) were used for each sample. Samples were homogenized in ice-cold HPLC-grade methanol in a 1:15 ratio, and 30 µL of the supernatant was used in the reaction mixture. Cumene hydroperoxide equivalents (CHPequiv./mg wet weight) were calculated using the following equation:

$$CHPE = \frac{ABS570}{ABS570+CHP} \times Volume\ CHP \times \frac{Total\ Volume}{Sample\ Volume} \times Dilution\ Factor$$
$$= \frac{ABS570}{ABS570+CHP} \times 1 \times \frac{200}{30} \times 15$$

2.8. Transciptomics

2.8.1. RNA Extraction

RNA was extracted from 100 mg of Arabidopsis seedling roots treated for 6 h and 7 d with 10 mg/L Au-SCTA or SCTA (SC 2.2 mM; TA 200 µM) in triplicate using the RNeasy Plant Mini Kit (QIAGEN, Hilden, Germany) followed by on-column DNA digestion with the RNase-Free DNase Set (QIAGEN, Hilden, Germany). The total RNA concentration,

RNA Integrity Number (RIN) value, and rRNA ratio (28S/18S) were evaluated using Agilent2100 Bionalyzer (RNA 6000 Nano Kit; Agilent, Waldbronn, Germany).

2.8.2. Transcriptome Sequencing Analysis

The BGI Group (Shenzhen, China) performed the total transcriptome sequencing (RNA-Seq) analysis. Samples were sequenced on the Illumina HiSeq platform. The internal software SOAPnuke v1.5.2 was used to filter low-quality reads, reads with adaptors, or those containing more than 5% of unknown bases (N). Genome mapping of clean reads was performed using HISAT v2.0.4 (Hierarchical Indexing for Spliced Alignment of Transcripts) software [72]. The assembler of RNA-Seq alignments into potential transcripts StringTie v1.0.4 was used to reconstruct transcripts [73]. Cuffcompare, a tool of Cufflinks [74], was used to identify novel transcripts by comparing reconstructed transcripts with genome reference annotation information. The coding ability of those new transcripts was predicted using CPC v0.9-r2 [75]. After novel transcript detection, novel coding transcripts were merged with reference transcripts to get a complete reference and clean reads were mapped to it using Bowtie2 v2.2.5 [76]. For each sample, the gene expression level was calculated with RSEM, a software package for estimating gene and isoform expression levels from RNA-Seq data [77]. Differentially expressed genes (DEGs) were detected with the nonparametric approach NOIseq method (parameters: fold change $\geq$ 2.00 and probability $\geq$ 0.8) as described by Tarazona et al. [78].

2.9. Mass Spectrometry Analysis

2.9.1. Total Protein Extraction

For total protein extraction from seedlings, 100 mg of material were ground in liquid nitrogen and mixed in a ratio of 1:3 with ice-cold extraction buffer (10% glycerol, 150 mM Tris/HCl, pH 7.5, 1 mM EDTA, 150 mM NaCl, 10 mM DTT, 0.2% Nonidet P-40, 2% PVPP, 1 tablet of proteinase inhibitor cocktail (Roche, Mannheim, Germany) per 10 mL solution). Protein extraction was performed on a rotor at 4 °C for 1 h and the extract was purified by a centrifuging at 4 °C, 5000× g for 20 min. The supernatant was then transferred through a one-layer Miracloth (Merck, Darmstadt, Germany) in a fresh pre-chilled 1.5 mL tube on ice.

2.9.2. NanoLC-MS/MS Analysis

The Proteome Center Tübingen performed the nanoscale liquid chromatography coupled to tandem mass spectrometry (LC-MS/MS) on total protein extracts as described.

Proteins were purified in a 12% NUPAGE Novex Bis-Tris Gel (Invitrogen, Karlsruhe, Germany) for 10 min at 200 V and stained with Colloidal Blue Staining Kit (Invitrogen, Karlsruhe, Germany). In-gel digestion of proteins was performed as previously described [79]. Extracted peptides were first desalted and then labeled using C18 StageTips [80] as described elsewhere [81]. Samples were labeled with dimethyl "light" $((CH_3)_2)$ and dimethyl "intermediate" $((CH_1D_2)_2)$. Complete incorporation levels of the dimethyl labels were achieved in all cases.

Eluted peptides were mixed in a 1:1 ratio according to the measured protein amounts. The analysis of the peptide mixture was performed on an Easy-nLC 1200 system coupled to an LTQ Orbitrap Elite or a QExactive HF mass spectrometer (all Thermo Fisher Scientific) as described elsewhere [82] with slight modifications: Peptides were injected onto the column in HPLC solvent A (0.1% formic acid) at a flow rate of 500 nL/min and subsequently eluted with a 227 min (Orbitrap Elite) or 127 min (QExactive HF) gradient of 10–33–50–90% HPLC solvent B (80% ACN in 0.1% formic acid). During peptide elution the flow rate was kept constant at 200 nL/min.

In each scan cycle, the 15 (Orbitrap Elite) or 12 (Q Exactive HF) most intense precursor ions were sequentially fragmented using collision-induced dissociation (CID) and higher energy collisional dissociation (HCD) fragmentation, respectively. In all measurements, sequenced precursor masses were excluded from further selection for 60 (Orbitrap Elite) or 30 s (Q Exactive HF). The target values for MS/MS fragmentation were 5000 and 10^5 charges, and for the MS scan 10^6 and 3×10^6 charges.

2.9.3. MS Data Processing

The MS data were processed with MaxQuant software suite v1.5.2.8 and v1.6.3.4 (Cox and Mann 2008), respectively. A database search was performed using the Andromeda search engine [83], which is a module of the MaxQuant. MS/MS spectra were searched against an *Arabidopsis thaliana* database obtained from Uniprot, and a database consisting of 285 commonly observed contaminants. In the database search, full tryptic specificity was required and up to two missed cleavages were allowed. Protein N-terminal acetylation and oxidation of methionine were set as variable modifications. Initial precursor mass tolerance was set to 4.5 ppm and to 0.5 Da at the MS/MS level (CID fragmentation), or 20 ppm (HCD fragmentation). Peptide, protein, and modification site identifications were filtered using a target-decoy approach at a false discovery rate (FDR) set to 0.01 [84]. For protein group quantitation a minimum of two quantified peptides were required.

Perseus software (v1.6.1.3), a module from the MaxQuant suite [85], was used for calculation of the significance B (p_{sigB}) for each protein ratio with respect to the distance of the median of the distribution of all protein ratios as well as the intensities. All proteins with a fold change ≥ 2.00- and $p_{sigB} < 0.01$ in a pairwise comparison were considered to be differentially expressed.

3. Results

3.1. Physicochemical Characterization of AuNPs Dispersed in Plant Growth Media

Two different types of gold nanoparticles (AuNPs) with an average diameter of about 12 nm were synthesized with the two seeded-growth methods reported by Bastús et al. [64] and Piella et al. [65], with the only difference being the addition of tannic acid (TA), which can interact with the NP surface, inferring higher colloidal stability. The physicochemical characterization of one of the used batches of AuNPs prepared in the presence of TA (AuNP-SCTA) is shown in Figure 1a,b, whereas the characterization of AuNP-SC is reported in Supplemental Figure S1a,b.

It is important to characterize the evolution of the AuNPs once dispersed in the working media to correctly correlate the pristine and the evolving NP features with the observed biological effects [86]. Thus, over time, physicochemical characterization of AuNP-SC and AuNP-SCTA in the used working media, i.e., $\frac{1}{2}$ MS and agar-solidified $\frac{1}{2}$ MS media, was performed. Once dispersed in $\frac{1}{2}$ MS, AuNP-SC underwent fast aggregation, pointed out by an immediate emergence of a second localized surface plasmon resonance (LSPR) peak at around 650 nm in the UV-Vis spectra (Supplemental Figure S1c) [87]. This aggregation was probably due to the increase in the ionic strength by mono- and divalent inorganic ions in the media ($\frac{1}{2}$ MS has a salinity of 23 mM). The ions in the media can screen the negative charges provided by the SC present on the surface of the AuNPs, responsible for the electrostatic repulsion between particles [88,89].

By contrast, the UV-Vis spectra of AuNP-SCTA dispersed in $\frac{1}{2}$ MS showed no changes until 6 h of exposure. After 9 h, changes in the spectrum shape were observed, showing the start of a typical aggregation profile that led to complete aggregation after 15 h, detectable by a drastic change in the UV-Vis spectrum (Figure 1c) [87]. This result indicates that AuNP-SCTA had a good colloidal stability up to 6 h of exposure to the hydroponic medium, whereas after 9 h the NPs started to slowly aggregate. Therefore, in this study all experiments carried out in hydroponic cultures were short time exposures, in a time range of 6 h. The presence of TA was the only difference between the two types of AuNPs. Thus, we hypothesize that this organic molecule functions as a NP stabilizer, increasing the particle stability against salt-driven aggregation. TA confers an effective higher surface charge or partial steric stabilization, preventing NP aggregation. Regarding the observed aggregation of the AuNP-SCTA in $\frac{1}{2}$ MS after 9 h, it could be speculated that organic molecules (e.g., sucrose), present in the medium in excess compared to the NP stabilizers, could progressively replace the NP stabilizers on the NP surface, conferring a negative effect on stabilization and supporting aggregation. However, further studies will be necessary to precisely understand the role and nature of TA in the stabilization of AuNP-SCTA.

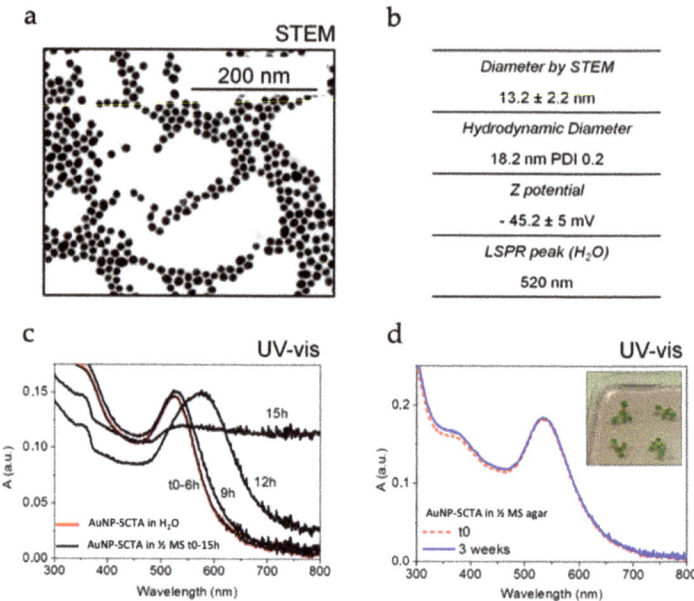

Figure 1. Physicochemical characterization of AuNP-SCTA dispersed in H_2O, $\frac{1}{2}$ MS, and $\frac{1}{2}$ MS agar. (**a**) Bright field—scanning transmission electron microscopy (STEM) of AuNP-SCTA. (**b**) NP average diameter measured by STEM; hydrodynamic diameters (in H_2O) measured by dynamic light scattering, reported as Z average and poly dispersity index (PDI); Z potential of the AuNP-SCTA dispersed in H_2O (pH 6.5, conductivity 0.85 mS/cm). (**c**) UV-Vis spectra of AuNP-SCTA dispersed in H_2O (red) and over time (from time 0 to 15 h) in $\frac{1}{2}$ MS (black). (**d**) UV-Vis spectra of AuNP-SCTA dispersed in $\frac{1}{2}$ MS agar at time 0 (red dashed) and after 3 weeks of exposure (blue); representative photograph of Arabidopsis seedlings germinated and grown for 1 week on an agar plate containing $\frac{1}{2}$ MS and AuNPs, showing a typical reddish color of non-aggregated AuNPs-SCTA. Absorbance A in arbitrary units (a.u.). All experiments were repeated twice with similar results.

UV-Vis spectroscopy of AuNP-SCTA exposed to $\frac{1}{2}$ MS agar showed high stability at least up to 3 weeks (Figure 1d), allowing for long-term exposure experiments. Conversely, AuNP-SC dispersed in $\frac{1}{2}$ MS agar showed an initial aggregation that, unlike in $\frac{1}{2}$ MS, did not evolve over time (Supplemental Figure S1d), probably due to the interaction with agar molecules and the fast viscosity increase due to medium jellification as well as to the reduced number of particles (aggregation is directly proportional to concentration). Note that below 10^{10} NP mL^{-1} the collision probability decreases to almost zero, so even if their surface is not passivated, NPs do not aggregate.

In light of these observations, the AuNP-SCTA were chosen for the following physiological and molecular studies, permitting all the experiments to be conducted with stable AuNPs, thereby allowing for the correct NP size to be correlated with the observed effects on Arabidopsis.

Several AuNP-SCTA batches with very similar physicochemical features were produced and tested. The results of the physiological studies after AuNP-SCTA treatment were fully reproducible between the different batches, showing that the synthesis protocol is very robust and produced reliable results.

3.2. AuNP-SCTA Sterilization

In order to grow seedlings under sterile conditions and to discriminate the AuNP effects from the possible physiological and molecular changes induced in plants by microbial contaminants such as, e.g., (pathogenic) bacteria and fungi, the sterility of the colloidal solution is a fundamental requirement. To sterilize AuNP-SCTA solutions, physical filtration methods were chosen. Two different filter materials, i.e., cellulose mixed ester (CME) and polyethersulfone (PES), both with a pore size of 0.2 µm, were tested. To analyze possible changes in the particle concentration or their aggregation state, UV-Vis spectra before and after filtration were acquired (Figure 2). Both filtering procedures were effective in removing all contaminating microorganisms and allowed plant cultivation under sterile conditions. The CME filter, a standard hydrophilic membrane commonly used for a broad range of applications, was shown to significantly affect the amplitude of the spectra, revealing a drastically reduced AuNP-SCTA concentration. By contrast, the PES filter, a hydrophilic and low protein-binding membrane, did not change the spectra and therefore did not affect the concentration of AuNP-SCTA. No changes in the overall shape of the UV-Vis spectrum were observed, indicating that no alterations of the physicochemical properties of the AuNPs occurred. Therefore, PES membranes were used in all subsequent experiments for NP sterilization.

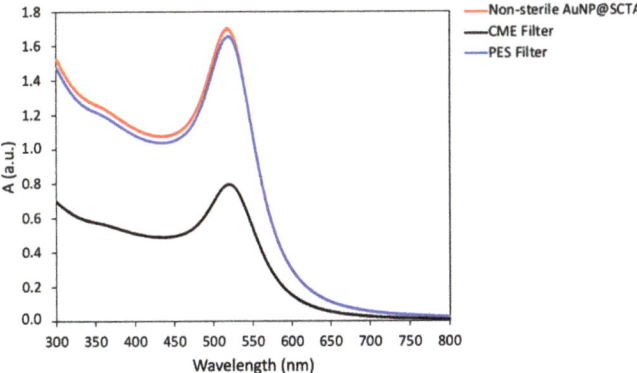

Figure 2. UV-Vis spectra of AuNP-SCTA before and after sterilization with different filter materials. UV-Vis spectra of AuNP-SCTA before (red dashed) and after sterilization with PES (blue) and CME (black) filters were acquired with a Shimadzu UV-2400 spectrophotometer. Absorbance A in arbitrary units (a.u.). The experiment was repeated twice with similar results.

3.3. Physiological Effects of AuNPs

Although gold (Au) can be present in the environment from natural sources, in the last decade the increased use and disposal of AuNPs has affected the level of this chemical element in soil and water [1]. Although many studies on the accumulation and physiological effects of Au in various plant species have been conducted [90], a comprehensive investigation on AuNP fate and action after their release into plant growth media and their effects on plants at the physiological, transcriptomic, and proteomic level is missing. In the present study, *Arabidopsis thaliana* was used as a model plant to investigate the effects of AuNPs on growth and development. As shown in Supplemental Figure S2b, AuNP-SCTA in a range from 0 to 20 mg/L affected Arabidopsis root growth in a dose-dependent manner with a maximal effect at 10 mg/L, whereas the NP stabilizer SCTA (SC 2.2 mM; TA 200 µM) did not affect the primary root length at any of the tested concentrations (Supplemental Figure S2a). For this reason, 10 mg/L AuNP-SCTA was chosen as the final concentration in all subsequent experiments.

Physiological analyses were performed in order to evaluate Arabidopsis responses to abiotic stress caused by AuNP-SCTA exposure. Seedlings, grown under controlled long day conditions, were harvested after 7 days, and representative parameters were recorded, i.e., primary root length, rosette diameter, number of lateral roots, and lateral root length. For each parameter, another set of plants was grown in the presence of SCTA (SC 2.2 mM; TA 200 µM) as a control.

Although SCTA did not affect plant growth and development, AuNP-SCTA had a positive influence on all parameters tested. Seedlings germinated and grown on AuNP-SCTA-containing medium developed a longer primary root, with an enhancement of 1.2 folds compared to control seedlings (Figure 3a). Furthermore, the lateral root number and length were positively affected upon AuNP-SCTA treatment, displaying, compared to the controls, an increase of 1.7- and 1.5-fold, respectively (Figure 3e,f). Shoot development was also influenced by AuNP-SCTA exposure in the same way as the root system (Figure 3c). The size of the rosette diameters was enhanced by 1.3-fold in comparison to the control seedlings. These data show that AuNP-SCTA is not acutely toxic to plants, but rather have a positive effect on plant growth.

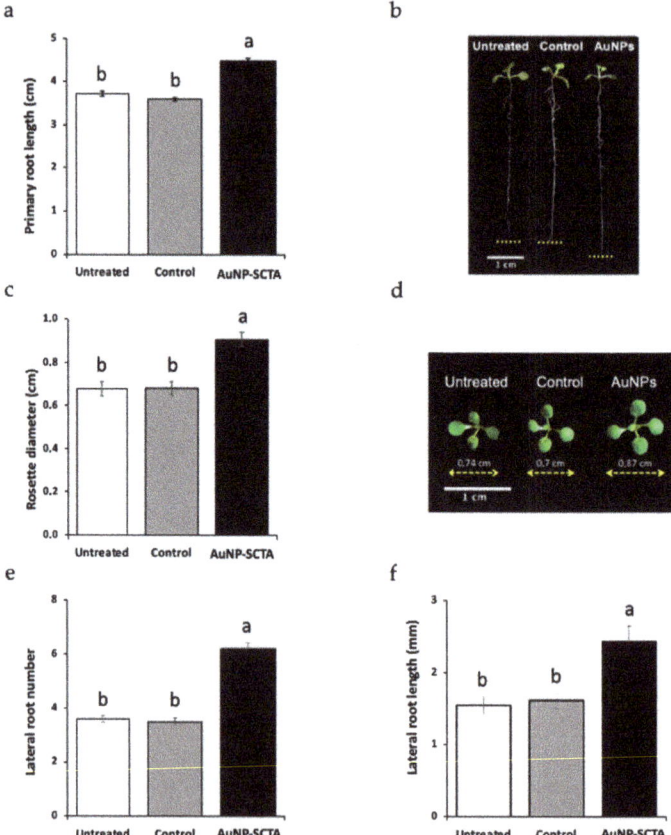

Figure 3. AuNP-SCTA enhances growth of Arabidopsis seedlings. Wild-type Arabidopsis seedlings were grown for 7 d on agar-solidified $\frac{1}{2}$ MS medium containing 10 mg/L of AuNP-SCTA or SCTA (SC 2.2 mM; TA 200 µM) (control) or on un-supplemented medium (untreated). Growth parameters were scored: (**a**) primary root length and (**b**) representative picture of (**a**). (**c**) Rosette diameter and (**d**) representative photograph of (**c**). (**e**) Lateral root number. (**f**) Lateral root length. Results shown are means ± SE with n = 20. Different labels a and b indicate statistically different groups according to multiple comparisons following one-way ANOVA analysis at a probability level of $p < 0.01$. All experiments were repeated twice with similar results.

3.4. Immune Responses upon AuNP Treatment

NPs have been reported to affect the innate immune system in animals [5]. To assess whether they have an influence on plant immune responses, different innate immune defensive reactions in plants were evaluated. The production of reactive oxygen species (ROS) in the apoplast and lipid peroxidation are typical cellular events triggered by the plant surveillance system that detects highly conserved microbe- or pathogen-associated molecular patterns (M/PAMPs) via cell surface-located pattern-recognition receptors (PRRs) in a process called pattern-triggered immunity (PTI) [91,92].

The cellular response of *Arabidopsis thaliana* to abiotic stress resulting from NP exposure was initially measured as reactive oxygen species (ROS) production or oxidative burst, using a luminol-based chemiluminescence assay. As shown in Figure 4a, no ROS production was detected after exposure to milliQ water (untreated control), AuNP-SCTA (100 mg/L), or coating solution SCTA (SC 2.2 mM; TA 200 µM) (control). This also confirms that the NP suspensions were free of endotoxins such as LPS that would induce ROS in plants [93]. As positive control, the PAMP flg22 was added at a final concentration of 100 nM. The same concentration of the elicitor was used as treatment also in combination with AuNP-SCTA (10 or 100 mg/L) or SCTA as control. Although the coating solution did not affect the level of ROS production caused by flg22 treatment, AuNP-SCTA influenced the level of recorded ROS. In particular, in the presence of 10 mg/L AuNP-SCTA the PAMP (flg22) signal decreased. Furthermore, a 10× higher NP concentration (100 mg/L) was tested, and a further decrease in the level of ROS was detected.

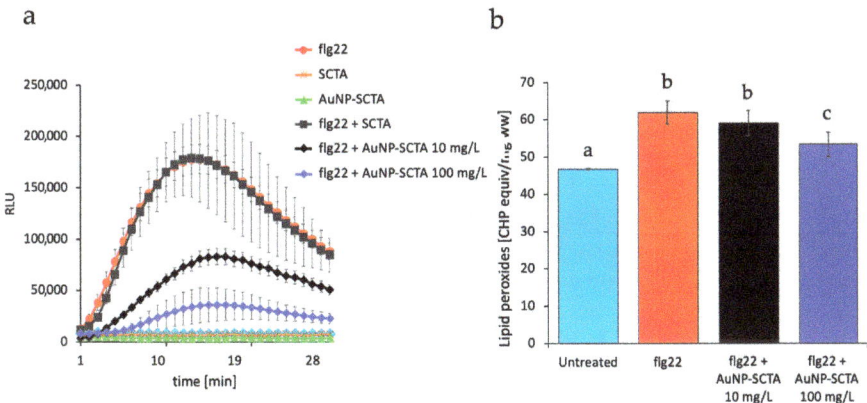

Figure 4. AuNP-SCTA decreases ROS production and lipid peroxidation levels. (**a**) ROS production measured with a luminol-based assay in leaf squares of Arabidopsis Col-0. ROS production is represented as relative light units (RLU) after elicitation with milliQ water (untreated control), flg22 (100 nM) (positive control), AuNPs-SCTA (100 mg/L), SCTA (control), flg22 + SCTA, or flg22 + AuNPs-SCTA 10 or 100 mg/L. Results are mean ± SE (n = 9). The experiment was repeated two times with similar results. (**b**) Lipid peroxides level, expressed as CHP equiv./mg ww, was measured in Arabidopsis leaves with the FOX assay. The results after treatment with milliQ water (untreated), flg22 (100 nM) (positive control), or flg22 + AuNPs-SCTA (10 or 100 mg/L) are presented as mean ± SE of three independent experiments. Based on two-way nested ANOVA followed by Dunnett's post-hoc test, data were normally distributed (Shapiro–Wilk test) and showed homogeneity of variances (Levene's test). Different letters indicate statistically significant differences at $p < 0.01$. Different labels a–c indicate statistically different groups according to multiple comparisons following two-way nested ANOVA analysis at a probability level of $p < 0.01$.

In order to discriminate between a real decrease in the ROS production and a mere technical interference with the light detection, a lipid peroxidation assay was performed. Cellular and organelle membranes, due to their high polyunsaturated fatty acid (PUFA) content, are particularly susceptible to ROS-induced peroxidation [94]. The applied colorimetric ferrous oxidation xylenol orange (FOX) assay was modified to quantify lipid hydroperoxides (LOOHs) in plant extracts. Upon treatment with 10 and 100 mg/L AuNP-SCTA plus flg22, the level of lipid peroxidation decreased significantly in comparison to flg22 alone (Figure 4b). Treatment with 100 mg/L AuNP-SCTA resulted in a more pronounced decrease in the lipid hydroperoxide level compared to 10 mg/L AuNP-SCTA. The FOX assay confirmed the oxidative burst assay results, clearly pointing out that co-exposure to PAMPs and AuNP-SCTA reduced the PAMP-induced ROS burst and subsequent lipid peroxidation. The underlying mechanism of this effect is still elusive, but the data suggest that AuNP-SCTA might be able to detoxify ROS and shift the balance between growth and immunity trade-off to the growth side.

3.5. Transcriptomics Analysis of AuNP-SCTA-Exposed Arabidopsis Seedlings

To untie the molecular nature of the plant–AuNP interaction, whole transcriptome analyses were performed on Arabidopsis seedling roots after short (6 h) and long (7 d) exposure to 10 mg/L AuNP-SCTA in hydroponic culture and agar-solidified medium (6 h and 7 d, respectively). As controls, the seedlings were treated with SCTA (2.2 mM SC; 200 µM TA). Samples were sequenced with an Illumina HiSeq platform. The average genome mapping rate was 94.66% and the average gene mapping rate was 92.04%. Raw data for both experimental conditions and all three replicates are shown in Supplemental Table S1.

As shown in Figure 5, a total of 651 differentially expressed genes (DEG) were identified after short-term treatment and 6 DEGs after long-term exposure. Whereas 121 genes were upregulated after 6 h of AuNP treatment, 530 genes were downregulated. After 7 d, 3 genes were upregulated and 3 genes were downregulated. DEGs with expression information are listed in Supplemental Table S2. Gene ontology (GO) (molecular biological function, cellular component, and biological process) and Kyoto Encyclopedia of Genes and Genomes (KEGG) pathway classification are reported in Supplemental Figures S3 and S4. In both conditions, genes involved in the response to external stimuli and cellular and metabolic processes are overrepresented within the DEGs. In particular, after short-term exposure the majority of genes involved in disease resistance, defense response, response to oxidative stress, and metal response were downregulated. This indicates that immune and oxidative stress responses were negatively affected during AuNP exposure.

DUF642 L-GalL-responsive gene 2 (DGR2, At5g25460), a gene involved in growth and development of Arabidopisis plants, was up-regulated. DGR2 has a key role in Arabidopsis root elongation and shoot development [95,96]. Downregulation of immune response genes and upregulation of growth factors indicate a shift in the trade-off between immune and growth effects and may explain the growth-promoting effects of AuNPs. The Nicotianamine synthase 2 gene, (NAS2, At5g56080), the only shared DEG between the two conditions, encodes for a protein involved in the synthesis of nicotianamin. Mutants in NAS2 show altered metal contents, indicating a role in metal uptake or response [97] (Supplemental Table S2). After 7 d of NP exposure, only 6 DEGs were detected, compared to the 651 genes identified after 6 h, clearly pointing out that transcriptome changes are relevant only at early time points after AuNP treatment.

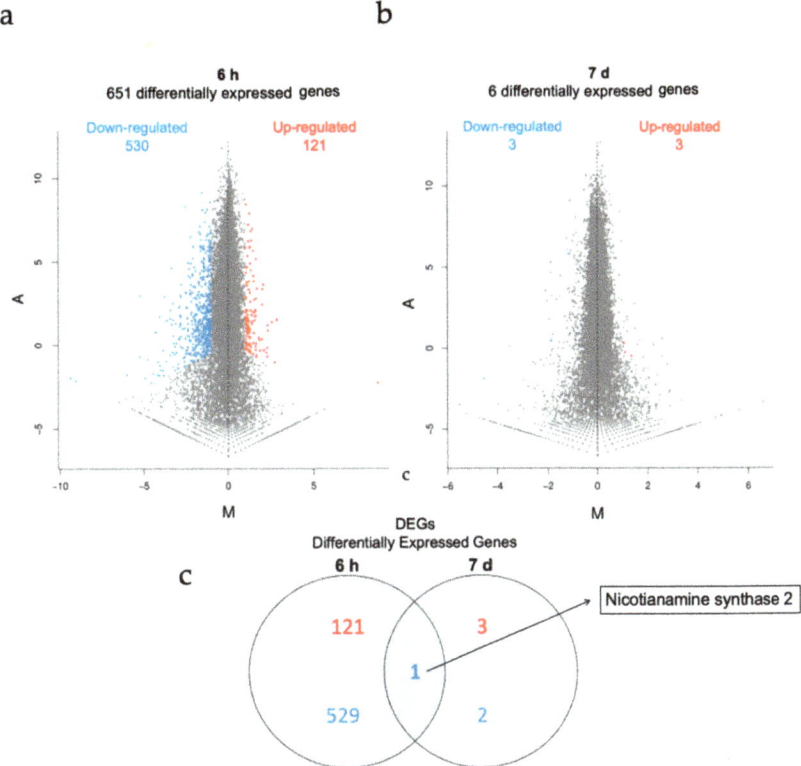

Figure 5. DEGs after AuNP-SCTA treatment. MA plot representing DEGs (upregulated genes: red dots; downregulated genes: blue dots) and non-DEGs (grey dots) in Arabidopsis seedling roots after (**a**) short- and (**b**) long-term AuNP-SCTA treatment (6 h and 7 d, respectively), detected by RNA-seq data analysis. The X-axis represents value M (log2 transformed fold change of a gene expression value) and the Y-axis represents value A (log2 transformed mean expression level). (**c**) Venn diagram displaying the total number of up- (red) and downregulated (blue) differentially expressed genes in both treatments and the name of the single overlapping gene.

3.6. Proteomic Analysis of the Effect of AuNP-SCTA in Arabidopsis

To further understand the mechanisms underlying the effects of AuNPs on *Arabidopsis thaliana* seedlings, proteomic analyses were performed on seedlings using mass spectrometry. Global changes in protein expression were investigated in Arabidopsis seedlings in the same experimental setup as used for the transcriptome analyses. Protein extracts were analyzed via nano-liquid chromatography double mass spectrometry (NanoLC-MS/MS-spectrometry).

As shown in Figure 6, from a total of 2727 detected proteins after 6 h exposure and 2503 after 7 d exposure, 119 and 59 differentially expressed proteins (DEPs), respectively, were identified. All identified up- and downregulated proteins, along with their expression profiles, are listed in Supplemental Table S3. Furthermore, we sorted the DEPs into gene ontology (GO) categories (molecular biological function, cellular component, and biological process) and KEGG pathways, as shown in Supplemental Figures S5 and S6. DEPs significantly overrepresented after both treatments were involved in metabolic processes, protein synthesis, and response to stimuli (Supplemental Table S3).

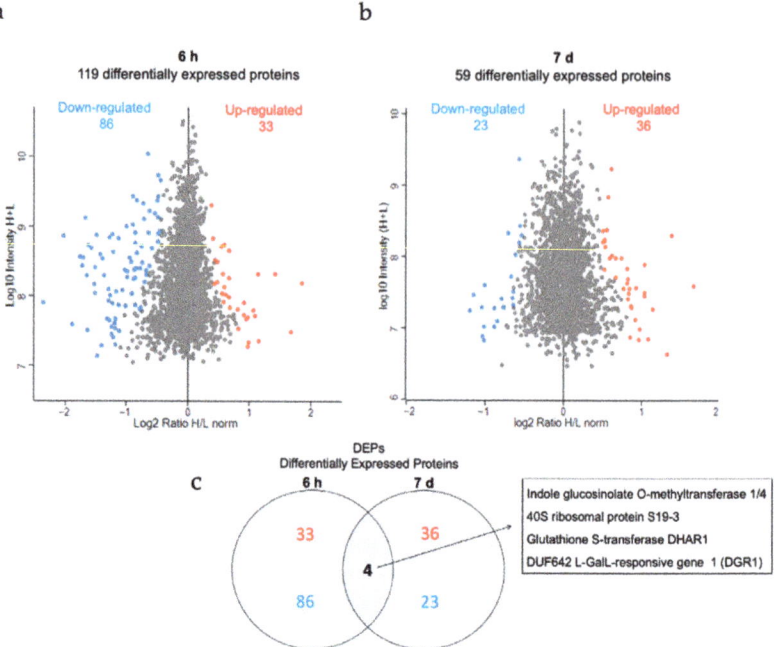

Figure 6. DEPs after AuNP-SCTA treatment. Volcano plots representing DEPs (upregulated proteins: red dots; downregulated proteins: blue dots) and non-DEPs (grey dots) in Arabidopsis seedlings after (**a**) short- and (**b**) long-term AuNP-SCTA treatment (6 h and 7 d, respectively) and detected by nano-liquid chromatography with tandem mass spectrometry (NanoLC-MS/MS) of total protein extracts. The X-axis represents the $\log_2$ transformed fold changes; the Y-axis represents the $\log_{10}$ transformed intensity (in log10), with H representing the treatment and L the control. (**c**) Venn diagram displaying the total number of up- (red) and downregulated (blue) differentially expressed proteins in both treatments and the protein names of the 4 overlapping proteins.

Oxidative stress-related proteins were mainly downregulated, as shown on the transcriptome level. The overlap analysis of the different timepoints revealed the protein DGR1 (DUF642 L-GalL-responsive gene 1, At1g80240), which was investigated for its role during the development of *Arabidopsis thaliana* [95]. After 7 d of treatment DGR1 and DGR2 were both upregulated, whereas after 6 h of treatment only DGR1 was initially downregulated. In the transcriptome analyses, the gene encoding for DGR2 was also detected to be upregulated. GSTF6 (Glutathione S-transferase F6, At1g02930), another DEG shared between treatments, encoded for a downregulated glutathione transferase involved in defense mechanisms (Supplemental Table S4). The finding of DGR2 and GSTF6 in both DEGs and DEPs indicates that these were reproducibly and robustly regulated genes/proteins upon AuNP exposure. As DGR1 and DGR2 have been previously described to be involved in growth and development, the differential regulation of these genes/proteins may explain why AuNPs have a positive effect on Arabidopsis growth. Our well-controlled transcriptome and proteome dataset provides a source for future analysis of the molecular mechanism underlying AuNP-induced growth-promotion.

4. Discussion

The widespread use of NP-containing products has led to the direct exposure of the terrestrial environment to these nanosized materials, raising concerns regarding their safety and biocompatibility with both living organisms and the environment [1,16,98–100]. Therefore, the risks and hazard assessment of NP exposure for plants, soil organisms, and consequently, humans, as a result of contamination of the food chain need to be addressed [1,101,102]. To date, despite recent developments in plant nanotoxicology, an unequivocal understanding of the effects of NPs on terrestrial plants is lacking, with fundamental information gaps about their mechanisms of action [103–105].

Plant-based nanosafety research focuses on a number of key aspects, i.e., the physicochemical properties of NPs such as material, size, and surface chemistry; the interaction of NPs with the surrounding environment; and the plant type and route of exposure [104–108]. Possible alterations in the properties and colloidal stability of NPs once released into an environment other than that of synthesis make studies under natural conditions difficult to interpret; thus, nanosafety assessments under reproducible and controlled conditions help to interpret investigations in ecotoxicological assays [24,86,109].

AuNPs, due to their unique intrinsic optical, biological, and catalytic properties [110–112] and their biocompatibility with mammalian systems, have been exploited in numerous medical and technological applications and used as model particles under laboratory conditions in nanotechnological research [113–116]. The effects on plants at the physiological and molecular level remain controversial [40,54,57,117]. In this light, this study aimed at studying the behavior of engineered AuNPs as a starting material and after dispersion in plant growth media, along with their physiological and molecular effects on the model plant *Arabidopsis thaliana*.

The high salt concentration of plant growth media may facilitate the aggregation of NPs and alterations in their bio-identity [118–121]; thus, surface-stabilizing agents are used to stabilize colloidal suspensions through electrostatic, steric, or electrosteric repulsion [122]. NP surface-stabilizing agents can play a key role in plant and animal toxicity tests [123,124]. In particular, the ionic charge conferred by particle coatings may influence the physical interaction between NPs and cell membranes, with positively charged NPs being more effective than negatively charged ones [125]. Barrena et al. [124] showed that, in germination tests of cucumber and lettuce seeds, toxic effects can be attributed to NP solvents rather than to NPs themselves. In this light, we showed that exposure of Arabidopsis seedlings to 10 mg/L of the negatively charged surface stabilizer SCTA did not influence Arabidopsis root growth.

Effects of electrostatically or sterically stabilized AuNPs have been studied in liquid and agar-solidified plant media, though their behavior and possible state of aggregation have not been further described in all cases [45,126–128]. By contrast, in their physiological and toxicological studies on Arabidopsis seedlings, Siegel et al. [41] dispersed SC-capped AuNPs in $1/16$-diluted low-salinity MS, detecting a slight aggregation of AuNPs and consequently suboptimal conditions of plant growth assays. In this study, we tested the overtime stability of SC-stabilized and SCTA-stabilized AuNPs. The presence of traces of TA, the only difference between the two types of synthetized NPs, increased the stability of the particles by conferring a higher surface charge or partial steric stabilization and providing the necessary stability against salt-driven aggregation. A comprehensive physicochemical characterization of newly synthesized NPs, prior to and during their use in Arabidopsis treatments, was carried out, showing that the NPs are stable, dispersed, and usable for reproducible plant exposure experiments.

Since contaminants in plant growth media allow for the growth of microorganisms, NPs need to be sterile before their use in plant assays. As shown by previous studies, autoclaving and radiation sterilization might result in the aggregation of the NPs, loss of the coating, and contamination with potential microbial toxins [129–133]. Sterile filtration has been shown not to directly affect the physical properties of NPs, but filter materials should be tested to exclude possible interactions with particle surfaces resulting in NP retention or coating removal [132]. We tested CME and PES filters and revealed that PES filters are suitable for sterilization of AuNPs, whereas CME filtering resulted in a significant reduction in the number of NPs in the filtered samples. Therefore, PES filters are considered suitable for AuNP sterilization to allow for sterile plant cultivation in the presence of AuNP-SCTA.

A number of studies have addressed AuNP responses in plants, reporting both positive and negative effects [40]. In this study, growth-promoting effects of AuNP-SCTA at a moderate concentration (10 mg/L) were revealed. As AuNP concentrations in the environment are very low, studies with lower concentrations might reflect more natural conditions [134]. Previous studies have found that AuNPs at high concentrations ($\geq$100 mg/L) cause detrimental effects on plants, whereas for lower concentrations of AuNPs larger than 5 nm growth-promoting effects have been shown, supporting our findings that AuNPs have positive effects on plant growth [45–47,57]. Furthermore, Siegel et al. [41] tested three different sizes of AuNPs (10, 14, and 18 nm) at increasing concentrations (1, 10, and 100 mg/L) and showed that at the highest concentration the smaller particles reduced the length of the *Arabidopsis thaliana* root more than the larger ones. It has been hypothesized that a high concentration of NPs negatively affects plant growth by particle adsorption onto the cell wall of the root system, decreasing pore size and inhibiting water transport [124,135,136]. On the other hand, some contradictory studies have been reported. Feichtmeier et al. [135] reported a decrease in the biomass of *Hordeum vulgare* after AuNP treatment at a final concentration of between 3 and 10 mg/L. Some of these discrepancies can be explained by differences in specific experimental settings and different behavior of NPs under test conditions, which make a clear assessment of AuNP responses more difficult. Therefore, a careful evaluation of each study is necessary to draw a complete picture of the effects of AuNPs on plants.

Although the mechanisms of action and effects of AuNPs on plants are not yet fully understood [40,54,57,117], for the Au bulk counterpart the results are clearer. As plants have revealed their potential in the green synthesis of AuNPs, many studies have been produced on the physiological responses of plants to Au salts [137], used as starting material in order to obtain NPs. Gold is required by plants in traces, but its absorption in higher amounts can cause drastic changes in plant growth [40]. A previous study demonstrated that Arabidopsis seedlings treated with 10 mg/L of potassium tetrachloroaurate(III) ($KAuCl_4$) showed the formation of AuNPs in the roots and shoots and enhanced vegetative growth [138], whereas higher amounts of $KAuCl_4$ or gold(III) chloride ($AuCl_3$) (100 mg/L) negatively affected the root length and shoot development [139].

Immune responses are reported to be activated upon NP exposure in many plant and animal models, including reactive oxygen species (ROS) production and lipid peroxidation [48,140–142]. Here, we found that AuNP-SCTA alone did not induce these classical plant defense responses. In addition, ROS production induced by the 22-amino acid peptide derived from bacterial flagellin (flg22), sensed in plants as a pathogen-associated molecular pattern (PAMP), was significantly reduced in the presence of increasing amounts of AuNP-SCTA. To exclude a biophysical quenching effect of the light emitted by luminol, we performed lipid peroxidation assays. The same results were obtained by measuring lipid peroxidation, an indicator of oxidative stress in animals and plants [143], showing that the PAMP-triggered ROS burst was indeed reduced. Kumar et al. [47] showed that AuNPs at 80 mg/L significantly improved the free radical scavenging activity of Arabidopsis seedlings by increasing the activity of enzymes involved in the defense system against ROS, whereas plants treated with AuNPs in the range of 100 to 400 mg/L showed reduced growth, which was considered to be a consequence of increased free radical stress [40,144]. After 6 h of treatment with 10 mg/L of AuNP-SCTA, we found 10 peroxidases to be downregulated on the transcript level and 6 at the protein level, which were likely involved in oxidative stress reactions. These data indicate a correlation between ROS production and AuNP effects and show that AuNPs can reduce stress responses triggered by immune stimulatory peptides. Whether this effect is based on a direct effect on the peptide, e.g., through adsorption to the NP surface or changes in the peptide accessibility (and consequent alteration of its mode of perception) [145], or on a protective effect of AuNPs on PAMP recognition or downstream signaling, will be interesting to study in the future.

We performed transcriptomics and proteomics analyses to study the alterations caused by short (6 h) and long (7 d) AuNP exposure at the molecular level. In particular, after short-term AuNP treatment, genes involved in disease resistance, defense response, oxidative stress, and auxin- and metal-response were downregulated. In the proteomic analysis after short treatment we detected two distinct categories of upregulated proteins, i.e., proteins involved in responses to oxidative stress and abiotic stimuli, whereas after long NP exposure all upregulated proteins were annotated as involved in development processes. To our knowledge, this is the only study analyzing the transcriptomic and proteomic changes after AuNP treatments in Arabidopsis, whereas such analyses have been performed on the roots of Arabidopsis seedlings upon gold ($KAuCl_4$) exposure, which leads to AuNP formation by the plant [138]. As for the physiological effects mentioned above, at the molecular level the changes induced by gold exposure also showed some effects similar to those induced by AuNP exposure. A comparative analysis between our transcriptomics data and Tiwari et al.'s [138] shows that there is a significant overlap of up- and downregulated genes (three common upregulated and 22 common downregulated genes, Figure S7). In particular, between the upregulated DEGs two metal response genes (MT1C, At1g07610 and ALMT1, At1g08430) and DGR2 (At5g25460) were found. In both studies, disease and defense response and oxidative stress genes were downregulated. By contrast, Tiwari et al. [138] found that developmental, auxin-responsive, and metal-responsive genes were upregulated after Au treatment, whereas in our study the same categories of genes were downregulated after AuNP treatment. These differences were likely caused by different effects caused by Au ion uptake compared to exposure to nanoparticles. As metal AuNPs are very inert, the significant overlap between Au salt and AuNP is potentially caused by NP effects in both experiments, as Au ions are taken up and converted into AuNPs inside the plant, where they may cause similar effects as external NP exposure.

An overlap analysis of our proteomic and transcriptomic studies revealed two particularly interesting candidates: DUF642 L-GalL-responsive genes 1 and 2 (DGR1, At1g80240 and DGR2, At5g25460), which were also found to be upregulated by Au salt exposure [138]. DGR1 and DGR2 encode for two proteins belonging to the DUF642 protein family, whose members are part of the cell wall proteome [96] and have shown in Arabidopsis a complementary expression pattern in young and developed roots, suggesting a similar but non-redundant function [95]. As Gao et al. reported in their study [95], DGRs are involved in the development processes of Arabidopsis, and in particular in root elongation. DGR2 seems to have a predominant role, as *dgr2* single mutants show a short, undeveloped root phenotype [95]. These results suggest the potential involvement of these proteins in the root growth-promoting effects induced by AuNPs and can be used as a starting point for further studies aimed at dissecting the pathways underlying the beneficial effects of AuNP-SCTA on Arabidopsis development.

5. Conclusions

NPs are released into the environment in increasing amounts and their high reactivity may cause problems that are not associated with the respective bulk material. Therefore, an ecotoxicological assessment is necessary to evaluate their risk in nature, but to understand the molecular mechanisms underlying the effects of NPs on the environment, controlled model systems are necessary. Here, we describe the establishment of a stable and reproducible system to study plant responses to AuNPs after short- and long-term exposure. Both initial and overtime characterization of NPs, especially after dispersal in new environments, is essential. The effects resulting from NP-plant interaction need stable, sterile, and reproducible colloidal solutions, ensured by the use of non-toxic NP surface stabilizing agents. In this study, we demonstrated that these AuNP-SCTAs positively influence the growth of Arabidopsis seedlings, while also conferring partial protection against oxidative stress caused by triggering immune-responses. Transcriptomics and proteomics studies show downregulation of (oxidative) stress and immune responses and upregulation of growth-promoting genes and support the scenario that the trade-off between growth and immune/stress responses are shifted to the growth side after AuNP exposure (Figure 7).

The identified DEGs and DEPs provide a useful data source for future analysis of the molecular mechanism underlying AuNP-induced growth stimulation.

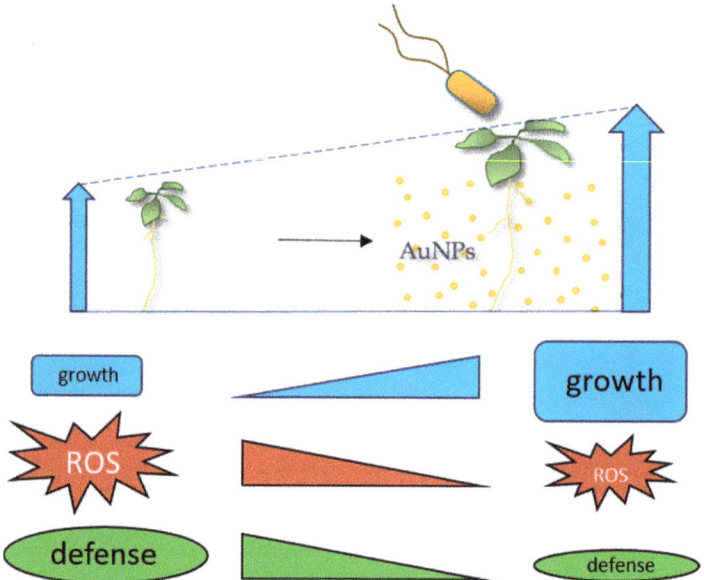

Figure 7. Model of AuNP effects on Arabidopsis seedlings. AuNPs stabilized with SCTA have growth-promoting effects on Arabidopsis seedlings and can reduce oxidative stress genes/proteins and ROS burst after triggering with the pathogen-associated molecular pattern (PAMP) flg22, indicating that the NPs can shift the trade-off between growth and defense responses to the growth side.

Supplementary Materials: The following information is available online at https://www.mdpi.com/article/10.3390/nano11123161/s1, Figure S1: Physicochemical characterization of AuNP-SC dispersed in H2O, $\frac{1}{2}$ MS, and $\frac{1}{2}$ MS agar; Figure S2: Growth of Arabidopsis seedlings in the absence and presence of AuNPs; Figure S3: GO classification of DEGs after AuNP-SCTA treatment; Figure S4: Pathway classification of DEGs after AuNP-SCTA treatment; Figure S5: GO classification of DEPs after AuNP-SCTA treatment; Figure S6: Pathway classification of DEPs after AuNP-SCTA treatment; Figure S7: Venn diagram of DEGs after AuNP-SCTA exposure (this study) and DEG after exposure to KAuCl4 resulting in in planta AuNP formation [140]. Table of the overlap between our DEGs and those published by Tiwari et al. (2016); Table S1: Clean reads quality metrics and summary of genome mapping; Table S2: DEGs list after short (6 h) and long (7 d) AuNP-SCTA treatment; Table S3: DEP list after short (6 h) and long (7 d) AuNP-SCTA treatment; Table S4: Transcriptomic and proteomic studies: overview and overlap.

Author Contributions: Conceptualization, E.F. and B.K.; methodology, E.F., F.B., M.B.-F., H.-R.K. and B.K.; validation, E.F. and B.K.; formal analysis, E.F.; investigation, E.F. and F.B.; resources, M.F.-W.; data curation, E.F., F.B. and M.F.-W.; writing—original draft preparation, E.F. and B.K.; writing—review and editing, all authors; visualization, E.F. and B.K.; supervision, V.P. and B.K.; project administration, B.K.; funding acquisition, B.K. All authors have read and agreed to the published version of the manuscript.

Funding: This research received funding from the European Union's Horizon 2020 research and innovation program under the Marie Sklodowska-Curie grant agreement PANDORA, no. 671881.

Institutional Review Board Statement: Not applicable.

Informed Consent Statement: Not applicable.

Acknowledgments: We thank Helene Eckstein for her support with the FOX assays and Silke Wahl and Irina Droste-Borel for their technical support with NanoLC-MS/MS analysis.

Conflicts of Interest: The authors declare no conflict of interest.

References

1. Bundschuh, M.; Filser, J.; Lüderwald, S.; McKee, M.S.; Metreveli, G.; Schaumann, G.E.; Schulz, R.; Wagner, S. Nanoparticles in the environment: Where do we come from, where do we go to? *Environ. Sci. Eur.* **2018**, *30*, 6. [CrossRef] [PubMed]
2. Nowack, B.; Bucheli, T.D. Occurrence, behavior and effects of nanoparticles in the environment. *Environ. Pollut.* **2007**, *150*, 5–22. [CrossRef] [PubMed]
3. Lespes, G.; Faucher, S.; Slaveykova, V.I. Natural Nanoparticles, Anthropogenic Nanoparticles, Where Is the Frontier? *Front. Environ. Sci.* **2020**, *8*. [CrossRef]
4. Hochella, M.F., Jr.; Mogk, D.W.; Ranville, J.; Allen, I.C.; Luther, G.W.; Marr, L.C.; McGrail, B.P.; Murayama, M.; Qafoku, N.P.; Rosso, K.M.; et al. Natural, incidental, and engineered nanomaterials and their impacts on the Earth system. *Science* **2019**, *363*, eaau8299. [CrossRef]
5. Boraschi, D.; Alijagic, A.; Auguste, M.; Barbero, F.; Ferrari, E.; Hernadi, S.; Mayall, C.; Michelini, S.; Navarro Pacheco, N.I.; Prinelli, A.; et al. Addressing Nanomaterial Immunosafety by Evaluating Innate Immunity across Living Species. *Small* **2020**, *16*, 2000598. [CrossRef]
6. Ramalingam, V. Multifunctionality of gold nanoparticles: Plausible and convincing properties. *Adv. Colloid Interface Sci.* **2019**, *271*, 101989. [CrossRef]
7. Alaqad, K.; Saleh, T. Gold and Silver Nanoparticles: Synthesis Methods, Characterization Routes and Applications towards Drugs. *J. Environ. Anal. Toxicol.* **2016**, *6*. [CrossRef]
8. Leso, V.; Fontana, L.; Iavicoli, I. Biomedical nanotechnology: Occupational views. *Nano Today* **2019**, *24*, 10–14. [CrossRef]
9. Ashraf, R.; Amna, T.; Sheikh, F.A. Unique Properties of the Gold Nanoparticles: Synthesis, Functionalization and Applications. In *Application of Nanotechnology in Biomedical Sciences*; Sheikh, F.A., Ed.; Springer: Singapore, 2020; pp. 75–98.
10. Spampinato, V.; Parracino, M.A.; La Spina, R.; Rossi, F.; Ceccone, G. Surface Analysis of Gold Nanoparticles Functionalized with Thiol-Modified Glucose SAMs for Biosensor Applications. *Front. Chem.* **2016**, *4*, 8. [CrossRef]
11. Singh, P.; Pandit, S.; Mokkapati, V.R.S.S.; Garg, A.; Ravikumar, V.; Mijakovic, I. Gold Nanoparticles in Diagnostics and Therapeutics for Human Cancer. *Int. J. Mol. Sci.* **2018**, *19*, 1979. [CrossRef]
12. Grisel, R.; Weststrate, K.-J.; Gluhoi, A.; Nieuwenhuys, B.E. Catalysis by Gold Nanoparticles. *Gold Bull.* **2002**, *35*, 39–45. [CrossRef]
13. Ojea-Jiménez, I.; López, X.; Arbiol, J.; Puntes, V. Citrate-Coated Gold Nanoparticles As Smart Scavengers for Mercury(II) Removal from Polluted Waters. *ACS Nano* **2012**, *6*, 2253–2260. [CrossRef]
14. Hua, Z.; Yu, T.; Liu, D.; Xianyu, Y. Recent advances in gold nanoparticles-based biosensors for food safety detection. *Biosens. Bioelectron.* **2021**, *179*, 113076. [CrossRef] [PubMed]
15. Li, L.; Zhang, M.; Chen, W. Gold nanoparticle-based colorimetric and electrochemical sensors for the detection of illegal food additives. *J. Food Drug Anal.* **2020**, *28*, 642–654. [CrossRef]
16. Mittal, D.; Kaur, G.; Singh, P.; Yadav, K.; Ali, S.A. Nanoparticle-Based Sustainable Agriculture and Food Science: Recent Advances and Future Outlook. *Front. Nanotechnol.* **2020**, *2*. [CrossRef]
17. Sundararajan, B.; Ranjitha Kumari, B.D. Novel synthesis of gold nanoparticles using *Artemisia vulgaris* L. leaf extract and their efficacy of larvicidal activity against dengue fever vector *Aedes aegypti* L. *J. Trace Elem. Med. Biol.* **2017**, *43*, 187–196. [CrossRef]
18. Thakur, R.K.; Dhirta, B.; Shirkot, P. Studies on effect of gold nanoparticles on Meloidogyne incognita and tomato plants growth and development. *bioRxiv* **2018**, *2*, 428144.
19. Giese, B.; Klaessig, F.; Park, B.; Kaegi, R.; Steinfeldt, M.; Wigger, H.; von Gleich, A.; Gottschalk, F. Risks, Release and Concentrations of Engineered Nanomaterial in the Environment. *Sci. Rep.* **2018**, *8*, 1565. [CrossRef]
20. Yokel, R.A.; Macphail, R.C. Engineered nanomaterials: Exposures, hazards, and risk prevention. *J. Occup. Med. Toxicol.* **2011**, *6*, 7. [CrossRef]
21. Mourdikoudis, S.; Pallares, R.M.; Thanh, N.T.K. Characterization techniques for nanoparticles: Comparison and complementarity upon studying nanoparticle properties. *Nanoscale* **2018**, *10*, 12871–12934. [CrossRef]
22. Albanese, A.; Tang, P.S.; Chan, W.C. The effect of nanoparticle size, shape, and surface chemistry on biological systems. *Annu. Rev. Biomed. Eng.* **2012**, *14*, 1–16. [CrossRef] [PubMed]
23. Powers, K.; Palazuelos, M.; Moudgil, B.; Roberts, S. Characterization of the size, shape, and state of dispersion of nanoparticles for toxicological studies. *Nanotoxicology* **2009**, *1*, 42–51. [CrossRef]
24. Barbero, F.; Moriones, O.H.; Bastús, N.G.; Puntes, V. Dynamic Equilibrium in the Cetyltrimethylammonium Bromide–Au Nanoparticle Bilayer, and the Consequent Impact on the Formation of the Nanoparticle Protein Corona. *Bioconjug. Chem.* **2019**, *30*, 2917–2930. [CrossRef] [PubMed]
25. Ai, H.; Jones, S.A.; Lvov, Y.M. Biomedical applications of electrostatic layer-by-layer nano-assembly of polymers, enzymes, and nanoparticles. *Cell Biochem. Biophys.* **2003**, *39*, 23. [CrossRef]
26. Wagner, S.; Gondikas, A.; Neubauer, E.; Hofmann, T.; von der Kammer, F. Spot the Difference: Engineered and Natural Nanoparticles in the Environment—Release, Behavior, and Fate. *Angew. Chem. Int. Ed.* **2014**, *53*, 12398–12419. [CrossRef] [PubMed]

27. Wu, H.; Huang, L.; Rose, A.; Grassian, V.H. Impact of surface adsorbed biologically and environmentally relevant coatings on TiO_2 nanoparticle reactivity. *Environ. Sci. Nano* **2020**, *7*, 3783–3793. [CrossRef]
28. Lopez-Chaves, C.; Soto-Alvaredo, J.; Montes-Bayon, M.; Bettmer, J.; Llopis, J.; Sanchez-Gonzalez, C. Gold nanoparticles: Distribution, bioaccumulation and toxicity. In vitro and in vivo studies. *Nanomedicine* **2018**, *14*, 1–12. [CrossRef]
29. Downs, T.R.; Crosby, M.E.; Hu, T.; Kumar, S.; Sullivan, A.; Sarlo, K.; Reeder, B.; Lynch, M.; Wagner, M.; Mills, T.; et al. Silica nanoparticles administered at the maximum tolerated dose induce genotoxic effects through an inflammatory reaction while gold nanoparticles do not. *Mutat. Res. Genet. Toxicol. Environ. Mutagen.* **2012**, *745*, 38–50. [CrossRef]
30. Khan, H.A.; Abdelhalim, M.A.K.; Alhomida, A.S.; Al-Ayed, M.S. Effects of Naked Gold Nanoparticles on Proinflammatory Cytokines mRNA Expression in Rat Liver and Kidney. *BioMed Res. Int.* **2013**, *2013*, 590730. [CrossRef]
31. Yang, C.; Yang, H.; Wu, J.; Meng, Z.; Xing, R.; Tian, A.; Tian, X.; Guo, L.; Zhang, Y.; Nie, G.; et al. No overt structural or functional changes associated with PEG-coated gold nanoparticles accumulation with acute exposure in the mouse heart. *Toxicol. Lett.* **2013**, *222*, 197–203. [CrossRef]
32. Piryazev, A.P.; Azizova, O.A.; Aseichev, A.V.; Dudnik, L.B.; Sergienko, V.I. Effect of gold nanoparticles on production of reactive oxygen species by human peripheral blood leukocytes stimulated with opsonized zymosan. *Bull. Exp. Biol. Med.* **2013**, *156*, 101–103. [CrossRef]
33. Mateo, D.; Morales, P.; Ávalos, A.; Haza, A.I. Oxidative stress contributes to gold nanoparticle-induced cytotoxicity in human tumor cells. *Toxicol. Mech. Methods* **2014**, *24*, 161–172. [CrossRef]
34. Li, J.J.; Hartono, D.; Ong, C.-N.; Bay, B.-H.; Yung, L.-Y.L. Autophagy and oxidative stress associated with gold nanoparticles. *Biomaterials* **2010**, *31*, 5996–6003. [CrossRef]
35. Li, T.; Albee, B.; Alemayehu, M.; Diaz, R.; Ingham, L.; Kamal, S.; Rodriguez, M.; Bishnoi, S.W. Comparative toxicity study of Ag, Au, and Ag-Au bimetallic nanoparticles on Daphnia magna. *Anal. Bioanal. Chem.* **2010**, *398*, 689–700. [CrossRef] [PubMed]
36. Falagan-Lotsch, P.; Grzincic, E.M.; Murphy, C.J. One low-dose exposure of gold nanoparticles induces long-term changes in human cells. *Proc. Natl. Acad. Sci. USA* **2016**, *113*, 13318–13323. [CrossRef] [PubMed]
37. Sousa, A.A.; Hassan, S.A.; Knittel, L.L.; Balbo, A.; Aronova, M.A.; Brown, P.H.; Schuck, P.; Leapman, R.D. Biointeractions of ultrasmall glutathione-coated gold nanoparticles: Effect of small size variations. *Nanoscale* **2016**, *8*, 6577–6588. [CrossRef] [PubMed]
38. Tiede, K.; Hassellöv, M.; Breitbarth, E.; Chaudhry, Q.; Boxall, A.B.A. Considerations for environmental fate and ecotoxicity testing to support environmental risk assessments for engineered nanoparticles. *J. Chromatogr. A* **2009**, *1216*, 503–509. [CrossRef]
39. Batley, G.E.; Kirby, J.K.; McLaughlin, M.J. Fate and Risks of Nanomaterials in Aquatic and Terrestrial Environments. *Acc. Chem. Res.* **2013**, *46*, 854–862. [CrossRef]
40. Siddiqi, K.; Husen, A. Engineered Gold Nanoparticles and Plant Adaptation Potential. *Nanoscale Res. Lett.* **2016**, *11*, 400. [CrossRef]
41. Siegel, J.; Záruba, K.; Švorčík, V.; Kroumanová, K.; Burketová, L.; Martinec, J. Round-shape gold nanoparticles: Effect of particle size and concentration on *Arabidopsis thaliana* root growth. *Nanoscale Res. Lett.* **2018**, *13*, 95. [CrossRef]
42. Pan, Y.; Leifert, A.; Ruau, D.; Neuss, S.; Bornemann, J.; Schmid, G.; Brandau, W.; Simon, U.; Jahnen-Dechent, W. Gold Nanoparticles of Diameter 1.4 nm Trigger Necrosis by Oxidative Stress and Mitochondrial Damage. *Small* **2009**, *5*, 2067–2076. [CrossRef]
43. Coradeghini, R.; Gioria, S.; García, C.P.; Nativo, P.; Franchini, F.; Gilliland, D.; Ponti, J.; Rossi, F. Size-dependent toxicity and cell interaction mechanisms of gold nanoparticles on mouse fibroblasts. *Toxicol. Lett.* **2013**, *217*, 205–216. [CrossRef]
44. Boyoglu, C.; He, Q.; Willing, G.; Boyoglu-Barnum, S.; Dennis, V.A.; Pillai, S.; Singh, S.R. Microscopic Studies of Various Sizes of Gold Nanoparticles and Their Cellular Localizations. *ISRN Nanomater.* **2013**, *2013*, 123838. [CrossRef]
45. Arora, S.; Sharma, P.; Kumar, S.; Nayan, R.; Khanna, P.K.; Zaidi, M.G.H. Gold-nanoparticle induced enhancement in growth and seed yield of Brassica juncea. *Plant Growth Regul.* **2012**, *66*, 303–310. [CrossRef]
46. Mahakham, W.; Theerakulpisut, P.; Maensiri, S.; Phumying, S.; Sarmah, A. Environmentally benign synthesis of phytochemicals-capped gold nanoparticles as nanopriming agent for promoting maize seed germination. *Sci. Total Environ.* **2016**, *573*, 1089–1102. [CrossRef] [PubMed]
47. Kumar, V.; Guleria, P.; Kumar, V.; Yadav, S.K. Gold nanoparticle exposure induces growth and yield enhancement in *Arabidopsis thaliana*. *Sci. Total Environ.* **2013**, *461–462*, 462–468. [CrossRef] [PubMed]
48. Marslin, G.; Sheeba, C.; Gregory, F. Nanoparticles Alter Secondary Metabolism in Plants via ROS Burst. *Front. Plant Sci.* **2017**, *8*, 832. [CrossRef]
49. Chandra, S.; Chakraborty, N.; Dasgupta, A.; Sarkar, J.; Panda, K.; Acharya, K. Chitosan nanoparticles: A positive modulator of innate immune responses in plants. *Sci. Rep.* **2015**, *5*, 15195. [CrossRef]
50. Iqbal, M.S.; Singh, A.K.; Singh, S.P.; Ansari, M.I. Nanoparticles and Plant Interaction with Respect to Stress Response. In *Nanomaterials and Environmental Biotechnology*; Bhushan, I., Singh, V.K., Tripathi, D.K., Eds.; Springer International Publishing: Cham, Switzerland, 2020; pp. 1–15.
51. Yang, L.; Kuang, H.; Zhang, W.; Aguilar, Z.P.; Wei, H.; Xu, H. Comparisons of the biodistribution and toxicological examinations after repeated intravenous administration of silver and gold nanoparticles in mice. *Sci. Rep.* **2017**, *7*, 3303. [CrossRef] [PubMed]
52. Zhao, L.; Lu, L.; Aodi, W.; Zhang, H.; Huang, M.; Wu, H.; Xing, B.; Wang, Z.; Ji, R. Nanobiotechnology in Agriculture: Use of Nanomaterials To Promote Plant Growth and Stress Tolerance. *J. Agric. Food Chem.* **2020**, *68*, 1935–1947. [CrossRef]

53. Milewska-Hendel, A.; Zubko, M.; Karcz, J.; Stróż, D.; Kurczyńska, E. Fate of neutral-charged gold nanoparticles in the roots of the *Hordeum vulgare* L. cultivar Karat. *Sci. Rep.* **2017**, *7*, 3014. [CrossRef]
54. Zhu, Z.J.; Wang, H.; Yan, B.; Zheng, H.; Jiang, Y.; Miranda, O.R.; Rotello, V.M.; Xing, B.; Vachet, R.W. Effect of surface charge on the uptake and distribution of gold nanoparticles in four plant species. *Environ. Sci. Technol.* **2012**, *46*, 12391–12398. [CrossRef] [PubMed]
55. Koelmel, J.; Leland, T.; Wang, H.; Amarasiriwardena, D.; Xing, B. Investigation of gold nanoparticles uptake and their tissue level distribution in rice plants by laser ablation-inductively coupled-mass spectrometry. *Environ. Pollut.* **2013**, *174*, 222–228. [CrossRef] [PubMed]
56. Judy, J.D.; Unrine, J.M.; Rao, W.; Wirick, S.; Bertsch, P.M. Bioavailability of Gold Nanomaterials to Plants: Importance of Particle Size and Surface Coating. *Environ. Sci. Technol.* **2012**, *46*, 8467–8474. [CrossRef] [PubMed]
57. Sabo-Attwood, T.; Unrine, J.M.; Stone, J.W.; Murphy, C.J.; Ghoshroy, S.; Blom, D.; Bertsch, P.M.; Newman, L.A. Uptake, distribution and toxicity of gold nanoparticles in tobacco (Nicotiana xanthi) seedlings. *Nanotoxicology* **2012**, *6*, 353–360. [CrossRef]
58. Carpita, N.; Sabularse, D.; Montezinos, D.; Delmer, D.P. Determination of the Pore Size of Cell Walls of Living Plant Cells. *Science* **1979**, *205*, 1144–1147. [CrossRef]
59. García-Sánchez, S.; Bernales, I.; Cristobal, S. Early response to nanoparticles in the Arabidopsis transcriptome compromises plant defence and root-hair development through salicylic acid signalling. *BMC Genom.* **2015**, *16*, 341. [CrossRef]
60. Kaveh, R.; Li, Y.S.; Ranjbar, S.; Tehrani, R.; Brueck, C.L.; Van Aken, B. Changes in *Arabidopsis thaliana* gene expression in response to silver nanoparticles and silver ions. *Environ. Sci. Technol.* **2013**, *47*, 10637–10644. [CrossRef] [PubMed]
61. Zhang, C.L.; Jiang, H.S.; Gu, S.P.; Zhou, X.H.; Lu, Z.W.; Kang, X.H.; Yin, L.; Huang, J. Combination analysis of the physiology and transcriptome provides insights into the mechanism of silver nanoparticles phytotoxicity. *Environ. Pollut.* **2019**, *252*, 1539–1549. [CrossRef]
62. Tumburu, L.; Andersen, C.P.; Rygiewicz, P.T.; Reichman, J.R. Molecular and physiological responses to titanium dioxide and cerium oxide nanoparticles in Arabidopsis. *Environ. Toxicol. Chem.* **2017**, *36*, 71–82. [CrossRef]
63. Simon, D.F.; Domingos, R.F.; Hauser, C.; Hutchins, C.M.; Zerges, W.; Wilkinson, K.J. Transcriptome sequencing (RNA-seq) analysis of the effects of metal nanoparticle exposure on the transcriptome of *Chlamydomonas reinhardtii*. *Appl. Environ. Microbiol.* **2013**, *79*, 4774–4785. [CrossRef]
64. Bastús, N.G.; Comenge, J.; Puntes, V. Kinetically controlled seeded growth synthesis of citrate-stabilized gold nanoparticles of up to 200 nm: Size focusing versus Ostwald ripening. *Langmuir* **2011**, *27*, 11098–11105. [CrossRef] [PubMed]
65. Piella, J.; Bastús, N.G.; Puntes, V. Size-Controlled Synthesis of Sub-10-nanometer Citrate-Stabilized Gold Nanoparticles and Related Optical Properties. *Chem. Mater.* **2016**, *28*, 1066–1075. [CrossRef]
66. Chen, Y.; Xianyu, Y.; Jiang, X. Surface Modification of Gold Nanoparticles with Small Molecules for Biochemical Analysis. *Acc. Chem. Res.* **2017**, *50*, 310–319. [CrossRef] [PubMed]
67. Ghosh, P.; Han, G.; De, M.; Kim, C.K.; Rotello, V.M. Gold nanoparticles in delivery applications. *Adv. Drug Deliv. Rev.* **2008**, *60*, 1307–1315. [CrossRef] [PubMed]
68. Hvolbæk, B.; Janssens, T.V.W.; Clausen, B.S.; Falsig, H.; Christensen, C.H.; Nørskov, J.K. Catalytic activity of Au nanoparticles. *Nano Today* **2007**, *2*, 14–18. [CrossRef]
69. Albert, M.; Butenko, M.A.; Aalen, R.B.; Felix, G.; Wildhagen, M. Chemiluminescence Detection of the Oxidative Burst in Plant Leaf Pieces. *Bio-protocol* **2015**, *5*, e1423. [CrossRef]
70. Hermes-Lima, M.; Willmore, W.G.; Storey, K.B. Quantification of lipid peroxidation in tissue extracts based on Fe(III)xylenol orange complex formation. *Free Radic. Biol. Med.* **1995**, *19*, 271–280. [CrossRef]
71. Schmieg, H.; Huppertsberg, S.; Knepper, T.P.; Krais, S.; Reitter, K.; Rezbach, F.; Ruhl, A.S.; Köhler, H.-R.; Triebskorn, R. Polystyrene microplastics do not affect juvenile brown trout (Salmo trutta f. fario) or modulate effects of the pesticide methiocarb. *Environ. Sci. Eur.* **2020**, *32*, 49. [CrossRef]
72. Kim, D.; Langmead, B.; Salzberg, S.L. HISAT: A fast spliced aligner with low memory requirements. *Nat. Methods* **2015**, *12*, 357–360. [CrossRef]
73. Pertea, M.; Pertea, G.M.; Antonescu, C.M.; Chang, T.-C.; Mendell, J.T.; Salzberg, S.L. StringTie enables improved reconstruction of a transcriptome from RNA-seq reads. *Nat. Biotechnol.* **2015**, *33*, 290–295. [CrossRef] [PubMed]
74. Trapnell, C.; Roberts, A.; Goff, L.; Pertea, G.; Kim, D.; Kelley, D.R.; Pimentel, H.; Salzberg, S.L.; Rinn, J.L.; Pachter, L. Differential gene and transcript expression analysis of RNA-seq experiments with TopHat and Cufflinks. *Nat. Protoc.* **2012**, *7*, 562–578. [CrossRef] [PubMed]
75. Kong, L.; Zhang, Y.; Ye, Z.Q.; Liu, X.Q.; Zhao, S.Q.; Wei, L.; Gao, G. CPC: Assess the protein-coding potential of transcripts using sequence features and support vector machine. *Nucleic Acids Res.* **2007**, *35*, W345–W349. [CrossRef] [PubMed]
76. Langmead, B.; Salzberg, S.L. Fast gapped-read alignment with Bowtie 2. *Nat. Methods* **2012**, *9*, 357–359. [CrossRef]
77. Li, B.; Dewey, C.N. RSEM: Accurate transcript quantification from RNA-Seq data with or without a reference genome. *BMC Bioinform.* **2011**, *12*, 323. [CrossRef]
78. Tarazona, S.; García-Alcalde, F.; Dopazo, J.; Ferrer, A.; Conesa, A. Differential expression in RNA-seq: A matter of depth. *Genome Res* **2011**, *21*, 2213–2223. [CrossRef]
79. Borchert, N.; Dieterich, C.; Krug, K.; Schütz, W.; Jung, S.; Nordheim, A.; Sommer, R.J.; Macek, B. Proteogenomics of Pristionchus pacificus reveals distinct proteome structure of nematode models. *Genome Res.* **2010**, *20*, 837–846. [CrossRef]

80. Rappsilber, J.; Mann, M.; Ishihama, Y. Protocol for micro-purification, enrichment, pre-fractionation and storage of peptides for proteomics using StageTips. *Nat. Protoc.* **2007**, *2*, 1896–1906. [CrossRef]
81. Boersema, P.J.; Raijmakers, R.; Lemeer, S.; Mohammed, S.; Heck, A.J.R. Multiplex peptide stable isotope dimethyl labeling for quantitative proteomics. *Nat. Protoc.* **2009**, *4*, 484–494. [CrossRef]
82. Kliza, K.; Taumer, C.; Pinzuti, I.; Franz-Wachtel, M.; Kunzelmann, S.; Stieglitz, B.; Macek, B.; Husnjak, K. Internally tagged ubiquitin: A tool to identify linear polyubiquitin-modified proteins by mass spectrometry. *Nat. Methods* **2017**, *14*, 504–512. [CrossRef]
83. Cox, J.; Mann, M. MaxQuant enables high peptide identification rates, individualized p.p.b.-range mass accuracies and proteome-wide protein quantification. *Nat. Biotechnol.* **2008**, *26*, 1367–1372. [CrossRef] [PubMed]
84. Elias, J.E.; Gygi, S.P. Target-decoy search strategy for increased confidence in large-scale protein identifications by mass spectrometry. *Nat. Methods* **2007**, *4*, 207–214. [CrossRef] [PubMed]
85. Tyanova, S.; Temu, T.; Sinitcyn, P.; Carlson, A.; Hein, M.Y.; Geiger, T.; Mann, M.; Cox, J. The Perseus computational platform for comprehensive analysis of (prote)omics data. *Nat. Methods* **2016**, *13*, 731–740. [CrossRef]
86. Barbero, F.; Russo, L.; Vitali, M.; Piella, J.; Salvo, I.; Borrajo, M.L.; Busquets-Fité, M.; Grandori, R.; Bastús, N.G.; Casals, E.; et al. Formation of the Protein Corona: The Interface between Nanoparticles and the Immune System. *Semin. Immunol.* **2017**, *34*, 52–60. [CrossRef] [PubMed]
87. Sepúlveda, B.; Angelomé, P.C.; Lechuga, L.M.; Liz-Marzán, L.M. LSPR-based nanobiosensors. *Nano Today* **2009**, *4*, 244–251. [CrossRef]
88. Cosgrove, T. *Colloid Science: Principles, Methods and Applications*; Wiley: Chichester, UK, 2010.
89. Abbott, S.; Holmes, N. *Nanocoatings: Principles and Practice: From Research to Production*; DEStech Publications: Lancaster, PA, USA, 2013.
90. Wilson-Corral, V.; Anderson, C.; Rodriguez, M. Gold phytomining. A review of the relevance of this technology to mineral extraction in the 21st century. *J. Environ. Manag.* **2012**, *111*, 249–257. [CrossRef]
91. Saijo, Y.; Loo, E.; Yasuda, S. Pattern recognition receptors and signaling in plant-microbe interactions. *Plant J.* **2017**, *93*, 592–613. [CrossRef]
92. Farmer, E.E.; Mueller, M.J. ROS-mediated lipid peroxidation and RES-activated signaling. *Annu. Rev. Plant Biol.* **2013**, *64*, 429–450. [CrossRef]
93. Ranf, S. Immune Sensing of Lipopolysaccharide in Plants and Animals: Same but Different. *PLoS Pathog.* **2016**, *12*, e1005596. [CrossRef]
94. Su, L.-J.; Zhang, J.-H.; Gomez, H.; Murugan, R.; Hong, X.; Xu, D.; Jiang, F.; Peng, Z.-Y. Reactive Oxygen Species-Induced Lipid Peroxidation in Apoptosis, Autophagy, and Ferroptosis. *Oxid. Med. Cell. Longev.* **2019**, *2019*, 5080843. [CrossRef]
95. Gao, Y.; Badejo, A.A.; Sawa, Y.; Ishikawa, T. Analysis of two L-Galactono-1,4-lactone-responsive genes with complementary expression during the development of *Arabidopsis thaliana*. *Plant Cell Physiol.* **2012**, *53*, 592–601. [CrossRef]
96. Cruz-Valderrama, J.E.; Gómez-Maqueo, X.; Salazar-Iribe, A.; Zúñiga-Sánchez, E.; Hernández-Barrera, A.; Quezada-Rodríguez, E.; Gamboa-deBuen, A. Overview of the Role of Cell Wall DUF642 Proteins in Plant Development. *Int. J. Mol. Sci.* **2019**, *20*, 3333. [CrossRef] [PubMed]
97. Klatte, M.; Schuler, M.; Wirtz, M.; Fink-Straube, C.; Hell, R.; Bauer, P. The Analysis of Arabidopsis Nicotianamine Synthase Mutants Reveals Functions for Nicotianamine in Seed Iron Loading and Iron Deficiency Responses. *Plant Physiol.* **2009**, *150*, 257–271. [CrossRef] [PubMed]
98. Gupta, R.; Xie, H. Nanoparticles in Daily Life: Applications, Toxicity and Regulations. *J. Environ. Pathol. Toxicol. Oncol.* **2018**, *37*, 209–230. [CrossRef] [PubMed]
99. Liu, J.; Williams, P.C.; Geisler-Lee, J.; Goodson, B.M.; Fakharifar, M.; Peiravi, M.; Chen, D.; Lightfoot, D.A.; Gemeinhardt, M.E. Impact of wastewater effluent containing aged nanoparticles and other components on biological activities of the soil microbiome, Arabidopsis plants, and earthworms. *Environ. Res.* **2018**, *164*, 197–203. [CrossRef]
100. Singh, D.; Kumar, A. Human Exposures of Engineered Nanoparticles from Plants Irrigated with Contaminated Water: Mixture Toxicity Issues and Challenges Ahead. *Adv. Sci. Lett.* **2014**, *20*, 1204–1207. [CrossRef]
101. Stampoulis, D.; Sinha, S.K.; White, J.C. Assay-Dependent Phytotoxicity of Nanoparticles to Plants. *Environ. Sci. Technol.* **2009**, *43*, 9473–9479. [CrossRef]
102. Chawla, J.; Singh, D.; Sundaram, B.; Kumar, A. Identifying Challenges in Assessing Risks of Exposures of Silver Nanoparticles. *Expo. Health* **2018**, *10*, 61–75. [CrossRef]
103. Zia-ur-Rehman, M.; Qayyum, M.F.; Akmal, F.; Maqsood, M.A.; Rizwan, M.; Waqar, M.; Azhar, M. Chapter 7—Recent Progress of Nanotoxicology in Plants. In *Nanomaterials in Plants, Algae, and Microorganisms*; Tripathi, D.K., Ahmad, P., Sharma, S., Chauhan, D.K., Dubey, N.K., Eds.; Academic Press: Cambridge, MA, USA, 2018; pp. 143–174.
104. Sanzari, I.; Leone, A.; Ambrosone, A. Nanotechnology in Plant Science: To Make a Long Story Short. *Front. Bioeng. Biotechnol.* **2019**, *7*, 120. [CrossRef]
105. Kranjc, E.; Drobne, D. Nanomaterials in Plants: A Review of Hazard and Applications in the Agri-Food Sector. *Nanomaterials* **2019**, *9*, 1094. [CrossRef]
106. Du, W.; Xu, Y.; Yin, Y.; Ji, R.; Guo, H. Risk assessment of engineered nanoparticles and other contaminants in terrestrial plants. *Curr. Opin. Environ. Sci. Health* **2018**, *6*, 21–28. [CrossRef]

107. Khan, I.; Saeed, K.; Khan, I. Nanoparticles: Properties, applications and toxicities. *Arab. J. Chem.* **2019**, *12*, 908–931. [CrossRef]
108. Sukhanova, A.; Bozrova, S.; Sokolov, P.; Berestovoy, M.; Karaulov, A.; Nabiev, I. Dependence of Nanoparticle Toxicity on Their Physical and Chemical Properties. *Nanoscale Res. Lett.* **2018**, *13*, 44. [CrossRef] [PubMed]
109. Kim, T.; Lee, C.H.; Joo, S.W.; Lee, K. Kinetics of gold nanoparticle aggregation: Experiments and modeling. *J. Colloid Interface Sci* **2008**, *318*, 238–243. [CrossRef] [PubMed]
110. Hu, X.; Zhang, Y.; Ding, T.; Liu, J.; Zhao, H. Multifunctional Gold Nanoparticles: A Novel Nanomaterial for Various Medical Applications and Biological Activities. *Front. Bioeng. Biotechnol.* **2020**, *8*, 990. [CrossRef]
111. Das, M.; Shim, K.H.; An, S.S.A.; Yi, D.K. Review on gold nanoparticles and their applications. *Toxicol. Environ. Health Sci.* **2011**, *3*, 193–205. [CrossRef]
112. Zhang, X. Gold Nanoparticles: Recent Advances in the Biomedical Applications. *Cell Biochem. Biophys.* **2015**, *72*, 771–775. [CrossRef]
113. Azzazy, H.; Mansour, M.; Samir, T.; Franco, R. Gold nanoparticles in the clinical laboratory: Principles of preparation and applications. *Clin. Chem. Lab. Med.* **2011**, *50*, 193–209. [CrossRef]
114. Connor, E.E.; Mwamuka, J.; Gole, A.; Murphy, C.J.; Wyatt, M.D. Gold Nanoparticles Are Taken Up by Human Cells but Do Not Cause Acute Cytotoxicity. *Small* **2005**, *1*, 325–327. [CrossRef]
115. Sperling, R.A.; Rivera Gil, P.; Zhang, F.; Zanella, M.; Parak, W.J. Biological applications of gold nanoparticles. *Chem. Soc. Rev.* **2008**, *37*, 1896–1908. [CrossRef]
116. Li, Y.; Italiani, P.; Casals, E.; Valkenborg, D.; Mertens, I.; Baggerman, G.; Nelissen, I.; Puntes, V.F.; Boraschi, D. Assessing the Immunosafety of Engineered Nanoparticles with a Novel in Vitro Model Based on Human Primary Monocytes. *ACS Appl. Mater. Interfaces* **2016**, *8*, 28437–28447. [CrossRef] [PubMed]
117. Rico, C.M.; Majumdar, S.; Duarte-Gardea, M.; Peralta-Videa, J.R.; Gardea-Torresdey, J.L. Interaction of Nanoparticles with Edible Plants and Their Possible Implications in the Food Chain. *J. Agric. Food Chem.* **2011**, *59*, 3485–3498. [CrossRef]
118. Fuller, M.; Köper, I. Polyelectrolyte-Coated Gold Nanoparticles: The Effect of Salt and Polyelectrolyte Concentration on Colloidal Stability. *Polymers* **2018**, *10*, 1336. [CrossRef] [PubMed]
119. Sun, M.; Liu, F.; Zhu, Y.; Wang, W.; Hu, J.; Liu, J.; Dai, Z.; Wang, K.; Wei, Y.; Bai, J.; et al. Salt-Induced Aggregation of Gold Nanoparticles for Photoacoustic Imaging and Photothermal Therapy of Cancer. *Nanoscale* **2016**, *8*, 4452–4457. [CrossRef] [PubMed]
120. Nierenberg, D.; Khaled, A.R.; Flores, O. Formation of a protein corona influences the biological identity of nanomaterials. *Rep. Pract. Oncol. Radiother.* **2018**, *23*, 300–308. [CrossRef]
121. Moore, T.; Rodriguez Lorenzo, L.; Hirsch, V.; Balog, S.; Urban, D.; Jud, C.; Rothen-Rutishauser, B.; Lattuada, M.; Fink, A. Nanoparticle colloidal stability in cell culture media and impact on cellular interactions. *Chem. Soc. Rev.* **2015**, *44*. [CrossRef] [PubMed]
122. Guerrini, L.; Alvarez-Puebla, R.A.; Pazos-Perez, N. Surface Modifications of Nanoparticles for Stability in Biological Fluids. *Materials* **2018**, *11*, 1154. [CrossRef]
123. Attarilar, S.; Yang, J.; Ebrahimi, M.; Wang, Q.; Liu, J.; Tang, Y.; Yang, J. The Toxicity Phenomenon and the Related Occurrence in Metal and Metal Oxide Nanoparticles: A Brief Review From the Biomedical Perspective. *Front. Bioeng. Biotechnol.* **2020**, *8*, 822. [CrossRef]
124. Barrena, R.; Casals, E.; Colón, J.; Font, X.; Sánchez, A.; Puntes, V. Evaluation of the ecotoxicity of model nanoparticles. *Chemosphere* **2009**, *75*, 850–857. [CrossRef]
125. El Badawy, A.M.; Silva, R.G.; Morris, B.; Scheckel, K.G.; Suidan, M.T.; Tolaymat, T.M. Surface Charge-Dependent Toxicity of Silver Nanoparticles. *Environ. Sci. Technol.* **2011**, *45*, 283–287. [CrossRef]
126. Avellan, A.; Schwab, F.; Masion, A.; Chaurand, P.; Borschneck, D.; Vidal, V.; Rose, J.; Santaella, C.; Levard, C. Nanoparticle Uptake in Plants: Gold Nanomaterial Localized in Roots of *Arabidopsis thaliana* by X-ray Computed Nanotomography and Hyperspectral Imaging. *Environ. Sci. Technol.* **2017**, *51*, 8682–8691. [CrossRef]
127. Lovecká, P.; Macůrková, A.; Záruba, K.; Hubáček, T.; Siegel, J.; Valentová, O. Genomic Damage Induced in *Nicotiana tabacum* L. Plants by Colloidal Solution with Silver and Gold Nanoparticles. *Plants* **2021**, *10*, 1260. [CrossRef] [PubMed]
128. Milewska-Hendel, A.; Zubko, M.; Stróż, D.; Kurczyńska, E.U. Effect of Nanoparticles Surface Charge on the *Arabidopsis thaliana* (L.) Roots Development and Their Movement into the Root Cells and Protoplasts. *Int. J. Mol. Sci.* **2019**, *20*, 1650. [CrossRef] [PubMed]
129. Masson, V.; Maurin, F.; Fessi, H.; Devissaguet, J.P. Influence of sterilization processes on poly(epsilon-caprolactone) nanospheres. *Biomaterials* **1997**, *18*, 327–335. [CrossRef]
130. Özcan, I.; Bouchemal, K.; Segura Sánchez, F.; Abaci, Ö.; Özer, Ö.; Güneri, T.; Ponchel, G. Effects of sterilization techniques on the PEGylated poly (γ-benzyl-L-glutamate) (PBLG) nanoparticles. *Acta Pharm. Sci.* **2009**, *51*, 211–218.
131. Memisoglu-Bilensoy, E.; Hincal, A.A. Sterile, injectable cyclodextrin nanoparticles: Effects of gamma irradiation and autoclaving. *Int. J. Pharm.* **2006**, *311*, 203–208. [CrossRef]
132. Bernal-Chávez, S.A.; Del Prado-Audelo, M.L.; Caballero-Florán, I.H.; Giraldo-Gomez, D.M.; Figueroa-Gonzalez, G.; Reyes-Hernandez, O.D.; González-Del Carmen, M.; González-Torres, M.; Cortés, H.; Leyva-Gómez, G. Insights into Terminal Sterilization Processes of Nanoparticles for Biomedical Applications. *Molecules* **2021**, *26*, 2068. [CrossRef]

133. França, Á.; Pelaz, B.; Moros, M.; Sánchez-Espinel, C.; Hernández, A.; Fernández-López, C.; Grazú, V.; de la Fuente, J.M.; Pastoriza-Santos, I.; Liz-Marzán, L.M.; et al. Sterilization Matters: Consequences of Different Sterilization Techniques on Gold Nanoparticles. *Small* **2010**, *6*, 89–95. [CrossRef]
134. Mahapatra, I.; Sun, T.Y.; Clark, J.R.A.; Dobson, P.J.; Hungerbuehler, K.; Owen, R.; Nowack, B.; Lead, J. Probabilistic modelling of prospective environmental concentrations of gold nanoparticles from medical applications as a basis for risk assessment. *J. Nanobiotechnol.* **2015**, *13*, 93. [CrossRef]
135. Feichtmeier, N.S.; Walther, P.; Leopold, K. Uptake, effects, and regeneration of barley plants exposed to gold nanoparticles. *Environ. Sci. Pollut. Res. Int.* **2015**, *22*, 8549–8558. [CrossRef]
136. Asli, S.; Neumann, P.M. Colloidal suspensions of clay or titanium dioxide nanoparticles can inhibit leaf growth and transpiration via physical effects on root water transport. *Plant Cell Environ.* **2009**, *32*, 577–584. [CrossRef] [PubMed]
137. Khan, T.; Ullah, N.; Khan, M.A.; Mashwani, Z.-u.-R.; Nadhman, A. Plant-based gold nanoparticles; a comprehensive review of the decade-long research on synthesis, mechanistic aspects and diverse applications. *Adv. Colloid Interface Sci.* **2019**, *272*, 102017. [CrossRef] [PubMed]
138. Tiwari, M.; Krishnamurthy, S.; Shukla, D.; Kiiskila, J.; Jain, A.; Datta, R.; Sharma, N.; Sahi, S.V. Comparative transcriptome and proteome analysis to reveal the biosynthesis of gold nanoparticles in Arabidopsis. *Sci. Rep.* **2016**, *6*, 21733. [CrossRef]
139. Taylor, A.F.; Rylott, E.L.; Anderson, C.W.N.; Bruce, N.C. Investigating the Toxicity, Uptake, Nanoparticle Formation and Genetic Response of Plants to Gold. *PLoS ONE* **2014**, *9*, e93793. [CrossRef] [PubMed]
140. Abdal Dayem, A.; Hossain, M.K.; Lee, S.B.; Kim, K.; Saha, S.K.; Yang, G.-M.; Choi, H.Y.; Cho, S.-G. The Role of Reactive Oxygen Species (ROS) in the Biological Activities of Metallic Nanoparticles. *Int. J. Mol. Sci.* **2017**, *18*, 120. [CrossRef] [PubMed]
141. Feidantsis, K.; Kalogiannis, S.; Marinoni, A.; Vasilogianni, A.M.; Gkanatsiou, C.; Kastrinaki, G.; Dendrinou-Samara, C.; Kaloyianni, M. Toxicity assessment and comparison of the land snail's Cornu aspersum responses against CuO nanoparticles and ZnO nanoparticles. *Comp. Biochem. Physiol. Part-C Toxicol. Pharmacol.* **2020**, *236*, 108817. [CrossRef]
142. Husen, A.; Iqbal, M.; Aref, I.M. Growth, water status, and leaf characteristics of Brassica carinata under drought and rehydration conditions. *Rev. Bras. Bot.* **2014**, *37*, 217–227. [CrossRef]
143. El-Beltagi, H.; Mohamed, H. Reactive Oxygen Species, Lipid Peroxidation and Antioxidative Defense Mechanism. *Not. Bot. Horti Agrobot. Cluj-Napoca* **2013**, *41*, 44–57. [CrossRef]
144. Bisht, G.; Zaidi, M.G.H.; Sandeep, A. Impact of Gold Nanoparticles on Physiological and Biochemical Characteristics of Brassica juncea. *J. Plant Biochem. Physiol.* **2014**, *2*, 3.
145. Barbero, F.; Mayall, C.; Drobne, D.; Saiz-Poseu, J.; Bastús, N.G.; Puntes, V. Formation and evolution of the nanoparticle environmental corona: The case of Au and humic acid. *Sci. Total Environ.* **2021**, *768*, 144792. [CrossRef]

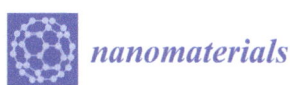

Article

In Vitro Interactions of TiO$_2$ Nanoparticles with Earthworm Coelomocytes: Immunotoxicity Assessment

Natividad Isabel Navarro Pacheco [1,2], Radka Roubalova [1], Jaroslav Semerad [1,3], Alena Grasserova [1,3], Oldrich Benada [1], Olga Kofronova [1], Tomas Cajthaml [1,3], Jiri Dvorak [1], Martin Bilej [1] and Petra Prochazkova [1,*]

[1] Institute of Microbiology of the Czech Academy of Sciences, Videnska 1083, 142 20 Prague 4, Czech Republic; natividad.pacheco@biomed.cas.cz (N.I.N.P.); r.roubalova@biomed.cas.cz (R.R.); jaroslav.semerad@biomed.cas.cz (J.S.); alena.grasserova@biomed.cas.cz (A.G.); benada@biomed.cas.cz (O.B.); kofra@biomed.cas.cz (O.K.); cajthaml@biomed.cas.cz (T.C.); dvorak@biomed.cas.cz (J.D.); mbilej@biomed.cas.cz (M.B.)
[2] First Faculty of Medicine, Charles University, Katerinska 1660/32, 121 08 Prague 2, Czech Republic
[3] Faculty of Science, Institute for Environmental Studies, Charles University, Benatska 2, 128 01 Prague 2, Czech Republic
* Correspondence: kohler@biomed.cas.cz

Abstract: Titanium dioxide nanoparticles (TiO$_2$ NPs) are manufactured worldwide. Once they arrive in the soil environment, they can endanger living organisms. Hence, monitoring and assessing the effects of these nanoparticles is required. We focus on the *Eisenia andrei* earthworm immune cells exposed to sublethal concentrations of TiO$_2$ NPs (1, 10, and 100 µg/mL) for 2, 6, and 24 h. TiO$_2$ NPs at all concentrations did not affect cell viability. Further, TiO$_2$ NPs did not cause changes in reactive oxygen species (ROS) production, malondialdehyde (MDA) production, and phagocytic activity. Similarly, they did not elicit DNA damage. Overall, we did not detect any toxic effects of TiO$_2$ NPs at the cellular level. At the gene expression level, slight changes were detected. Metallothionein, fetidin/lysenin, lumbricin and MEK kinase I were upregulated in coelomocytes after exposure to 10 µg/mL TiO$_2$ NPs for 6 h. Antioxidant enzyme expression was similar in exposed and control cells. TiO$_2$ NPs were detected on coelomocyte membranes. However, our results do not show any strong effects of these nanoparticles on coelomocytes at both the cellular and molecular levels.

Keywords: earthworm; coelomocyte; TiO$_2$ nanoparticles; reactive oxygen species; innate immunity; lipid peroxidation; alkaline comet assay; phagocytosis; apoptosis; gene expression

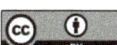

1. Introduction

Titanium dioxide nanoparticles (TiO$_2$ NPs) are commonly used in different industries because of their physico-chemical properties. TiO$_2$ NPs have photocatalytic properties, protect against UV radiation, are used as semiconductors, etc. These nanoparticles are used, e.g., in cosmetics, food industry, paints, ceramics, devices development, and the agriculture industry [1–3]. In the last decade, TiO$_2$ NPs have been used in wastewater treatment plants for their ability to degrade some organic pollutants [1]. Thus, TiO$_2$ NPs reach the soil system from different sources including sludge, nanofertilizers, and nanopesticides. These nanoparticles then interact with the soil biota. It is therefore very important to assess the potential risk of TiO$_2$ NPs to soil organisms.

Earthworms are dominant soil invertebrate animals. They possess a strong immune system because of their permanent contact with soil bacteria, viruses, and fungi. Defense mechanisms are used in earthworm protection against soil pollutants including nanoparticles. Earthworms *Eisenia andrei* and *E. fetida* are used as model organisms to monitor ecotoxicity according to OECD guidelines [4–6]. TiO$_2$ NPs do not affect earthworm viability and growth [2,3]. In some cases, reproductive inhibition was observed [7]. Further, these nanoparticles can induce, e.g., oxidative stress, DNA damage, apoptosis, and affect gene expression [3]. Earthworm cellular defense mechanisms are based on coelomocytes present in the coelomic fluid. Coelomocytes can be divided into free chloragogen cells called eleocytes, with a mainly nutritive function, and amoebocytes, which are the immune effector cells [8]. Amoebocytes can be further divided into granular (GA) and hyaline (HA) amoebocytes.

Various nanoparticles were described to impair earthworm defense mechanisms. Hayashi et al. showed that Ag NPs altered the expression of some genes involved in coelomocyte oxidative stress and immune reactions [9]. Further, Ag nanowires detected on coelomocyte membranes increased intracellular esterase activity [10]. ZnO NPs were internalized by coelomocytes, with consequent DNA damage [11]. However, similar mechanisms were not described for TiO_2 NPs in earthworms. TiO_2 NPs cause significant mitochondrial dysfunction by increasing mitochondrial ROS levels and decreasing ATP generation in macrophages. Moreover, TiO_2 NPs exposure activated inflammatory responses and attenuated macrophage phagocytic function [12]. TiO_2 NPs interacted with sea urchin immune cells and increased the antioxidant metabolic pathway in vitro [13]. In earthworms, only increased apoptosis was observed following TiO_2 nanocomposites exposure [7,14–16].

A compromised immune system may result in a decreased reproductive rate and increased mortality of earthworms. Thus, nanoparticle toxicity risk assessment is extremely important, as the adverse health effects remain poorly characterized for many nanomaterials. We aimed to assess the potentially dangerous impact of TiO_2 NPs exposure on earthworms' cellular function, including the immune responses to harmful stimuli.

E. andrei coelomocytes were exposed to 1, 10, and 100 µg/mL of TiO_2 NPs for 2, 6, and 24 h in vitro. After exposure, viability, oxidative stress (reactive oxygen species and malondialdehyde production), immune functions (phagocytosis), and genotoxicity (DNA damage) were assessed. Further, electron microscopy (transmission and scanning) enabled TiO_2 NPs localization on the cell surface. Gene expression changes were also followed to better understand the underlying cellular mechanisms.

2. Materials and Methods

2.1. Animal Handling, Sample Collection, and Culture Medium Preparation

Clitelate, adult *Eisenia andrei* earthworms were obtained from the laboratory compost breeding. Earthworms were first kept on moist filter paper for 48 h to depurate their guts. Coelomocytes were harvested by applying 2 mL of extrusion buffer (5.37 mM EDTA (Sigma-Aldrich, Steinheim, Germany); 50.4 mM guaiacol glyceryl ether (GGE; Sigma-Aldrich, Steinheim, Germany) in Lumbricus Balanced Salt Solution (LBSS; [17]) per earthworm for 2 min. The cells were then centrifuged and washed twice in LBSS ($200\times g$, 4 °C, 10 min). Subsequently, cells were counted and diluted to 10^6 cells/well for scanning electron microscopy (SEM) and lipid peroxidation assessment. 1×10^5 cells/well, 2×10^5 cells/well, and 3×10^5 cells/well were used for the ROS production analysis, apoptosis detection, and phagocytosis assay, respectively.

RPMI 1640 culture medium supplemented with 5% heat-inactivated fetal bovine serum (FBS; Life technologies, Carlsbad, USA), 1 M HEPES (4-(2-hydroxyethyl)-1-piperazineethane sulfonic acid; pH 7.0–7.6, Sigma-Aldrich; Gillingham, UK), 100 mM sodium pyruvate (Sigma-Aldrich, Steinheim, Germany), 100 mg/mL gentamycin (Corning, Manassas, VA, USA), and antibiotic–antimycotic solution (Sigma-Aldrich, Steinheim, Germany) was diluted with autoclaved MilliQ-water to 60% (v/v) to obtain R-RPMI 1640 medium [18]. Subsequently, TiO_2 NPs were dispersed in R-RPMI 1640 medium and incubated with cells in darkness at 20 °C for 2, 6, and 24 h in triplicate.

2.2. TiO₂ NPs Characterization

Aeroxide TiO_2 P25 nanoparticles (irregular and semi-spherical shape; mexoporous NPs, anatase, and rutile 4:1; primary size between 10 and 65 nm) were purchased from Evonik Degussa (Essen, Germany). TiO_2 NPs were previously characterized in several aqueous solutions, as described by Brunelli et al. [19]. Nanoparticle physico-chemical properties were determined by ZetaSizer Ultra (Panalytical Malvern; Malvern, UK), transmission electron microscope (TEM), and TECAN 200 Pro plate reader. Powder TiO_2 NPs were weighed and dispersed in distilled water. Then, diluted TiO_2 NPs were vortexed thoroughly for 5 min prior to further dilution [20]. TiO_2 NPs were diluted either in R-RPMI 1640 medium or distilled water to a concentration of 1, 10, and 100 µg/mL, and incubated for 2, 6, and 24 h. Experiments were carried out in triplicate. Culture medium and distilled water without NPs were used as negative controls.

2.3. Electron Microscopy Analyses

2.3.1. Cell Preparation

Coelomocytes were exposed to 1, 10, and 100 µg/mL TiO_2 NPs for 2, 6, and 24 h. Cell viability was measured by propidium iodide (PI; 1 µg/mL) staining using flow cytometer. Then, samples were collected and fixation solution (5% glutaraldehyde in PBS) was added in a 1:1 ratio (v:v). Fixed cells were shaken gently for 15 min and kept overnight at 4 °C.

2.3.2. Scanning Electron Microscopy (SEM)

For SEM, fixed cells were washed with LBSS buffer three times at room temperature for 20 min, and centrifuged at 150× g for 10 min. Then, they were allowed to adhere onto poly-L-lysine coated round 13 mm Thermanox Plastic Coverslips (Nunc, Thermo Fisher Scientific; Roskilde, Denmark) overnight at 4 °C. The coverslips with attached cells were washed with ddH_2O and fixed with 1% OsO_4 for one hour at room temperature. The coverslips were then washed three times for 20 min, dehydrated through an alcohol series (25, 50, 75, 90, 96, and 100%), and were critical-point dried from liquid CO_2 in a K850 Critical Point Dryer (Quorum Technologies Ltd., Ringmer, UK). The dried coverslips were sputter-coated using a high-resolution Turbo-Pumped Sputter Coater Q150T (Quorum Technologies Ltd., Ringmer, UK) with 3 nm of platinum. Alternatively, for EDS microanalysis, the samples were coated with 10 nm of silver or 5 nm of carbon. The final samples were examined in a FEI Nova NanoSEM scanning electron microscope (FEI, Brno, Czech Republic) at 5 kV using CBS and TLD detectors. An electron beam deceleration [21] mode of the Nova NanoSEM scanning electron microscope performed at a StageBias of 883.845 V and accelerating voltage of 5 kV was used for high-resolution imaging. The EDS microanalysis was performed at 15 kV using an Ametek® EDAX Octane Plus SDD detector and TEAM™ EDS Analysis Systems (AMETEK B. V.; Tilburg, The Netherlands).

2.3.3. Transmission Electron Microscopy (TEM)

For TEM, a TiO_2 NPs suspension (500 µg/mL; 5 µL) was applied onto glow-discharge-activated [22] carbon-coated 400-mesh copper grids (G400, SPI Supplies, Structure Probe, Inc., West Chester, PA, USA). Nanoparticles were sedimented for 1 min and the remaining solution was then blotted with filter paper and the grids were air-dried. A Philips CM100 electron microscope (Philips EO, Eindhoven, The Netherlands; Thermo Fisher Scientific) equipped with a Veleta slow-scan CCD camera (EMSIS GmbH, Muenster, Germany) was used to examine the grids. TEM images were processed in the proprietary iTEM software (EMSIS GmbH, Muenster, Germany).

2.4. Flow Cytometry Assays

Coelomocytes were incubated with TiO_2 NPs (1, 10, and 100 µg/mL) for 2, 6, and 24 h. Cells were then treated as described below and analyzed with a laser scanning flow cytometer. Through flow cytometry, coelomocytes were subdivided into eleocytes, granular (GA), and hyaline amoebocytes (HA). The coelomocytes subset detection was based on the cell size (FSC) and the cell inner complexity/granularity (SSC). Cell viability was assessed for every assay. All flow cytometry assays were performed by three independent experiments with three replicates per each treatment and time interval. The minimum collected events were 1000 per population. Event counts per each gate were calculated by Flowjo (9.9.4 version, BD Biosciences, San Jose, CA, USA). In each flow cytometry assay, coelomocytes were exposed to H_2O_2 as a positive control (Sigma-Aldrich, Steinheim, Germany; 10 mM H_2O_2 for 30 min incubation for apoptosis and phagocytosis, and 1 mM H_2O_2 for ROS production assesment). Controls with and without PI (1 mg/L; Sigma-Aldrich, Steinheim, Germany) were included in each experiment. Further, control analysis of 1, 10, and 100 µg/mL TiO_2 NPs incubated with or without cells for 2, 6, and 24 h were performed (Figure S1).

For ROS production determination, 20.6 µM 2′,7′-dichlorofluorescin diacetate (DCF-DA; Sigma-Aldrich, Steinheim, Germany) was added to the washed cell suspension (LBSS, 200× g, 4 °C, 10 min) for 15 min in darkness. Subsequently, the cell suspension was washed twice with LBSS (200× g, 4 °C, 10 min) and stained with PI.

To detect the apoptotic process a cell suspension was washed twice with Annexin V buffer (200× g, 4 °C, 10 min; 0.01 M HEPES (pH 7.4), 0.14 M NaCl, and 2.5 mM $CaCl_2$ solution), and subsequently stained with 5 µL of Alexa Fluor 647-Annexin V (15 min in darkness; Thermo Fisher Scientific, Eugene, OR, USA). PI was then added to the cell suspension and measured by flow cytometry. The apoptosis % represented the apoptotic cell number out of each subpopulation. The necrosis % represented the necrotic cell number out of each subpopulation.

The phagocytosis assay was performed using latex beads (Fluoresbrite® Plain YG; 1 µm microspheres diameter; Polysciencies Inc., Warrington, PA, USA) added to the incubation plates in a 1:100 ratio (cells:beads) and kept in darkness at 17 °C for 18 h. Then, cell suspensions were washed twice with LBSS (200× g, 4 °C, 10 min), stained with PI, and analyzed by flow cytometry. The % phagocytic activity was determined by the % of alive cells, which were able to engulf at least one bead out of each subpopulation. Each experiment included samples with NPs dispersed in the medium in order to detect effects exerted by NPs alone.

2.5. Malondialdehyde (MDA) Production and Alkaline Comet Assay

Coelomocytes were incubated with TiO_2 NPs (10 and 100 µg/mL) or $CuSO_4$ (100 µg/mL; positive control) for 2, 6, and 24 h. Afterward, cell suspensions were collected and MDA production was measured. MDA production was detected by high-performance liquid chromatography with fluorescence detection (HPLC/FLD) using derivatized MDA-TBA2 [23]. MDA analysis was performed in three independent experiments with 3 replicates for each treatment and time interval.

For the alkaline comet assay, 1.5×10^4 cells exposed to 1, 10, and 100 µg/mL TiO_2 NPs for 2, 6, and 24 h were mixed with 2% 2-hydroxyethyl agarose (Sigma-Aldrich, Steinheim, Germany) at 37 °C. Glass slides containing agarose with cells were kept at 4 °C for 10 min. Subsequently, samples were incubated for 2 h in lysis buffer (2.5 M NaCl, 10 mM Tris-HCl, 100 mM EDTA, 1% Triton X-100, pH 10). Then, slides were immersed three times in unwinding buffer (0.03 M NaOH, 2 mM EDTA, pH 12.7) for 20 min. Gel electrophoresis was carried out at 24 V, 300 mA for 25 min. Subsequently, slides were rinsed with neutralizing buffer (0.4 M Tris, pH 7.5) and stained with PI (3 µg/mL) for 20 min. The excess dye was removed with distilled water (5 min). Then, samples were stored in humidified chambers until the analysis by LUCIA Comet Assay software. One hundred cells per replicate of each treatment and time interval were analyzed, and the mean of DNA content in 100 comet tails (%) was calculated as a parameter of DNA damage. Positive control (100 mM H_2O_2; 30 min incubation; Sigma-Aldrich, Steinheim, Germany) was included with the assay. The comet assay was repeated in three independent experiments with three replicates for each treatment and time interval.

2.6. mRNA Levels Quantification

Cells were incubated with TiO_2 NPs (1 and 10 µg/mL) for 2, 6, and 24 h. Cellular RNA was isolated using the RNAqueous®-Micro Kit (Invitrogen, Vilnius, Lithuania). RNA (500 ng) was reverse-transcribed with the Oligo(dT)12–18 primer and Superscript

IV Reverse Transcriptase (Life Technologies). Non-RT controls were included to show the elimination of gDNA contamination.

Quantitative PCR (CFX96 Touch™ Real-Time PCR detection System, Bio-Rad) was performed to detect changes in mRNA levels encoding proteins participating in metal detoxification (metallothionein, phytochelatin), oxidative stress (manganese superoxide dismutase, Mn-SOD; copper-zinc-superoxide dismutase CuZn-SOD; catalase), immunity (endothelial monocyte-activating polypeptide II, EMAPII; fetidin/lysenin, and lumbricin), and signal transduction (MEK kinase I, MEKK I; and protein kinase C I, PKC I). Sequences of primers used in qPCR assays are referred in Table S1. The PCR reactions were performed in a 25 µL volume containing 4 µL of cDNA (dilution 1:10, except for 1:5 dilution for SODs). The cycling parameters were similar to Roubalova et al., with slight changes [24]: 4 min at 94 °C, 35 cycles of 10 s at 94 °C, 25 s at 60 °C (at 58 °C for MEKK I, PKC I, and catalase), 35 s at 72 °C, and a final extension for 7 min at 72 °C. Gene expression changes were calculated according to the 2−ΔΔCT (Livak) method. Two reference genes (RPL13, RPL17) were selected as internal controls for gene expression normalization. Non-template control was included in each experiment. The fold change in the mRNA level was related to the change of the corresponding controls. The results were expressed as the mean ± SEM of the values. mRNA levels quantification was performed by three independent experiments with duplicates per each treatment and time interval.

2.7. Statistical Analyses

Statistical analyses were performed using GraphPad Prism (8.3.1 version, San Diego, CA, USA). Flow cytometry assays, lipid peroxidation, alkaline comet assay, and gene expression were analyzed by two-way ANOVA with Bonferroni post-test.

3. Results

3.1. TiO$_2$ NPs Characterization

TiO$_2$ NPs were dispersed and stabilized in distilled water and in R-RPMI 1640 culture medium evenly. However, differences in NPs characteristics were observed between both mediums along the exposure time (2, 6, and 24 h) (Table 1). In the UV/Vis spectra, NPs exerted a similar wavelength range: 300–370 nm for distilled water; 320–380 nm for R-RPMI 1640 medium. Although NPs absorbed similar UV/Vis wavelengths, differences were observed in the hydrodynamic size distribution. TiO$_2$ NPs dispersed in R-RPMI 1640 medium were not stabilized and tended to aggregate. The aggregation was detected between 6 and 24 h of incubation. After 6 h, the hydrodynamic size distribution was 35.5 ± 3.94 nm, and it increased to 597 ± 447 nm after 24 h. At 2–6 h, the hydrodynamic size of TiO$_2$ NPs was stable (31.34 ± 1.55 to 35.5 ± 3.94 nm, respectively). In distilled water, the hydrodynamic size distribution was stable between 2–24 h 581 ± 23.30 and 480 ± 64.3 nm, respectively. Regarding zeta potential, TiO$_2$ NPs dispersed in both distilled water and R-RPMI 1640 did not change significantly over time (Table 1).

Table 1. Characterization of 100 µg/mL TiO$_2$ nanoparticles (NPs) suspension in milliQ water and R-RPMI 1640 medium.

	UV/Vis (nm) [a]			Z-Avg. (nm) [b]			ζ (mV) [c]		
	2 h	6 h	24 h	2 h	6 h	24 h	2 h	6 h	24 h
Distilled water	300–370	300–370	300–370	581 ± 23.30	570 ± 2.75	480 ± 64.3	−26.8 ± 2.99	−31.7 ± 0.921	−32.9 ± 2.59
R-RPMI 1640 medium	320–380	320–380	320–380	31.34 ± 1.55	35.5 ± 3.94	597 ± 447	−16.9 ± 0.60	−7.87 ± 0.631	−5.94 ± 0.45

(a) ultraviolet-visible = UV/Vis spectra absorbance (nm), (b) Z-Avg = Hydrodynamic size determined by multi-angle dynamic light scattering (MADLS), and (c) ζ = zeta potential values are expressed as mean of 3 measurements ± SD.

3.2. Electron Microscopy

The TiO$_2$ NPs size given by the manufacturer was 10–65 nm. However, we were not able to verify this information because of a great aggregation of TiO$_2$ NPs in concentrations detectable by TEM. According to our measurements, the nanoparticles ranged between 20 and 100 nm. The TiO$_2$ NPs were rode/spherical (Figure 1).

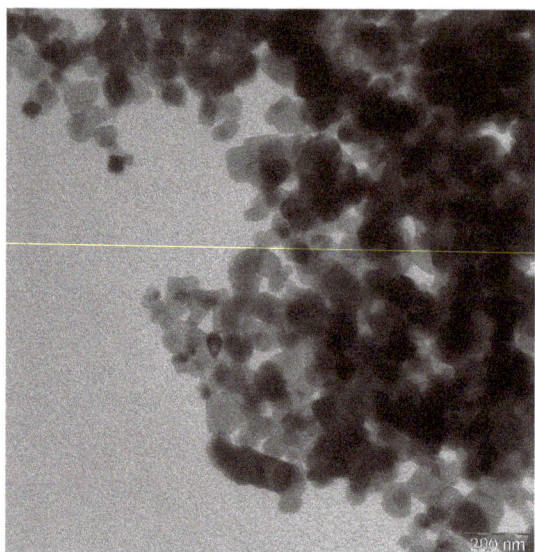

Figure 1. Transmission electron microscopy of 500 µg/mL TiO$_2$ NPs clustered in distilled water. The scale bar represents 200 nm.

In coelomocytes exposed to 100 µg/mL TiO$_2$ NPs, nanoparticles were observed on cell membranes by scanning electron microscopy (Figure 2). Moreover, EDS microanalysis confirmed Ti presence in nanoparticle clusters on the cell surface (Figure 3). At 10 µg/mL TiO$_2$ NPs exposure, nanoparticles were also detected on the coelomocyte surface but with lower frequency. EDS microanalysis of non-treated cells is shown in Figure S2.

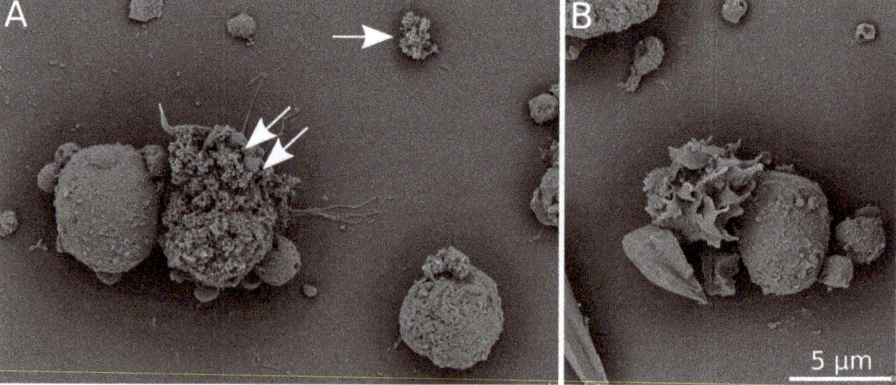

Figure 2. Scanning electron microscopy of coelomocytes. (**A**) cells exposed to 100 µg/mL TiO$_2$ NPs for 2 h; (**B**) control cells cultured in the medium. Images recorded with B + C segments of a CBS detector at 3 kV. White arrow indicates a TiO$_2$ NPs cluster on sample support. Clusters of the same morphology can be seen on the cell surface (white double arrow). The scale bar represents 5 µm.

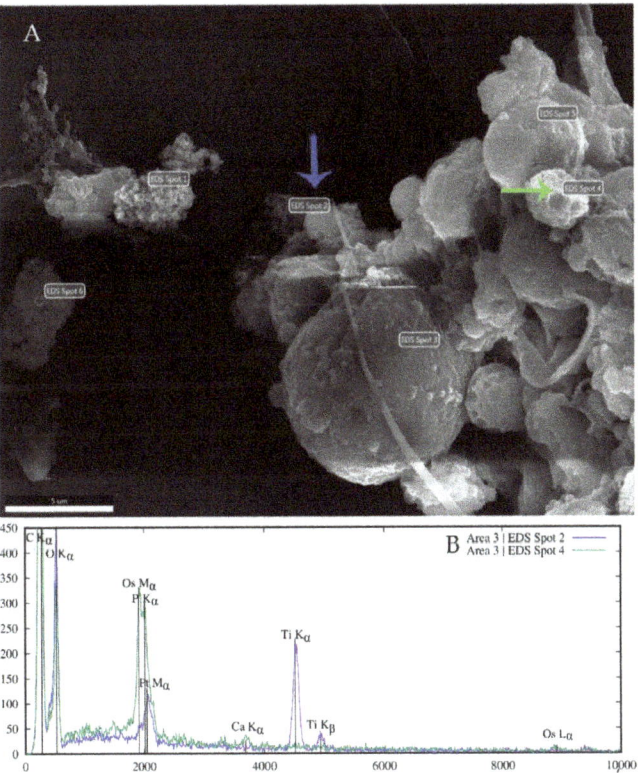

Figure 3. EDS microanalysis of coelomocytes incubated with 100 μg/mL TiO$_2$ NPs. (**A**) An image showing the area of interest taken with EDX TEAM software at 15 kV using a SED detector. The spectra collection places are marked with EDS labels. Increased charging effects caused by the non-conductive nature of Thermanox coverslips used for sample preparation deteriorated image quality. (**B**) EDS microanalysis confirmed Ti in NPs clusters found on the cell surface (e.g., EDS Spot 2 label) and also in the cluster labeled EDS spot 1. Blue arrow indicates TiO$_2$ NPs cluster (EDS Spot 2 label), green arrow points to the cell surface without NPs clusters (EDS Spot 4 label). Corresponding EDS spectra in matching colors are shown in B. The scale bar represents 5 μm.

3.3. Flow Cytometry Assays

Coelomocyte subpopulations were differentiated by flow cytometry (Figure S3). Thus, the viability of HA and GA were analyzed. The eleocyte subpopulation was excluded from the results because of the interaction between their autofluorescence and the fluorescences used in the assays.

HA and GA viability (the percentage of alive cells in each subpopulation) was similar in non-treated cells and TiO$_2$ NPs-exposed cells. No differences in viability were observed between amoebocyte subpopulations.

We did not observe any significant changes in ROS production in HA or in GA after exposure to any of the TiO$_2$ NPs concentrations (Figure 4). HA population exerted two times lesser fluorescence intensity in comparison to the GA population. This suggests that HA population is less potent to produce ROS than GA population (Figure 4). Illustrative histograms of ROS production between control samples and positive control (1 mM H$_2$O$_2$), indicating a clear shift in sample fluorescence, are shown in Figure S4.

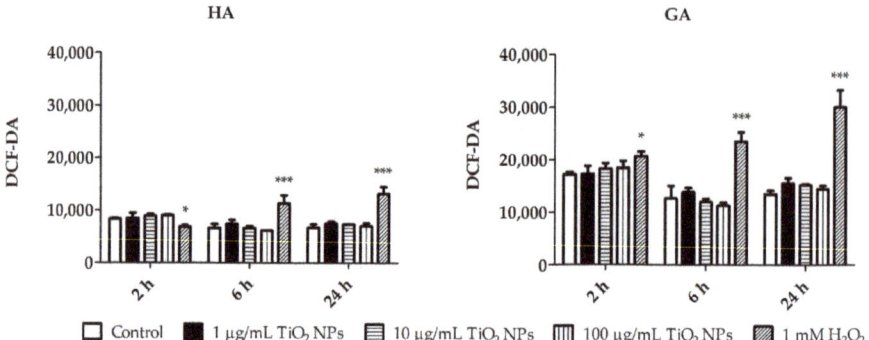

Figure 4. ROS production by hyaline (HA) and granular (GA). ROS production was measured in HA and GA after incubation with 1, 10, and 100 µg/mL TiO$_2$ NPs for 2, 6, and 24 h using a cell-permeant tracer 2′,7′-dichlorofluorescein diacetate (DCF-DA). Coelomocytes were also exposed to 1 mM H$_2$O$_2$ (positive control) for 30 min. The results are shown as the mean of fluorescence intensity (DCF-DA) ± SEM of three independent experiments with 3 replicates in each. *** $p < 0.001$, and * $p < 0.05$ according to two-way ANOVA and Bonferroni post-test.

Similarly, we did not detect any significant differences in the apoptosis level between TiO$_2$ NPs exposed and control cells (both in HA and GA; Figures 5 and 6). In both populations, the early apoptosis percent is similar over time, while late apoptosis slightly decreased after 24 h (Figures 5 and 6). Necrosis increased along the exposure time in GA (Figure 6). However, statistically significant differences were not detected between treated and control cells. Representative distributions of the apoptotic/necrotic cell stages in GA and HA cell subpopulations are shown in Figures S5 and S6, respectively.

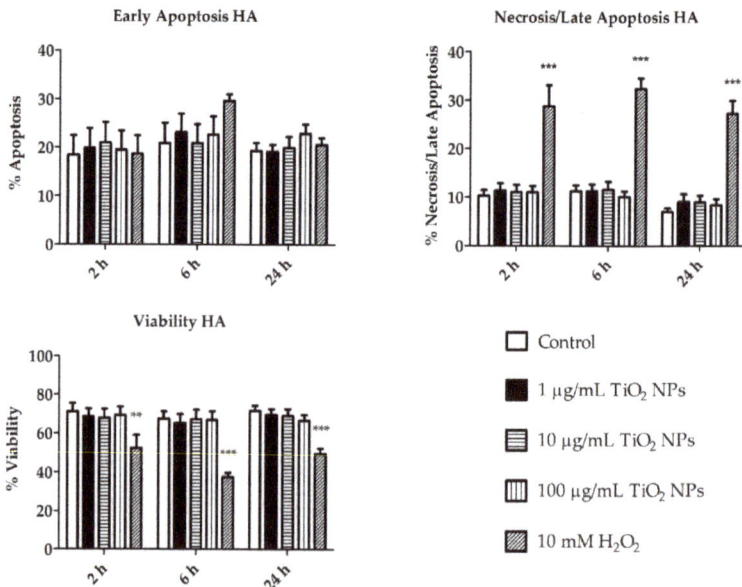

Figure 5. Early and late apoptosis, viability and necrosis of hyaline amoebocytes (HA). Early and late apoptosis, viability and necrosis of HA of non-treated cells, cells exposed to 1, 10, and 100 µg/mL TiO$_2$ NPs after 2, 6, and 24 h. 10 mM H$_2$O$_2$ was used as positive control for 30 min exposure. The results are shown as mean (%) ± SEM of three independent experiments with 3 replicates in each. *** $p < 0.001$, and ** $p < 0.01$ according to two-way ANOVA and Bonferroni post-test.

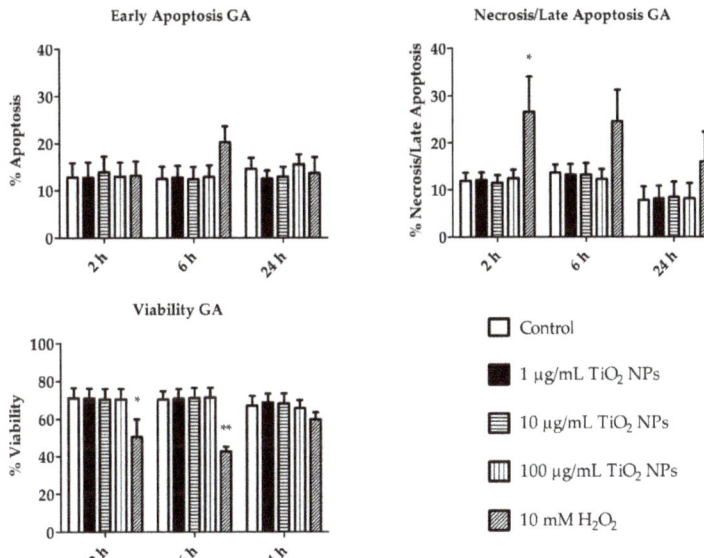

Figure 6. Early and late apoptosis, viability and necrosis of granular amoebocytes (GA). Early and Late apoptosis, viability and necrosis of GA of non-treated cells, cells exposed to 1, 10, and 100 µg/mL TiO$_2$ NPs after 2, 6, and 24 h. 10 mM H$_2$O$_2$ was used as positive control for 30 min exposure. The results are shown as mean (%) ± SEM of three independent experiments with 3 replicates in each. ** $p < 0.01$, and * $p < 0.05$ according to two-way ANOVA and Bonferroni post-test.

The viable amoebocyte phagocytic activity was measured in both amoebocyte subsets (HA and GA). Representative phagocytic activity density plots of GA and HA cell subpopulations are shown in Figures S7 and S8, respectively. The phagocytic activity was similar in both amoebocyte subpopulations (GA and HA; Figure 7). A decrease in the phagocytic activity of HA control cells and TiO$_2$ NPs-exposed cells occurred after 24 h (Figure 7). This slight decrease may indicate the greater sensitivity of HA to external conditions. However, phagocytic activity was not significantly affected by NPs treatment or by the incubation time. Phagocytic activity of untreated cells with and without Fluoresbrite® YG Plain 1µm microspheres was also compared (Figure S9).

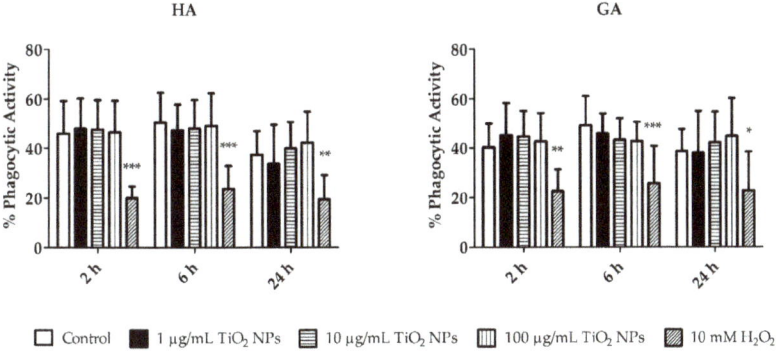

Figure 7. Phagocytic activity of HA and GA. Phagocytic activity was measured after incubation with TiO$_2$ NPs (1, 10, and 100 µg/mL) for 2, 6, and 24 h. Coelomocytes were also exposed to 10 mM H$_2$O$_2$ (positive control) for 30 min. Results are represented as the mean ± SEM of three independent experiments with 3 replicates in each. *** $p < 0.001$, ** $p < 0.01$, and * $p < 0.05$ according to two-way ANOVA and Bonferroni post-test.

3.4. MDA and Alkaline Comet Assay

Malondialdehyde (MDA) is a lipid peroxidation subproduct, and it is therefore used as an oxidative stress biomarker in cells. We did not detect any significant increase in MDA production in cells exposed to TiO$_2$ NPs (10 and 100 µg/mL) at the tested timepoints (2, 6, and 24 h; Figure 8).

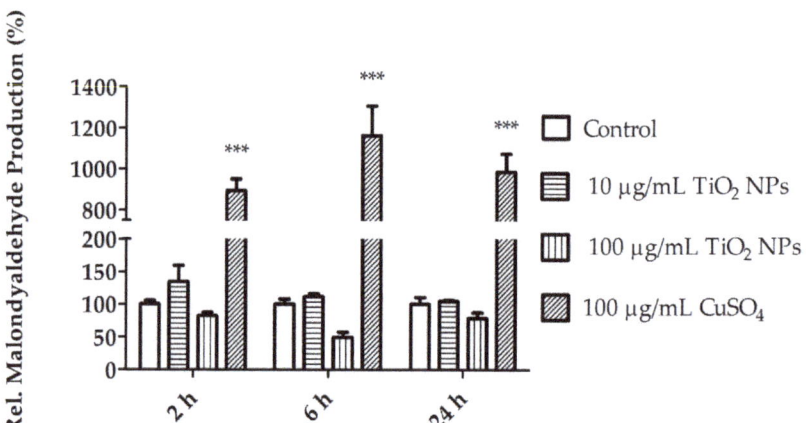

Figure 8. Relative malondialdehyde (MDA) production in coelomocytes exposed to 10, 100 µg/mL TiO$_2$ NPs and positive control (100 µg/mL CuSO$_4$) for 2, 6, and 24 h. Values are expressed as mean (%) ± SEM of three independent experiments each with three replicates. *** $p < 0.001$ according to two-way ANOVA and Bonferroni post-test.

The DNA damage in coelomocytes exposed to 1, 10, and 100 µg/mL TiO$_2$ NPs for 2, 6, and 24 h was assessed by the alkaline comet assay. DNA damage was evaluated by the mean tail intensity (% DNA in tail) of 100 comets in each incubation. The observed DNA damage was not greater than 40% during exposure with TiO$_2$ NPs and the non-treated cells (Figure 9).

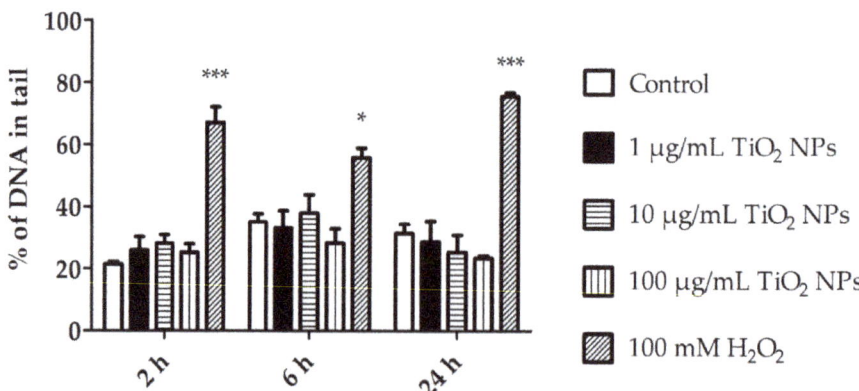

Figure 9. DNA damage in coelomocytes after their exposure to 1, 10, and 100 µg/mL TiO$_2$ NPs for 2, 6, and 24 h. Coelomocytes were also exposed to 100 mM H$_2$O$_2$ (positive control) for 30 min. Values are expressed as the mean of DNA content in tail (%) ± SEM of three experiment with three replicates. *** $p < 0.001$ and * $p < 0.05$ according to two-way ANOVA and Bonferroni post-test.

3.5. mRNA Levels of Detoxification, Immune, Antioxidant, and Signal Transduction Molecules

The change in mRNA levels of appropriate molecules after coelomocyte exposure to TiO$_2$ NPs was assessed (Table 2). Metallothioneins involved in metal detoxification were significantly upregulated in coelomocytes exposed to 1 µg/mL TiO$_2$ NPs for 2, 6 and 24 h, and in coelomocytes exposed to 10 µg/mL TiO$_2$ NPs for 6 h. Further, significant Mn-SOD downregulation was detected in coelomocytes incubated with 10 µg/mL TiO$_2$ NPs for 6 h. Then, fetidin/lysenin and lumbricin were upregulated upon coelomocyte exposure to 10 µg/mL TiO$_2$ NPs for 6 h. MEKK I upregulation after 1 µg/mL TiO$_2$ NPs exposure for 24 h, and PKC I downregulation after 10 µg/mL TiO$_2$ NPs exposure for 6 and 24 h were detected. Surprisingly, the mRNA levels of catalase and CuZn-SOD (antioxidant enzymes) were not significantly altered.

Table 2. The mRNA levels of distinct molecules in coelomocytes exposed to 1 and 10 µg/mL TiO$_2$ NPs.

Function	Gene	TiO$_2$ NPs (µg/mL)	Normalized Gene Expression		
			2 h	6 h	24 h
Metal detoxification	Metallothionein	1	5.16 ± 1.73 **	2.00 ± 0.32 *	2.71 ± 0.20 *
		10	1.11 ± 0.2	1.97 ± 0.22 **	1.00 ± 0.25
Heavy metal detoxification	Phytochelatin	1	1.38 ± 0.09	1.02 ± 0.04	1.18 ± 0.08
		10	1.00 ± 0.02	0.82 ± 0.02	0.80 ± 0.01
Oxidative stress	Mn-SOD	1	1.47 ± 0.12	0.85 ± 0.19	0.58 ± 0.05
		10	0.93 ± 0.09	0.53 ± 0.01 *	0.72 ± 0.01
	CuZn-SOD	1	0.68 ± 0.05	0.84 ± 0.22	0.98 ± 0.04
		10	0.96 ± 0.07	0.71 ± 0.04	0.87 ± 0.01
	Catalase	1	1.41 ± 0.19	0.87 ± 0.03	0.66 ± 0.03
		10	1.04 ± 0.13	0.71 ± 0.02	0.8 ± 0.2
Immunity	EMAP II	1	0.90 ± 0.07	0.94 ± 0.1	0.86 ± 0.02
		10	0.84 ± 0.09	1.21 ± 0.01	1.33 ± 0.20
	Fetidin/lysenin	1	0.64 ± 0.08	0.62 ± 0.13	0.70 ± 0.04
		10	0.65 ± 0.05	2.20 ± 0.2 **	0.81 ± 0.19
	Lumbricin	1	1.33 ± 0.05	0.75 ± 0.10	1.84 ± 0.02
		10	0.84 ± 0.10	2.10 ± 0.43 *	1.92 ± 0.55
Signal Transduction	MEKK I	1	1.40 ± 0.19	1.47 ± 0.44	1.73 ± 0.04 *
		10	1.00 ± 0.15	1.96 ± 0.11 *	1.33 ± 0.03
	PKC I	1	1.52 ± 0.30	1.08 ± 0.19	1.43 ± 0.06
		10	1.10 ± 0.16	0.33 ± 0.04 **	0.58 ± 0.11 *

Values were normalized to two reference molecules (RPL13 and RPL17). Fold changes (±SEM) in mRNA levels in TiO$_2$ NPs exposed coelomocytes are relative to the mRNA levels in control cells. Two-way ANOVA and Bonferroni post-test were performed to evaluate data significance (* $p < 0.05$, ** $p < 0.01$). mRNA levels quantification was performed by three independent experiments with duplicates per each treatment and time interval. Mn-SOD: manganese superoxide dismutase; CuZN-SOD: copper-zinc-superoxide dismutase; EMAP II: endothelial monocyte-activating polypeptide-II; MEKK I: MEK kinase I; PKC I: protein kinase C I.

4. Discussion

The physico-chemical properties of TiO$_2$ NPs were analyzed in R-RPMI 1640 medium to understand their behavior in cell cultures. The analyses in distilled water were performed to observe possible changes in nanoparticles behavior in the stock over time. UV/Vis spectra, hydrodynamic size, zeta potential, and TEM were used for the NPs characterization. TiO$_2$ NPs dispersed in distilled water showed an aggregation behavior at the greatest concentration (100 µg/mL), and the size remained approximately the same between 2 and 24 h. The zeta potential was also stable at all TiO$_2$ NPs concentrations (Table 1). However, different NPs behavior was observed when dispersed in the R-RPMI 1640 culture medium. Between 2 and 6 h of incubation, changes were not observed in the size distribution, while zeta potential indicated instability (Table 1). Between 6 and 24 h, we observed a great increase in particle size distribution in comparison with previous intervals. These changes indicate that NPs were dispersed in R-RPMI 1640 medium, and they started to precipitate only after 6 h of incubation. Magdolenova and colleagues assessed the relationship between the cytotoxic effects and the dispersion of TiO$_2$ NPs [25]. They showed that tested cell culture medium types did not influence TiO$_2$ NPs dispersion. However, they observed that different dispersion protocols and the use of serum in stock solution affected nanoparticles aggregation and size distribution. Accordingly, Ji et al. showed the improvement in TiO$_2$ NPs dispersion upon addition of bovine serum albumin (BSA), although the dispersion also depended on cell culture media phosphate concentration [26]. TiO$_2$ NPs tended to aggregate in R-RPMI 1640 medium (Table 1), which may be related to the low FBS concentration or the effect of phosphate ions in the cell culture medium.

By TEM, the aggregation of 500 µg/mL TiO$_2$ NPs was also observed in distilled water (Figure 1). Therefore, it was not possible to determine the nanoparticles' size. UV/Vis spectra were similar in exposed and control samples in both distilled water and R-RPMI 1640, as well as during the experiment, indicating that NPs properties did not change. Previously, the addition of HEPES and FBS into RPMI-1640 medium led to NPs re-dispersion [14].

Scanning electron microscopy showed the NPs cluster in contact with the cell membranes (Figure 2). EDS spectra showed TiO$_2$ NPs that are present on cells at the 100 µg/mL concentration (Figure 3), but not at the lesser concentration (10 µg/mL). This may be because of the EDS microanalysis detection limit. TiO$_2$ NPs are internalized by *E. fetida* coelomocytes. Bigorgne et al. determined their presence in the cell cytoplasm, but not in the nucleus or mitochondria [14]. However, we were unable to detect TiO$_2$ NPs inside coelomocytes. This could be because TiO$_2$ NPs aggregates are large. Earthworm coelomocytes are probably unable to engulf large NP clusters via phagocytosis and/or endocytosis, the most probable routes of TiO$_2$ NPs entry into coelomocytes [1,14]. Phagocytic cells are potentially the most affected because they engulf NPs. Coelomocyte viability was not affected by exposure to 1, 10, and 100 µg/mL TiO$_2$ NPs for 2, 6, and 24 h. Similar results were observed in *E. fetida* coelomocytes exposed to TiO$_2$ NP [14]. Nanoparticles often trigger reactive oxygen species (ROS) production in cells, resulting in biomolecule oxidative damage [27,28]. We did not detect any statistically significant differences in ROS production in TiO$_2$ NPs-exposed cells in comparison with control cells (Figure 4). Cells exposed to other nanoparticles, such as Ag NPs, nZVI NPs or ZnO NPs release significantly greater ROS amounts. Contrary to TiO$_2$ NPs, ROS production could be elicited by the metal ions released from these nanoparticles [11,29,30].

We evaluated the apoptotic process in cells treated with TiO$_2$ NPs, and did not detect any significant differences between exposed and control coelomocytes (Figures 5 and 6). Late apoptosis was similar in GA and HA, with the greatest difference observed after 24 h of incubation. HA population exerted relatively greater early apoptosis than GA. Excess ROS production led to decreased cell viability and apoptosis [31,32]. Homa et al. suggested that coelomocytes are susceptible to bacterial or fungal products that may induce programmed cell death [31]. TiO$_2$ NPs did not increase ROS production, and simultaneously, apoptosis was not increased as compared to control cells (Figures 4–6). We suggest that TiO$_2$ NPs do not affect ROS production, and thus do not trigger the apoptotic pathway in amoebocyte subpopulations (HA and GA).

Amoebocytes are earthworm immune effector cells with the ability to phagocytose. At the phagocytic activity level, control cells and cells exposed to TiO$_2$ NPs (1, 10, and 100 µg/mL) did not show any statistically significant changes (Figure 7). The results are in accordance with Bigorgne et al., who reported that there were no phagocytic activity changes in coelomocytes exposed to 1, 5, 10, and 25 µg/mL of TiO$_2$ NPs, although TEM images demonstrated that TiO$_2$ NPs were engulfed by the coelomocytes [14]. Thus, we can confirm that phagocytic activity is not compromised due to TiO$_2$ NPs exposure.

ROS production initiates harmful radical chain reactions on cellular macromolecules, including DNA mutation, protein denaturation, and lipid peroxidation. At the lipid peroxidation level, MDA production was similar in both exposed and control cells. MDA is a subproduct derived from the reaction of free radical species with fatty acids [33]. We did not observe elevated lipid peroxidation (Figure 8). Ayala et al. explained that MDA is more stable and has a greater lifespan than ROS, and therefore it is more toxic [33]. Therefore, it could be a better biomarker for cellular oxidative stress detection. Excess ROS leads to MDA production [34]. Two oxidative stress markers, ROS and MDA, were produced at similar levels in control cells and TiO_2 NPs-exposed cells (Figures 4 and 8). The same results were also observed after THP1 human cells and sea urchin cells were exposed to TiO_2 NPs [20,35]. UVA light could also enhance ROS production and increase toxicity several fold [36]. However, in this instance, the cells were mimicking the environmental conditions in the soil ecosystem, where UVA light was not present.

Significant differences between exposed and control cells were not detected regarding DNA damage. The alkaline comet assay results showed that there is no significant DNA damage in coelomocytes exposed to 1, 10, and 100 µg/mL of TiO_2 NPs for 2, 6, and 24 h (Figure 9). A relationship between ROS, MDA, and DNA damage has been suggested. As mentioned previously, ROS may induce MDA production, which, in turn, affects nucleosides and results in DNA damage [33,34]. This mechanism has been described in coelomocytes exposed to pollutants, antibiotics, or pathogens [34]. Reeves et al. showed that GFSk-S1 cells (primary cell line from goldfish skin) exposed to different doses of TiO_2 NPs (1, 10, and 100 µg/mL) could result in slight DNA damage, whereas co-exposure with UVA caused a significant increase in toxicity [36]. In vitro analysis described in this study did not reveal substantial changes in cellular physiologic activities, but the long-term exposure experiments can reveal different findings [37]. Zhu et al. described transcriptomic and metabolomic changes in earthworms as a global response to TiO_2 NPs exposure that cannot be observed by conventional toxicity endpoints [38].

Treatment of coelomocytes with TiO_2 NPs induced slight changes in the mRNA levels of distinct molecules. Metallothioneins are proteins protecting against metal-induced oxidative stress [9]. Metallothionein was upregulated in coelomocytes exposed to 10 µg/mL TiO_2 NPs for 6 h, respectively (Table 2). This is in agreement with Bigorgne et al., who immunostimulated coelomocytes with lipopolysaccharides (LPS) (500 ng/mL) for 5 h prior to TiO_2 NPs addition. After 12 h of incubation with 10 and 25 µg/mL TiO_2 NPs, metallothioneins were upregulated [14]. We determined that even 1 µg/mL TiO_2 NPs concentration upregulated metallothionein expression during the whole experiment (Table 2). Interestingly, the highest upregulation was detected in coelomocytes incubated with 1 µg/mL TiO_2 NPs already after 2 h. Further, the induction of metallothionein expression in cells exposed to 10 µg/mL TiO_2 NPs started at 6 h, and afterward decreased after 24 h (Table 2). Bigorgne et al. similarly showed increased metallothioneins expression after 12 h of incubation, with a subsequent decrease after 24 h [14].

Further, the antioxidant enzymes were not affected, except for Mn-SOD, which was downregulated after 6 h of coelomocyte exposure to 10 µg/mL TiO_2 NPs (Table 2). Mn-SOD is a mitochondrial protein that protects cells against oxidative stress [39]. It seems that macrophages (RAW 264.7 cell line) and coelomocytes can engulf TiO_2 NPs. These nanoparticles affect mitochondria even if they are not located inside the mitochondria [12,14]. Moreover, TiO_2 NPs decreased ATP production in the macrophage RAW 264.7 cell line [12]. Thus, engulfed TiO_2 NPs could target mitochondria and cause mitochondrial malfunction [12]. Mn-SOD downregulation and loss in mitochondrial oxidative phosphorylation function was also reported in primary rat hepatocytes [40].

Elevated levels of the antimicrobial proteins fetidin/lysenin and lumbricin were detected in cells exposed to 10 µg/mL TiO_2 NPs for 6 h (Table 2). Similarly, Bigorgne et al. observed that fetidin was upregulated in cells exposed to 10 µg/mL TiO_2 NPs after 12 h [14]. As previously described in related earthworm species *E. fetida*, lysenin regulation is changed rapidly by environmental stressors and it is suggested as an early biomarker of stress [41]. However, we cannot exclude that the increase in antimicrobial protein mRNA levels could be caused by used TiO_2 NPs that were not LPS-free.

Referring to the signal transduction molecules, PKC I was strongly downregulated after coelomocyte exposure to 10 µg/mL TiO_2 NPs for 6 and 24 h (Table 2). PKC I is important in cellular homeostasis and is involved in the cell proliferation signaling cascade [42,43]. This downregulation could suggest a coelomocyte homeostasis destabilization upon TiO$_2$ NPs exposure. Another signal transduction molecule, MEKK, was upregulated in coelomocytes exposed to 1 µg/mL TiO$_2$ NPs for 24 h and in coelomocytes exposed to 10 µg/mL TiO$_2$ NPs for 6 h (Table 2). This molecule is involved in the MAPK cascade participating in many cellular processes, besides others in stress signaling [9,43]. Generally, coelomocyte exposure to TiO$_2$ NPs results in slight changes in the mRNA levels of various molecules, however, these changes seem not to be significant enough to affect the observed cellular functions.

5. Conclusions

Coelomocytes exposed to TiO$_2$ NPs (1, 10, and 100 µg/mL) did not show any impaired cellular responses as compared to control cells. The oxidative stress pathway and phagocytic activity were not affected as well. Nanoparticles do not cause greater DNA damage in treated cells than in non-treated cells. We also detected some gene expression alterations involved in metal detoxification, oxidative stress, defense reactions, and signal transduction. However, these changes do not seem to affect the observed cellular functions. In summary, we did not determine any detrimental effects of TiO$_2$ NPs on *E. andrei* coelomocytes.

Supplementary Materials: The following are available online at https://www.mdpi.com/2079-4991/11/1/250/s1, Figure S1. Illustrative figure of NPs distribution incubated without and with the cells. Figure S2. EDS spectra from standard non-treated cells. Figure S3. Illustrative figure of coelomocytes subpopulations detected by flow cytometry. Figure S4. Illustrative histogram of ROS production between control samples and positive control. Figure S5. Illustrative figure of apoptosis of GA after 24 h of exposure to 100 µg/mL TiO$_2$ NPs. Figure S6. Illustrative figure of apoptosis of HA after 24 h of exposure to 100 µg/mL TiO$_2$ NPs. Figure S7. Illustrative figure of phagocytic activity of GA after 2 h. Figure S8. Illustrative figure of phagocytic activity of HA after 2 h. Figure S9. Detection of Fluoresbrite® YG Plain 1µm microsphere. Table S1: Primer sequences used for qPCR.

Author Contributions: Conceptualization, N.I.N.P. and P.P.; methodology and data curation, N.I.N.P., J.S., J.D., O.B., A.G. and O.K.; writing—original draft preparation, N.I.N.P., J.S., R.R.; writing—review and editing, N.I.N.P., J.S., O.B., R.R. and P.P.; supervision, R.R. and P.P.; project administration, P.P., M.B. and T.C.; funding acquisition, P.P. and T.C. All authors have read and agreed to the published version of the manuscript.

Funding: This work was supported by Grant QK1910095 of the Ministry of Agriculture of the Czech Republic and by the Center for Geosphere Dynamics (UNCE/SCI/006). This project also received funding from the European Union's Horizon 2020 research and innovation programme under the Marie Skłodowska-Curie grant agreement No. 67188.

Institutional Review Board Statement: Not applicable.

Informed Consent Statement: Not applicable.

Data Availability Statement: Data is contained within the article or supplementary material.

Acknowledgments: The authors gratefully acknowledge the access to the electron microscopy facility, supported by the project LO1509 of the Ministry of Education, Youth and Sports of the Czech Republic. The authors also acknowledge the Cytometry and Microscopy Facility at the Institute of Microbiology of the ASCR, v.v.i. for the support of the staff and the use of their equipment, and we acknowledge the support of CMS-Biocev Biophysical techniques (LM2015043 funded by MEYS CR).

Conflicts of Interest: The authors declare no conflict of interest. The funders had no role in the design of the study; in the collection, analyses, or interpretation of data; in the writing of the manuscript, or in the decision to publish the results.

References

1. Gupta, S.M.; Tripathi, M. A review of TiO$_2$ nanoparticles. *Chin. Sci. Bull.* **2011**, *56*, 1639. [CrossRef]
2. Gautam, A.; Ray, A.; Mukherjee, S.; Das, S.; Pal, K.; Das, S.; Karmakar, P.; Ray, M.; Ray, S. Immunotoxicity of copper nanoparticle and copper sulfate in a common Indian earthworm. *Ecotoxicol. Environ. Saf.* **2018**, *148*, 620–631. [CrossRef] [PubMed]

3. Kwak, J.I.; An, Y.-J. Ecotoxicological Effects of Nanomaterials on Earthworms: A Review. *Hum. Ecol. Risk Assess.* **2015**, *21*, 1566–1575. [CrossRef]
4. OECD. Guideline for the Testing of Chemicals. In *No. 207, Earthworm, Acute Toxicity Tests*; Organisation for Economic Cooperation and Development: Paris, France, 1984.
5. OECD. Guideline for the Testing of Chemicals. In *No. 222, Earthworm Reproduction Test (Eisenia Fetida/Eisenia Andrei)*; Organisation for Economic Cooperation and Development: Paris, France, 2004.
6. OECD. Guidelines for the testing of chemicals. In *No. 317, Bioaccumulation in Terrestrial Oligochaetes*; Organisation for Economic Cooperation and Development: Paris, France, 2010.
7. Valerio-Rodríguez, M.F.; Trejo-Téllez, L.I.; Aguilar-González, M.A.; Medina-Pérez, G.; Zúñiga-Enríquez, J.C.; Ortegón-Pérez, A.; Fernández-Luqueño, F. Effects of ZnO, TiO$_2$ or Fe$_2$O$_3$ Nanoparticles on the Body Mass, Reproduction, and Survival of *Eisenia fetida*. *Pol. J. Environ. Stud.* **2020**, *29*, 2383–2394. [CrossRef]
8. Šíma, P. Annelid coelomocytes and haemocytes: Roles in cellular immune reactions. In *Immunology of Annelids*; CRC Press: Boca Raton, FL, USA, 1994; pp. 115–165.
9. Hayashi, Y.; Engelmann, P.; Foldbjerg, R.; Szabo, M.; Somogyi, I.; Pollak, E.; Molnar, L.; Autrup, H.; Sutherland, D.S.; Scott-Fordsmand, J.; et al. Earthworms and humans in vitro: Characterizing evolutionarily conserved stress and immune responses to silver nanoparticles. *Environ. Sci. Technol.* **2012**, *46*, 4166–4173. [CrossRef]
10. Kwak, J.I.; Park, J.-W.; An, Y.-J. Effects of silver nanowire length and exposure route on cytotoxicity to earthworms. *Environ. Sci. Pollut. Res.* **2017**, *24*, 14516–14524. [CrossRef]
11. Gupta, S.; Kushwah, T.; Yadav, S. Earthworm coelomocytes as nanoscavenger of ZnO NPs. *Nanoscale Res. Lett.* **2014**, *9*, 259. [CrossRef]
12. Chen, Q.; Wang, N.; Zhu, M.; Lu, J.; Zhong, H.; Xue, X.; Guo, S.; Li, M.; Wei, X.; Tao, Y.; et al. TiO$_2$ nanoparticles cause mitochondrial dysfunction, activate inflammatory responses, and attenuate phagocytosis in macrophages: A proteomic and metabolomic insight. *Redox Biol.* **2018**, *15*, 266–276. [CrossRef]
13. Alijagic, A.; Gaglio, D.; Napodano, E.; Russo, R.; Costa, C.; Benada, O.; Kofronova, O.; Pinsino, A. Titanium dioxide nanoparticles temporarily influence the sea urchin immunological state suppressing inflammatory-relate gene transcription and boosting antioxidant metabolic activity. *J. Hazard. Mater.* **2020**, *384*, 121389. [CrossRef]
14. Bigorgne, E.; Foucaud, L.; Caillet, C.; Giamberini, L.; Nahmani, J.; Thomas, F.; Rodius, F. Cellular and molecular responses of *E. fetida* coelomocytes exposed to TiO$_2$ nanoparticles. *J. Nanopart. Res.* **2012**, *14*. [CrossRef]
15. Bigorgne, E.; Foucaud, L.; Lapied, E.; Labille, J.; Botta, C.; Sirguey, C.; Falla, J.; Rose, J.; Joner, E.J.; Rodius, F.; et al. Ecotoxicological assessment of TiO$_2$ byproducts on the earthworm *Eisenia fetida*. *Environ. Pollut.* **2011**, *159*, 2698–2705. [CrossRef] [PubMed]
16. Lapied, E.; Nahmani, J.Y.; Moudilou, E.; Chaurand, P.; Labille, J.; Rose, J.; Exbrayat, J.M.; Oughton, D.H.; Joner, E.J. Ecotoxicological effects of an aged TiO$_2$ nanocomposite measured as apoptosis in the anecic earthworm *Lumbricus terrestris* after exposure through water, food and soil. *Environ. Int.* **2011**, *37*, 1105–1110. [CrossRef] [PubMed]
17. Stein, E.; Cooper, E.L. The Role of Opsonins in Phagocytosis by Coelomocytes of the Earthworm, *Lumbricus Terrestris*. *Dev. Comp. Immunol.* **1981**, *5*, 415–425. [CrossRef]
18. Hayashi, Y.; Miclaus, T.; Scavenius, C.; Kwiatkowska, K.; Sobota, A.; Engelmann, P.; Scott-Fordsmand, J.J.; Enghild, J.J.; Sutherland, D.S. Species Differences Take Shape at Nanoparticles: Protein Corona Made of the Native Repertoire Assists Cellular Interaction. *Environ. Sci. Technol.* **2013**, *47*, 14367–14375. [CrossRef] [PubMed]
19. Brunelli, A.; Pojana, G.; Callegaro, S.; Marcomini, A. Agglomeration and sedimentation of titanium dioxide nanoparticles (n-TiO$_2$) in synthetic and real waters. *J. Nanoparticle Res.* **2013**, *15*. [CrossRef]
20. Alijagic, A.; Benada, O.; Kofronova, O.; Cigna, D.; Pinsino, A. Sea Urchin Extracellular Proteins Design a Complex Protein Corona on Titanium Dioxide Nanoparticle Surface Influencing Immune Cell Behavior. *Front. Immunol.* **2019**, *10*. [CrossRef]
21. Müllerová, I. Imaging of specimens at optimized low and very low energies in scanning electron microscopes. *Scanning* **2001**, *23*, 379–394. [CrossRef]
22. Benada, O.; Pokorný, V. Modification of the Polaron sputter-coater unit for glow-discharge activation of carbon support films. *J. Electron Microsc. Tech.* **1990**, *16*, 235–239. [CrossRef]
23. Semerad, J.; Cvancarova, M.; Filip, J.; Kaslik, J.; Zlota, J.; Soukupova, J.; Cajthaml, T. Novel assay for the toxicity evaluation of nanoscale zero-valent iron and derived nanomaterials based on lipid peroxidation in bacterial species. *Chemosphere* **2018**, *213*, 568–577. [CrossRef]
24. Roubalova, R.; Prochazkova, P.; Hanc, A.; Dvorak, J.; Bilej, M. Mutual interactions of *E. andrei* earthworm and pathogens during the process of vermicomposting. *Environ. Sci. Pollut. Res. Int.* **2019**. [CrossRef]
25. Magdolenova, Z.; Bilaničová, D.; Pojana, G.; Fjellsbø, L.M.; Hudecova, A.; Hasplova, K.; Marcomini, A.; Dusinska, M. Impact of agglomeration and different dispersions of titanium dioxide nanoparticles on the human related in vitro cytotoxicity and genotoxicity. *J. Environ. Monit.* **2012**, *14*, 455–464. [CrossRef] [PubMed]
26. Ji, Z.; Jin, X.; George, S.; Xia, T.; Meng, H.; Wang, X.; Suarez, E.; Zhang, H.; Hoek, E.M.V.; Godwin, H.A.; et al. Dispersion and Stability Optimization of TiO$_2$ Nanoparticles in Cell Culture Media. *Environ. Sci. Technol.* **2010**, *44*, 7309–7314. [CrossRef] [PubMed]

27. Huerta-García, E.; Pérez-Arizti, J.A.; Márquez-Ramírez, S.G.; Delgado-Buenrostro, N.L.; Chirino, Y.I.; Iglesias, G.G.; López-Marure, R. Titanium dioxide nanoparticles induce strong oxidative stress and mitochondrial damage in glial cells. *Free Radic. Biol. Med.* **2014**, *73*, 84–94. [CrossRef]
28. Semerad, J.; Moeder, M.; Filip, J.; Pivokonsky, M.; Filipova, A.; Cajthaml, T. Oxidative stress in microbes after exposure to iron nanoparticles: Analysis of aldehydes as oxidative damage products of lipids and proteins. *Environ. Sci. Pollut. Res.* **2019**, *26*, 33670–33682. [CrossRef] [PubMed]
29. Garcia-Velasco, N.; Gandariasbeitia, M.; Irizar, A.; Soto, M. Uptake route and resulting toxicity of silver nanoparticles in *Eisenia fetida* earthworm exposed through Standard OECD Tests. *Ecotoxicology* **2016**, *25*, 1543–1555. [CrossRef] [PubMed]
30. Semerad, J.; Pacheco, N.I.N.; Grasserova, A.; Prochazkova, P.; Pivokonsky, M.; Pivokonska, L.; Cajthaml, T. In Vitro Study of the Toxicity Mechanisms of Nanoscale Zero-Valent Iron (nZVI) and Released Iron Ions Using Earthworm Cells. *Nanomaterials* **2020**, *10*, 2189. [CrossRef] [PubMed]
31. Homa, J.; Stalmach, M.; Wilczek, G.; Kolaczkowska, E. Effective activation of antioxidant system by immune-relevant factors reversely correlates with apoptosis of *Eisenia andrei* coelomocytes. *J. Comp. Physiol. B* **2016**, *186*, 417–430. [CrossRef]
32. Tumminello, R.A.; Fuller-Espie, S.L. Heat stress induces ROS production and histone phosphorylation in celomocytes of *Eisenia hortensis*. *Invertebr. Surviv. J.* **2013**, *10*, 50–57.
33. Ayala, A.; Muñoz, M.F.; Argüelles, S. Lipid peroxidation: Production, metabolism, and signaling mechanisms of malondialdehyde and 4-hydroxy-2-nonenal. *Oxid. Med. Cell. Longev.* **2014**, *2014*, 360438. [CrossRef]
34. Zhang, C.; Zhu, L.; Wang, J.; Wang, J.; Du, Z.; Li, B.; Zhou, T.; Cheng, C.; Wang, Z. Evaluating subchronic toxicity of fluoxastrobin using earthworms (*Eisenia fetida*). *Sci. Total Environ.* **2018**, *642*, 567–573. [CrossRef]
35. Poon, W.-L.; Lee, J.C.-Y.; Leung, K.S.; Alenius, H.; El-Nezami, H.; Karisola, P. Nanosized silver, but not titanium dioxide or zinc oxide, enhances oxidative stress and inflammatory response by inducing 5-HETE activation in THP-1 cells. *Nanotoxicology* **2020**, *14*, 453–467. [CrossRef] [PubMed]
36. Reeves, J.F.; Davies, S.J.; Dodd, N.J.F.; Jha, A.N. Hydroxyl radicals (OH) are associated with titanium dioxide (TiO_2) nanoparticle-induced cytotoxicity and oxidative DNA damage in fish cells. *Mutat. Res.-Fund. Mol. Mech. Mut.* **2008**, *640*, 113–122. [CrossRef] [PubMed]
37. Hu, C.W.; Li, M.; Cui, Y.B.; Li, D.S.; Chen, J.; Yang, L.Y. Toxicological effects of TiO_2 and ZnO nanoparticles in soil on earthworm *Eisenia fetida*. *Soil Biol. Biochem.* **2010**, *42*, 586–591. [CrossRef]
38. Zhu, Y.; Wu, X.; Liu, Y.; Zhang, J.; Lin, D. Integration of transcriptomics and metabolomics reveals the responses of earthworms to the long-term exposure of TiO_2 nanoparticles in soil. *Sci. Total Environ.* **2020**, *719*, 137492. [CrossRef] [PubMed]
39. Candas, D.; Li, J.J. MnSOD in oxidative stress response-potential regulation via mitochondrial protein influx. *Antiox. Redox. Sign.* **2014**, *20*, 1599–1617. [CrossRef]
40. Natarajan, V.; Wilson, C.L.; Hayward, S.L.; Kidambi, S. Titanium Dioxide Nanoparticles Trigger Loss of Function and Perturbation of Mitochondrial Dynamics in Primary Hepatocytes. *PLoS ONE* **2015**, *10*, e0134541. [CrossRef]
41. Bernard, F.; Brulle, F.; Douay, F.; Lemiere, S.; Demuynck, S.; Vandenbulcke, F. Metallic trace element body burdens and gene expression analysis of biomarker candidates in *Eisenia fetida*, using an "exposure/depuration" experimental scheme with field soils. *Ecotoxicol. Environ. Saf.* **2010**, *73*, 1034–1045. [CrossRef]
42. Homa, J.; Zorska, A.; Wesolowski, D.; Chadzinska, M. Dermal exposure to immunostimulants induces changes in activity and proliferation of coelomocytes of *Eisenia andrei*. *J. Comp. Physiol. B* **2013**, *183*, 313–322. [CrossRef]
43. Bodó, K.; Ernszt, D.; Németh, P.; Engelmann, P. Distinct immune-and defense-related molecular fingerprints in sepatated coelomocyte subsets of *Eisenia andrei* earthworms. *Invertebr. Surviv. J.* **2018**, *15*, 338–345.

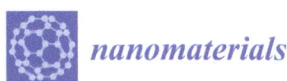

Article

Stressor-Dependant Changes in Immune Parameters in the Terrestrial Isopod Crustacean, *Porcellio scaber*: A Focus on Nanomaterials

Craig Mayall [1], Andraz Dolar [1], Anita Jemec Kokalj [1], Sara Novak [1], Jaka Razinger [2], Francesco Barbero [3], Victor Puntes [3] and Damjana Drobne [1,*]

[1] Biotechnical Faculty, University of Ljubljana, 1000 Ljubljana, Slovenia; craig_mayall@hotmail.co.uk (C.M.); Andraz.Dolar@bf.uni-lj.si (A.D.); anita.jemec@bf.uni-lj.si (A.J.K.); Sara.Novak@bf.uni-lj.si (S.N.)
[2] Plant Protection Department, Agricultural Institute of Slovenia, Ljubljana, Slovenia; jaka.razinger@kis.si
[3] Institut Català de Nanociència i Nanotecnologia (ICN2), CSIC and The Barcelona Institute of Science and Technology (BIST), Campus UAB, 08193 Bellaterra, Barcelona, Spain; fra.barbero@gmail.com (F.B.); victor.puntes@icn2.cat (V.P.)
* Correspondence: damjana.drobne@bf.uni-lj.si

Abstract: We compared the changes of selected immune parameters of *Porcellio scaber* to different stressors. The animals were either fed for two weeks with Au nanoparticles (NPs), CeO_2 NPs, or Au ions or body-injected with Au NPs, CeO_2 NPs, or lipopolysaccharide endotoxin. Contrary to expectations, the feeding experiment showed that both NPs caused a significant increase in the total haemocyte count (THC). In contrast, the ion-positive control resulted in a significantly decreased THC. Additionally, changes in phenoloxidase (PO)-like activity, haemocyte viability, and nitric oxide (NO) levels seemed to depend on the stressor. Injection experiments also showed stressor-dependant changes in measured parameters, such as CeO_2 NPs and lipopolysaccharide endotoxin (LPS), caused more significant responses than Au NPs. These results show that feeding and injection of NPs caused an immune response and that the response differed significantly, depending on the exposure route. We did not expect the response to ingested NPs, due to the low exposure concentrations (100 µg/g dry weight food) and a firm gut epithelia, along with a lack of phagocytosis in the digestive system, which would theoretically prevent NPs from crossing the biological barrier. It remains a challenge for future research to reveal what the physiological and ecological significance is for the organism to sense and respond, via the immune system, to ingested foreign material.

Keywords: gold nanoparticles; cerium nanoparticles; woodlice; immune response; haemocyte

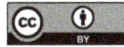

1. Introduction

The role of the immune system is to distinguish between the self and non-self and to choose the most effective response to exogenous or endogenous threats, in order to maintain the integrity and homeostasis of the organism [1–3]. The immune recognition and response mechanisms of crustaceans depend entirely on the innate immune system.

The most prominent and well-studied cellular effector reactions of the innate immune system are phagocytosis, nodulation, encapsulation, cell-mediated cytotoxicity, and clotting. Cellular responses act in conjunction with humoral factors [4].

In crustaceans, in response to natural infections and challenges that mimic natural infections, such as lipopolysaccharide endotoxin (LPS), the response mechanisms and the recognition system that governs them are well -studied [5–10]. However, much less is known about the immune effector reactions in response to other challenges, such as pollutants [11]. Recently, the research on adverse or beneficial interactions between engineered nanomaterials and model organisms has provided a new model system to study if and how organisms sense and respond to novel engineered material of sizes comparable to those of viruses or bacteria [3].

Terrestrial isopods are a valuable model organism to study defences against challenges to homeostasis, as isopoda are the only order of crustacean able to occupy freshwater, marine, and terrestrial environments, which indicates that they have been exposed to a large variety of stressors during their evolution [12].

Isopods, as well as other arthropods, primarily rely on the cuticle as a sensing and defence system and the innate immune system to cope with different challenges to homeostasis. The cuticle is the relatively thin but tough and flexible layer of noncellular material that is capable of inducing many biochemical processes and able to respond to different environmental cues [13].

Haemocytes play a central role in the internal defence of the animal, although their role and function are not solely limited to purely immunogenic responses. In oysters, haemocytes were seen to participate in calcium carbonate shell crystal production, transportation, and shell regeneration [14,15]. Moreover, haemocytes in a range of organisms have been found to be involved in muscle fibre degeneration and regeneration; adult neurogenesis; and the digestion, storage, and distribution of nutrients [16–19]. The total haemocyte count (THC) is traditionally taken as a measure of an organism's change in immunocompetence and is used in assessing the stress or health status in crustaceans [20–23]. It has been shown that the THC can vary not only in response to infection but also due to environmental stresses and endocrine activity during the moulting cycle [24,25].

An integral component of the innate immune system is the extracellular phenoloxidase (PO) cascade, which is part of humoral response that catalyses the formation of cytotoxic intermediates quinones, essential precursors for melanisation and sclerotisation [26–29]. Melanin accumulates at wound sites and around invading microorganisms [30]. It is not only involved in innate immune responses through melanotic encapsulation, it is also critical for cuticle tanning, which has been extensively studied in insects [19]. The PO cascade also has a role is ecdysis and exoskeleton formation [28].

The primary source of PO activity comes from the haemocytes [8,31]. However, prophenoloxidase (proPO) transcripts have been detected in nonhaemocyte cells too, including the hepatopancreas, stomach epithelium, anterior midgut caecum, glia cells in the nervous cord, and neurosecretory cells in ganglions [27,32]. Besides the plasma PO enzyme, literature also reports the existence of haemocyanin-derived PO (Hd–PO) activity [33,34]. Therefore, in isopods, PO-like activity in the haemolymph is usually shown, because, at this point, it is impossible to distinguish whether the observed activity is purely due to the plasma PO enzyme or haemocyanin-derived [5,33].

Activity of PO is taken as one of most frequently used parameters of assessing immune system activity. Phenoloxidase (PO) activity is increased as a result of clotting process's, phagocytosis, encapsulation of foreign material, antimicrobial action, and cell agglutination [35]. The moult cycle, for example, is also a source of variation of phenoloxidase activity and correlates with the presence of large granular cells, although this appears to be species-specific [36,37]. Correlative measures of phenoloxidase (PO) activity and resistance to infection against vibriosis have been also investigated during the moult cycle [38]. In addition, it is documented in insects that, when soft cuticles are damaged, the pro-enzymes can become activated, [39] and the active enzymes can take part in both wound healing and in defending against invading microorganisms. The PO cascade not only results in the formation of cytotoxic pigment precursors, including quinones, quinone methides, and semiquinones, but also reactive oxygen species (ROS) and reactive nitric species (RNS), such as nitric oxide (NO) [40].

The concentration of NO is another well-studied and often used measure of immune system activity. The first evidence for NO to have a role as an humoral molecule in an invertebrate was provided by Radomski et al. (1991) [41]. Both RNS and ROS are produced by activated phagocytic cells. These molecules are involved in the breaking down of phagocytosed infectious agents such as viruses and bacteria, as well as dead and dying cells [42–44]. Otherwise, at lower concentrations, NO is involved in diverse housekeeping functions, such as neurotransmission, mucus secretion, and in controlling certain activities of the circulatory system, while at higher concentrations, NO is cytotoxic [45].

In the work presented here, we have used different types of immune challenges, i.e., lipopolysaccharide (LPS) and two types of nanoparticles and metal salt. LPS is a constituent of the cell membrane of Gram-negative bacteria. It has been widely used in investigating the immune function of a spectrum of model organisms [46–49]. For nanoparticles (NPs), two particles with well-known and frequently studied biological interactions were selected. Metal salt was used as a positive control to compare the effect of different forms of a metal (ions and nanoparticles).

Gold nanoparticles (Au NPs) have been used extensively in different experimental studies as their size, shape, and surface chemistry can be readily manipulated [50]. Due to their unique properties, they have a wide potential for applications in industry and biomedicine [50,51]. Numerous previous studies have found Au NPs to be relatively inert and nonharmful to organisms [52,53]. While some authors have suggested Au NPs have anti-inflammatory and antiangiogenic effects [54–56], others have shown Au NPs have toxic potential and can modulate immune processes in vitro and in vivo in some studies [50,54,57].

CeO_2 NPs also represent nanoparticles with great industrial potential, due to their catalytic and redox properties [58,59]. Compared to Au NPs, they are more often considered as biologically potent and can induce oxidative stress; inflammation; DNA damage; and affect reproductive capability, growth, and the survival of exposed animals [59,60]. In the study of Kos et al. (2017), honeybees were exposed to the very same CeO_2 NPs as in the present study. Significant alterations in Acetylcholinesterase and glutathione-S-transferase activities were evidenced at concentration 2 mg/L. However, in another experiment testing the toxicity of Au NPs and CeO_2 NPs on earthworms, where the same exposure duration (as this paper) was used, CeO_2 NPs showed a low toxic potential [59]. CeO_2 NPs also possess dual properties, contrary to adverse effects some studies report on their antioxidant and anti-inflammatory properties [61,62].

Both CeO_2 NPs and Au NPs have low dissolution rate [54,58]; therefore, the particles, and not the dissolved ions, are primarily responsible for the biological effect.

We provide a comparison of the responses of the innate immune system of terrestrial isopod *P. scaber* to different types of challenges to homeostasis (Au and Ce nanoparticles, salt, and LPS). We have analysed and compared some well-studied immune parameters (THC, haemocyte viability, PO-like activity, and NO concentration) after dietary exposure and in the case of body injection [63].

The aim of our work was to investigate if and how the most well-known and studied parameters of the immune system respond to nanomaterials in the food and to compare this response to that when nanomaterials are injected directly into the haemolymph of a terrestrial isopod, *Porcellio scaber*. Our focus was also directed towards comparing the response to nanoparticles vs. ions in the feeding experiment and towards comparing the response to nanoparticles vs. LPS in body injection experiments. We hypothesise that the response to NPs directly injected into the haemolymph or consumed with food is substantially different. We discuss the differences in response to the selected types of noninfectious immune system challenges in a model terrestrial invertebrate species.

2. Materials and Methods

2.1. Nanoparticle Synthesis and Characterisation

Au NPs were synthesised by the Catalan Institute of Nanoscience and Nanotechnology (ICN2). Au NPs (26.4 ± 3 nm) were synthesised according to the seeded-growth method developed and detailed in Bastús et al. (2011) [64]. Au NPs were purified and surface coated in PVP following the procedure outlined in Alijagic (2020) to produce PVP–Au NPs, referred to in this paper as Au NPs [65]. Dynamic light scattering (DLS) analysis showed the particles had an average hydrodynamic diameter of 67.2 nm, and laser doppler anemometry showed a Z potential of −3.9 ± 0.8 mV (pH 5.5, conductivity 0.9 mS/cm)

(Malvern Zetasizer Nano ZS, Malvern Panalytical Ltd, Worcester, UK). Diameters were reported as distribution by intensity calculated by non-negative least squares (NNLS). A typical UV–Vis spectrum profile with a surface plasmon resonance band peaking at 525 nm showed the particles were monodispersed (Agilent Cary 60 spectrophotometer, Santa Clara, CA, USA). Tetrachloroauric (III) acid trihydrate (99.9% purity), sodium citrate tribasic dihydrate ($\geq$99%), and polyvinylpyrrolidone (55 KDa) were purchased from Sigma–Aldrich. Particle characterisation can be found in Figure A1.

Stabiliser-free, uncoated spherical CeO_2 NPs as an aqueous dispersion in dH_2O (batch number PROM-CeO2-20 nm-2306/5a) were supplied by NanoMILE PROM (Promethean Particles, Nottingham, UK, http://www.prometheanparticles.co.uk/ 2 April 2021) within the framework of the EU FP7 NanoMILE project. The CeO_2 NPs were synthesised using supercritical fluid synthesis, followed by a washing step postsynthesis to remove unreacted species. The mean particle diameter (TEM) was 4.7 $\pm$ 1.4 nm (JEOL JEM2100F, Tokyo, Japan), the Z-average size was 172.1 $\pm$ 1.705 nm, the polydispersity index (PDI) was 0.272 $\pm$ 0.009, and the zeta potential was 50.3 $\pm$ 0.719 mV (Malvern Zetasizer 5000, Malvern Panalytical Ltd, Worcester, UK). Further particle characterisation can be found in Kos et al. (2017) [66].

2.2. Experimental Animals

Porcellio scaber were collected from a compost heap in noncontaminated, pollution-free garden in Kamnik, Slovenia. Prior to the experiment, animals were cultured for a several months under constant temperature (20 $\pm$ 2 °C) and illumination (light:dark 16:8 h) regime in a climate-controlled chamber at the University of Ljubljana. Animals were kept in a glass terrarium filled up with a humus soil (moistened at 40% of the water holding capacity; WHC) and fed with dry leaves of common hazel (*Corylus avellana*), common alder (*Alnus glutinosa*), and carrots, as described by Jemec Kokalj et al. (2018) [67]. Adult animals of both sexes with body mass greater than 25 mg were selected for the experiment, while individuals with evident signs of moulting, gravid females, and those with symptoms of bacterial or viral infection were excluded [5]. We have followed the the ARRIVE (Animal Research: Reporting of *In Vivo* Experiments) guidelines (http://www.nc3rs.org.uk/page.asp?id=1357) for reporting experiments with using living animals. Experiments with terrestrial isopods do not need to be approved by the ethics committee.

2.3. Feeding Experiment

The feeding experiment was carried out for 14 days in petri dishes with a single animal at constant temperature (20 $\pm$ 2 °C), illumination (light:dark 16:8 h) regime, and moisture in a climate-controlled chamber, a semichronic exposure period. The animals were fed dried leaves covered with either cerium oxide nanoparticles (CeO_2 NPs), gold nanoparticles (Au NPs), or ionic gold ($AuCl_3$) as salt control or pure dried leaves, which served as controls. Nanoparticles and metal ions were spread on a leaf at a concentration of 100 µg/g of dry weight (d.w.) leaf. This concentration was chosen, as it is lower than the previously observed lowest effect concentration yet higher than the estimated soil compartment concentration, in order to provide an example of the model response [68–71]. Animals' weights were taken before and after the experiment; additionally, dry leaf weights after nanoparticle application at the start and end of the experiment were taken. During the experiment, animal faeces were removed from the petri dishes every 48 h in order to measure defecation rate and to reduce coprophagy. At the end of the 14-day experiment, fresh haemolymph was collected from the animals, according to Dolar et al. (2020), to measure the selected immune parameters [5]. Details on the number of animals used can be found in Table A1.

2.4. Injection Experiment

For injection experiments, animals were injected with 0.5 µL of the lipopolysaccharide (LPS), CeO_2 NPs, Au NPs or Milli-Q water as a trauma control, using a 25 µL Hamilton microsyringe (700 series, 33 gauge, blunt tip) and a repeating dispenser (PB 600-1, Hamilton, Bonaduz, Switzerland). Cerium and Au NPs were suspended in Milli-Q water at a concentration of 0.3 µg/µL. A nonlethal dose of LPS (from *E. coli* O111:B4, Sigma-Aldrich, St. Louis, MO, USA) was used as a positive control for reference immune response (50 µg/µL). Injected animals were left for 48 h in a petri dish with a dry leaf for food at a constant temperature (20 ± 2 °C) and illumination (light: dark 16:8 h) regime and moisture in a climate-controlled chamber. Afterwards, fresh haemolymph was collected from the animals to measure the selected immune parameters. Details on the number of animals used can be found in Table A2.

2.5. Haemolymph Collection

A sterile syringe needle was used to puncture the intersegmental membrane on the dorsal side of the animal between the 5th and 6th segment; then a drop of haemolymph was withdrawn using glass microcapillary pipette. Where not enough haemolymph could be collected from a single animal, a pooled sample was prepared for nitric oxide and phenoloxidase-like measurements.

2.6. Immune Parameters

To determine haemocyte viability and total haemocyte count (THC), 3–5 µL of freshly collected haemolymph was diluted in 100 mM PPB (pH 7) up to a volume 28 µL, and then 2 µL of nigrosin dye was added (final concentration of 80 µg/mL), which stains dead cells, while viable haemocytes remain unstained. After that, ten microliters of haemocyte suspension was loaded on to each chamber of the Neubauer haemocytometer to assess haemocyte viability and THC under a phase contrast microscope (Axio Vert.A1, Zeiss; magnification: 40×, Oberkochen, Germany). In order to fulfil the requirement for a statistically significant count, at least 100 cells per square were counted (according to the instructions of the haemocytometer). Each haemolymph sample measurement was performed in duplicate.

Nitric oxide (NO) levels in the haemolymph were measured using Griess reagent after a modified protocol Faraldo et al. (2005) [72]. Twenty microliters of a pooled haemolymph sample, collected from an average of 4 animals, was placed into 28 µL of 1% sulphanilamide dissolved in 5% phosphoric acid (H_3PO_4) and kept on ice. After that, 20 µL of this solution was diluted at a ratio of 1:1 (v:v) with 1% naphthylethylenediamine dihydrochloride (NEED, Sigma). The absorbance of NO was measured in a 384-well assay plate at 543 nm after a 5-min incubation period using a Cytation 3 imaging reader (Biotek, Winooski, VT, USA). Each haemolymph sample measurement was done in duplicate. NO concentrations (µM) were calculated from a standard curve for $NaNO_2$ (2.5–200 µM).

Phenoloxidase (PO)-like activity was assessed photometrically in the haemolymph obtained from 1–3 animals, after a modified protocol described by Jaenicke et al. (2009) [34]. Five microliters of haemolymph was placed into 200 µL of Dulbecco's phosphate buffered saline buffer (DPBS, pH 7.1–7.5), containing 4 mM dopamine hydrochloride (Sigma-Aldrich, St. Louis, MO, USA) and 2 mM sodium dodecyl sulphate (SDS, Sigma), necessary for in vitro PO activation. Forty microliters of this reaction mixture was pipetted into 384-well plate (Greiner Bio-One, Kremsmünster, Austria). The formation of a reddish–brown pigment, which is nonenzymatically synthesised from the dopamine catalytic product dopaquinon, was measured using a Cytation 3 imaging reader (Biotek, Winooski, VT, USA) at 475 nm and 25 °C for at least three hours. Haemolymph PO-like activity was calculated as the change in absorbance from the linear part of the absorbance slope per minute per haemolymph volume, normalised to control and expressed as a percentage [73]. PO-like activity assessment was done in duplicate for each haemolymph sample.

2.7. Statistical Analysis

Statistical analysis of the data was performed using OriginPro v2020 software program OriginLab, Northampton, MA, USA). The data was tested using Kruskal–Wallis test, followed by pairwise comparison of treatments with control group, using Mann–Whitney U-test. Values of $p < 0.001$ (***), $p < 0.01$ (**) and $p < 0.05$ (*) were considered as significantly different.

3. Results

3.1. Feeding Activity of Isopods and Mortality

The feeding activity of isopods, calculated as the mass of leaves ingested per each animal's mass, in two weeks, was not significantly altered in animals that were fed CeO_2 NP- or Au NP-spiked leaves. In addition, Au ions ($AuCl_3$) as a salt control for Au NPs did not induce any changes in feeding activity. No signs of animal mortality were evidenced (data not shown) (Figure 1). These data show that the tested concentration (100 µg/g d.w. leaf) did not induce significant adverse effects and can be considered not toxic.

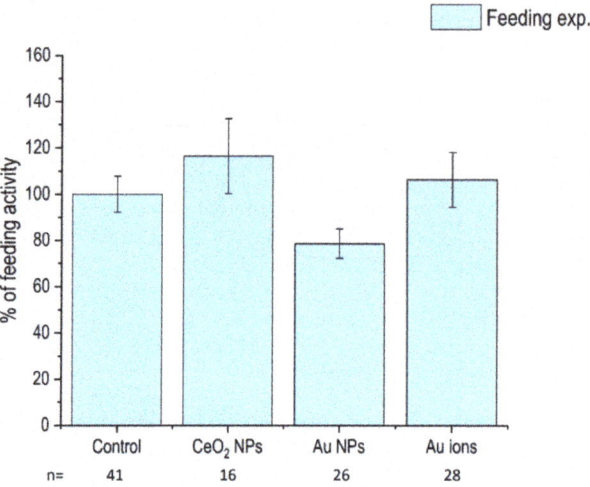

Figure 1. Feeding activity of isopods in comparison to control (%) after 14 days of feeding on CeO_2 nanoparticle (NP)-, Au NP-, and Au ions-spiked leaves. Columns represent the mean (±SE). n = number of biological repeats in each column.

3.2. NO Levels and PO-Like Activity

Nitric oxide (NO) levels were significantly increased after the animals were fed or injected with CeO_2 NPs, while Au NPs caused increases in NO levels only when injected. The observed increase was more significant in the case of CeO_2 NPs, in comparison to Au NPs (Figure 2a).

PO-like activity was significantly increased in the case of both CeO_2 NPs and Au NPs after feeding and injection. The increase was again more significant in response to CeO_2 NPs (Figure 2b). The injection procedure, itself, had no effect on NO levels or PO-like activity, as evidenced by no significant changes in the trauma controls. Injection with LPS, a positive control, significantly increased the NO levels and caused a decrease in PO-like activity.

3.3. Haemocyte Count

The total haemocyte count (THC) was significantly increased in the case of CeO_2 NPs and Au NPs, in comparison to control after feeding, but decreased in the case of Au ions. However, after injections, neither CeO_2 NPs nor Au NPs affected the THC. The viability of the haemocytes was decreased after both feeding and injection CeO_2 NP exposures, but Au treatments had no effect on viability after either exposure route. Injection, itself (evidenced as trauma control), had no effect on the THC or viability of haemocytes; however, both THC and viability were affected after LPS injection, serving as a positive control (Figure 3).

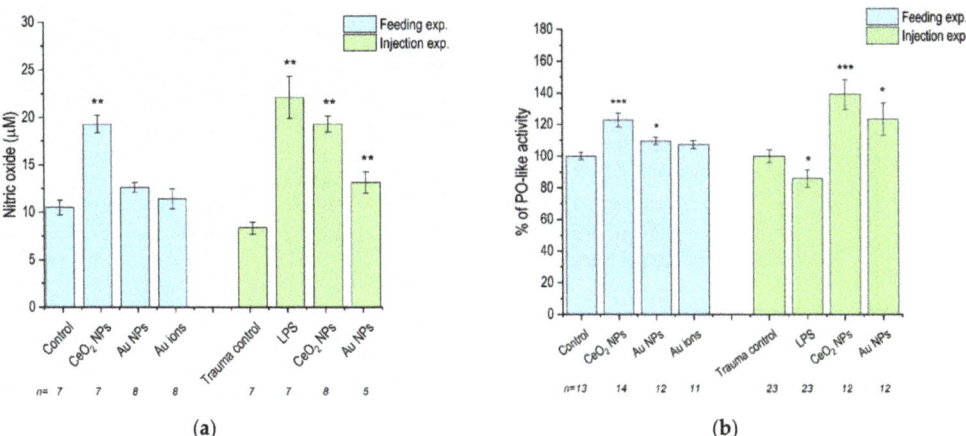

Figure 2. (a) Nitric oxide concentrations and (b) phenoloxidase (PO)-like activity in *P. scaber* exposed to CeO_2 NP- and Au NP-spiked leaves (Feeding exp.) and injected with CeO_2 NPs and Au NPs dispersion (Injection exp.). Au ions correspond to $AuCl_3$, trauma control are animals injected with dH_2O and lipopolysaccharide endotoxin (LPS); animals injected with 50 µg/µL LPS. Columns represent the mean (±SE). n represents the number of analysed samples. For nitric oxide (NO) measurements, on average, 4–5 animals were grouped into one sample, and for the PO-like measurements, 1–3 animals were grouped into 1 sample. (*) $p < 0.05$, (**) $p < 0.01$, (***) $p < 0.001$ in comparison to control (Kruskal–Wallis test followed by Mann–Whitney U-test).

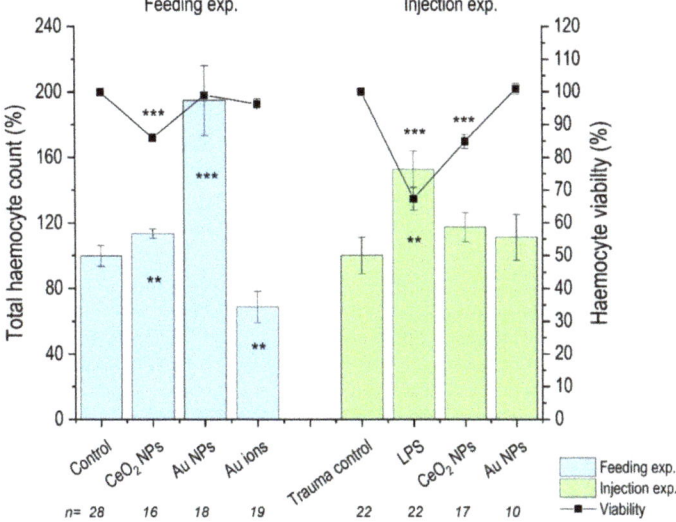

Figure 3. Total haemocyte count (THC) and haemocyte viability in *P. scaber* exposed to CeO_2 NP- and Au NP-spiked leaves (Feeding exp.) and injected with CeO_2 NPs and Au NPs dispersion (Injection exp.). Au ions correspond to $AuCl_3$, trauma control are animals injected with dH_2O and LPS; animals injected with 50 µg/µL. Columns represents mean (±SE). n represents the number of biological repeats. (**) $p \leq 0.01$, (***) $p \leq 0.001$ in comparison to control (Kruskal–Wallis test followed by Mann–Whitney U-test). When * is drawn inside the column, it refers to THC values.

4. Discussion

We report a comparison of the responses of well-studied immune parameters (THC, haemocyte viability, PO-like enzyme activity, and NO concentration) of the terrestrial isopod *P. scaber* to different types of stressors (Au and CeO$_2$ nanoparticles, salt, and LPS) after feeding exposure and after direct injection into the animal's body. While injection is not a realistic exposure route for NPs, it can help to study consequences of direct biological interactions between NPs and isopod haemocytes inside the body (in vivo).

4.1. Feeding on Au NP-Dosed Diet

In animals fed for 14 days on a Au NP-dosed diet, we detected a significant increase in the THC, no effect on haemocyte viability, a slight increase in PO-like activity, and no change in the NO concentration. Literature explains such a response as immunostimultion by oral administration [74] or an indication of increased immune capacity [75]. Setyawan et al. (2018) also provided evidence that diet composition (crude fucoidan from three tropical brown algae i.e., Sargassum, Padina, and Turbinaria) was able to provoke increased PO, THC, and relative superoxide dismutase (SOD) activity in white shrimp [74]. In addition, in lobster, haemocyte levels, as well as the haemolymph protein levels, were found to be influenced by diet more than by temperature [76]. Pascual et al. (2004) reported that the amounts of dietary protein were positively corelated to the TCH response in *L. vannamei* juveniles [77]. In their study, shrimp fed an optimal level of protein had an elevated concentration of haemocytes, indicating that optimal dietary protein levels promoted blood cell synthesis [77]. In contrast, shrimp fed suboptimal protein had more proPO per cell, showing that shrimps could be enhancing the content of the haemocytes (i.e., proPO) as a response of cell deficit induced by imbalanced dietary protein [77]. There are also reports in different insect species that the THC increased when they were withheld food [78,79]. Furthermore, Matozzo et al. (2011) observed a positive relationship between the THC and PO activity in starved crabs. They hypothesised that the number of circulating haemocytes increased in starved crabs to allow them to mobilise energy reserves during starvation [80]. In addition, Sequeira et al. (1996) suggested that increases in the THC in Crustacea may be either due to a more active mobilisation of haemocytes from tissues into the haemolymph or a faster division of circulating haemocytes [81]. In line with our findings are reports of Muralisankar et al. (2014), who found an elevated THC and haemocyte production after ZnNP exposure to the freshwater prawn, *Macrobrachium rosenbergii*, within a certain exposure dose range [82]. We can conclude that increases of the THC or in PO-like activity are the result of a complex response of the organism responding to ingested material that is different from its usual diet but one that is not necessarily an indication of adverse effect. What this complex response is and why it has physiological or ecological consequences needs to be discovered.

There are only a few studies on the mechanism of how components in the diet challenge immune processes. In crustaceans, for example, the hepatopancreas, which comes into direct contact with ingested material (not protected by cuticle or peritrophic membrane), produces many proteins that contribute to humoral immunity, including the two most abundant proteins in the haemolymph, clotting protein and haemocyanin [83,84]. Both of these proteins play roles in the immune response [83,84], especially haemocyanin, which is believed to carry out phenoloxidase-like functions in *P. scaber* [34].

We suggest that ingested Au NPs could come into contact with hepatopancreatic cells, and the NPs' environmental corona could be recognised by hepatopancreatic cells [85]. Since a feeding rate reduction was not detected in this study, food quality, and not food deprivation, must be the explanation for the increased THC or PO activity. As ingested Au NPs did not cause an increase in the NO concentration, we conclude that there is a lack of evidence of phagocytic activity of damaged material (damaged-self) [86]. In addition, with no changes in haemocyte viability, we speculate that the changes in immune parameters via hepatopancreas–humoral immunity communication/signalling are primarily not damage-related (damaged-self-related).

4.2. Feeding on CeO$_2$ NP-Dosed Diet

In animals fed for 14 days on the CeO$_2$ NP-dosed diet, increased PO-like activity and reduced viability of haemocytes was accompanied by a significant increase of NO activity, suggesting phagocytic activity of damaged or non-self material. However, NO is also produced in the PO cascade, which results in the formation of cytotoxic pigment precursors (quinones, quinone methides, and semiquinones) as well as reactive oxygen intermediates (ROI) and reactive nitrogen intermediates (RNI) [40].

In CeO$_2$ NP-fed animals, we explain the increased THC, reduced haemocyte viability, increased PO-like activity, and increased NO concentration as an immune response, indicating either increased melanisation via increased PO-like activity and/or increased production of toxic radicals (via NO), which could occur either during haemocyte phagocytic activity or melanisation. This response to CeO$_2$ NPs could be provoked due to cuticle (external surfaces) damage and subsequent melanisation of the cuticle either on the body surface or in the digestive system [13]. It is assumed that hepatopancreatic cells, as a possible contact site between cells and NPs, have probably not been damaged. If damage had occurred here, it would likely have been reflected in a reduced feeding rate, which was not seen in this study.

We speculate that the organism responded to microdamages or changes in the cuticle structure, which surrounds the gut epithelium, when exposed to CeO$_2$ NP-dosed food. As reported by Parle et al. (2017), for insects, an injury that penetrates the epidermis results in a scab which is never resorbed [87].

In the case of the CeO$_2$ NP-fed animals in our study, the increased THC and PO-like activity was accompanied by a significant reduction in the viability of haemocytes and a significant elevation in NO levels, suggesting phagocytosis [88], which may indicate a (micro)damage-related response. The response pattern of *P. scaber* to CeO$_2$ NPs is significantly different from that in Au NP-fed animals, indicating a different type of interaction between the two particles and *P. scaber*. The Au NPs appeared more biologically inert than CeO$_2$ NPs.

Even if CeO$_2$ NPs demonstrated some biological reactivity, according to Giese et al. (2018), environmentally relevant concentrations of CeO$_2$ NPs are those 100-fold lower that the one recorded to provoke toxicity—concentrations ranging from 100 to 3000 mg/kg or mg/L [89].

4.3. Feeding on Au Ions-Dosed Diet

As expected, the Au ions provoked a different type of response, as measured via the selected immune parameters, than the Au NP consumption. We detected a significant decline in the THC but no change in feeding, mortality, haemocyte viability, PO-like activity, or NO concentration. It is interesting that feeding on Au NPs provoked a completely opposite response compared to Au ions. Au NP particles in the diet caused significant increases in the THC and of PO-like activity, while Au ions in the diet resulted in a THC decline.

Similarly, a decrease in the number of circulating haemocytes (TCH) was demonstrated in mercury-exposed prawns [90] and in crabs after bacterial infection [91] or after temperature stress [92]. A decrease in the number of circulating haemocytes is explained as a consequence of haemocyte immobilisation in different tissues, as demonstrated in mercury-exposed prawns [90] and in crabs after bacterial infection [92,93]. Consequently, this leads to a stress-induced decrease in immunocompetence [94] and renders organisms more susceptible to disease. Le Moullac et al. (2000) reported that environmental stress from pollutants induced immunosuppression in crustaceans, in terms of haemocyte number, phagocytosis, and a change in PO activity [21]. Further, Quin et al. (2012) reported that the total haemocyte count in Cd-exposed groups was decreased significantly, when compared with the control groups of freshwater crab, *Sinopotamon henanense* [22]. In addition, Singaram et al. (2013) reported that 14 days of exposure to Hg at environmentally relevant concentrations suppressed THC, superoxide generation, phagocytosis, and PO activity, among other immune parameters [95].

Matozzo et al. (2011) hypothesised that increased PO activity in haemolymph from temperature-stressed crabs was a physiological response of animals to compensate for the lower THC, in order to increase immunosurveillance in both haemolymph and peripheral tissues [92], corroborating findings by Hauton et al. (1997) [96]. In our study, the PO-like activity was not changed to potentially compensate for the decreased THC. However, we confirm negative consequences of Au ion exposure on the THC, which is in line with findings after mercury exposure.

4.4. Injection of Stimuli into Blood

The second approach in our study to challenge the immune parameters of isopods was by the injection of different stimuli (LPS or NPs) directly into the haemocoel and to leave the animals for 48 h to develop a response. A lipopolysaccharide (LPS) is an endotoxin, which is an integral component of the outer membrane of Gram-negative bacteria and, thus, can be used to mimic a bacterial infection [97].

In our study, injected LPS resulted in an increased THC, decreased haemocyte viability, the generation of NO, and reduced PO-like activity. Other authors have also reported alterations in the THC after LPS injection. In insects, adult male *Acheta domesticus* crickets, an LPS injection caused a significant decrease in the number of circulating haemocytes 2 h post injection, which was followed by an increase in haemocyte numbers 1 day after injection and then maintained levels for at least 7 days [73]. Similarly, Bogolio et al. (2000) reported that, after an initial decrease in haemocyte counts in juvenile prawns, a sublethal infection with *V. alginolyticus* induced higher haemocyte counts than controls at 8 days post-infection [98]. In an experiment by Lorenzon et al. (1999), multiple shellfish were injected with an LD50 dose of LPS *E. coli* [99]. In most of the species, the LPS caused an initial decrease in haemocytes (40% at 3–5 hpi), then an increase in haemocytes to control animal levels after 48 hpi (*Palaemon elegans*, *Crangon crangon*, and *Squilla mantis*). A challenge with LPS injection is also reported by Chiaramonte et al. (2019) on the sea urchin *Paracentrotus lividus* [100]. Here, LPS treatment significantly increased the number of coelomocytes after the first hour of treatment. At 6 and 24 h post-LPS treatment, values obtained did not significantly differ from the untreated controls. LPS injection in crayfish [48] caused an increase in haemocytes 2 h post-LPS injection, as well as a significant decrease in haemocyte viability. Furthermore, Xu et al. (2015), who exposed crab haemocytes to LPS, reported that LPS causes a decrease in haemocyte viability, due to the increase apoptosis rate [101]. They found that LPS damaged DNA and caused morphological changes in the haemocytes, resulting in cell shrinkage, nucleus membrane and chromatin fracturing, and the formation of apoptotic bodies [101].

Similar to our work is a study conducted with juvenile *Litopenaeus stylirostris*, which evaluated the impact of the injection of (1) formalin-killed *Vibrio penueicida* cells (vaccine) and (2) a sublethal infection with a moderately pathogenic strain of *Vibrio alginolyticus* on total haemocyte counts. After an initial decrease in haemocyte counts, both the vaccination and the sublethal infection induced higher haemocyte counts than controls. In order to investigate the possibility of increasing the number of circulating haemocytes in pond-reared juvenile shrimp, the vaccine was added to the diet. No effect on the haemocyte counts was observed over a 20-day feeding period [98].

Contrary to our expectations, only LPS injection caused changes in the TCH. However, the level of NO was increased in all three injection treatments: LPS, CeO_2 NPs, and Au NPs. Literature reports that LPS stimulates non-self-induced nitric oxide generation involving nitric oxide synthase in haemocytes and the production of nitric oxide during phagocytosis as a cellular immune reaction to fight the pathogen [6]. Yeh et al. (2006) also postulate that the observed increase in nitric oxide synthase (NOS) and NO generation increases bacterial adhesion to haemocytes, and as such, LPS increases both haemocyte adhesion and the phagocytic activity of the haemocytes [102]. Gopalakrishnan et al. (2011) found that, in the crab *Scylla paramamosain,* LPS stimulation caused the levels of NO to increase from 3 h to 96 h post-injection [6]. In crayfish injected with LPS, after 1 h, a two-fold increase in NO levels was found, compared to animals injected with only saline [102]. Similarly, NP injection may also provoke phagocytic activity of the haemocytes, but only the CeO_2 NPs affected their viability.

We also evidenced alterations of PO-like activity in all cases of injected stimuli. LPS injection caused a reduction of PO-like activity, while both injected NPs increased the PO-like activity. Our results are in line with those reported by Charles & Killian (2015), who found that, in crickets, LPS caused an increased THC and decreased PO activity at 7 days [73]. However, these results were with LPS from *S. marcensces* and not *E. coli* [73]. Contrary to our study, Gopalakrishnan et al. (2011) found that, in the crab *Scylla paramamosain,* LPS injection stimulation caused an increase in PO activity from 3 h to 48 h, while at the same time causing a decrease in the THC [6]. Salawu et al. (2016) suggested that the role of activated PO in the crab *Uca tangeri* was to limit the survival of Gram-negative bacteria upon entry into the haemolymph, and the PO is immediately necessary upon the LPS being identified, with there being an increase in activated PO in the haemolymph 10 min after exposure to LPS [103]. In our study, LPS caused increases in the THC but no increase in PO-like activity; in fact, PO-like activity was decreased again, showing a complex response to a stimulus, as evidenced also in the ingestion exposure.

To sum up, our results show that haemocyte viability and NO response is more severe in case of LPS and least in case of Au NPs (LPS > CeO_2 NPs > Au NPs). Excessive NO production is explained by increased phagocytosis activity of cells [88]. Injection of CeO_2 NPs and Au NPs resulted in the significant increase in PO-like activity and NO concentration. CeO_2 NPs also caused a significant decrease in haemocyte viability, a response also seen after LPS injection, suggesting CeO_2 NPs were causing more damage than the Au NPs to the haemocytes, with the former causing a higher instance of haemocyte death. The same, CeO_2 NPs being more biologically potent than Au NPs, was observed in feeding exposure.

5. Conclusions

There are significant differences in the immune response after feeding or injection exposure to different stressors. In both types of exposure, feeding or injection of both NPs, increased the PO-like activity. However, injected LPS caused a reduction of PO-like activity. Increased PO-like activity is interpreted to lead to increased melanisation, which is needed for wound healing [29] but may have other functions, as well. Furthermore, NO was increased in all cases of injection, but only in the case of CeO_2 NPs in the feeding experiment and was most significantly increased after LPS injection. NO is associated with the phagocytosis of non-self and damaged-self [86,104]. Therefore, we conclude that CeO_2 NPs, and not Au NPs, were causing (micro)damage/alterations to the isopods' tissues and cells, resulting in the increase in phagocytosis, as evidenced by NO levels increasing, to remove the cell debris.

Next, the THC was observed to increase after feeding of both NPs and LPS injection, but feeding on a diet with Au ions caused the THC to decrease. The number of circulating haemocytes can change dramatically over the course of an infection. In other crustaceans exposed to LPS, haemocyte numbers have been found to increase [81,105] in the hours and days after exposure. However, many studies have also reported significant decreases in the haemocyte count and PO activity after exposure of different crustacean species to environmental pollutants [106]. A low number of circulating haemocytes in crustaceans is strongly correlated with a greater sensitivity to pathogens [107] and, hence, a low THC indicates a higher susceptibility to infectious disease [21]. On the other hand, recruitment of haemocytes, as well as increased phagocytic, phenoloxidase, and antioxidant enzymatic activities, among others, are described as a result of immunostimulantion [63,108]. It remains a challenge for the future research what are the physiological and ecological significances for the organism to sense foreign material in the food.

Author Contributions: Conceptualisation, C.M., D.D., and A.J.K.; methodology, C.M., A.J.K., A.D., and S.N.; investigation, resources, J.R., F.B., and V.P.; writing, review, and editing, C.M., D.D., A.J.K., A.D., and S.N. All authors have read and agreed to the published version of the manuscript.

Funding: This research has received funding from the European Union's Horizon 2020 research and innovation programme under the Marie Skłodowska-Curie grant agreement PANDORA No 671881 (Probing safety of nano-objects by defining immune responses of environmental organisms).

Informed Consent Statement: Not applicable.

Data Availability Statement: Not applicable.

Conflicts of Interest: The authors declare no conflict of interest. The funders had no role in the study design; in the collection, analyses, and interpretation of the data; in the writing of the manuscript; or in the decision to publish results.

Appendix A

Figure A1: Physiochemical characterisation of PVP-coated Au NPs and scanning electron microscopy (SEM) of dried leaves covered with PVP–Au NPs. Table A1: Details the number of animals used in the feeding experiment. Table A2: Details the number of animals used in the injection experiment.

Table A1. Details the number of animals used in the feeding experiment, the mortality rate, and the stages of the investigation. *, pooled from 4–5 animals; **, pooled from 1–3 animals.

Treatment (Feeding)		Number of Animals (Start of 2 Weeks)	Mortality	Removed (Gravid/Molting/Infected)	Feeding Activity	Haemocyte Count	Nitric Oxide *	Phenoloxidase-Like Activity **
Control	Total	50	4	5	41	28	7 (32)	13 (27)
		30	2	4	24	11		
		20	2	1	17	17	1 (5)	2 (4)
							6 (27)	
								11 (23)
Cerium NPs	Total	20	3	1	16	16	7 (32)	14 (29)
		20	3	1	16	16	2 (9)	2 (5)
							5 (23)	
								12 (24)
Gold NPs	Total	30	2	2	26	18	8 (34)	12 (20)
		30	2	2	26	18		
							8 (34)	
								12 (20)
Gold Ions	Total	30	2	0	28	19	8 (33)	11 (15)
		30	2	0	28	19		
							8 (33)	
								11 (15)

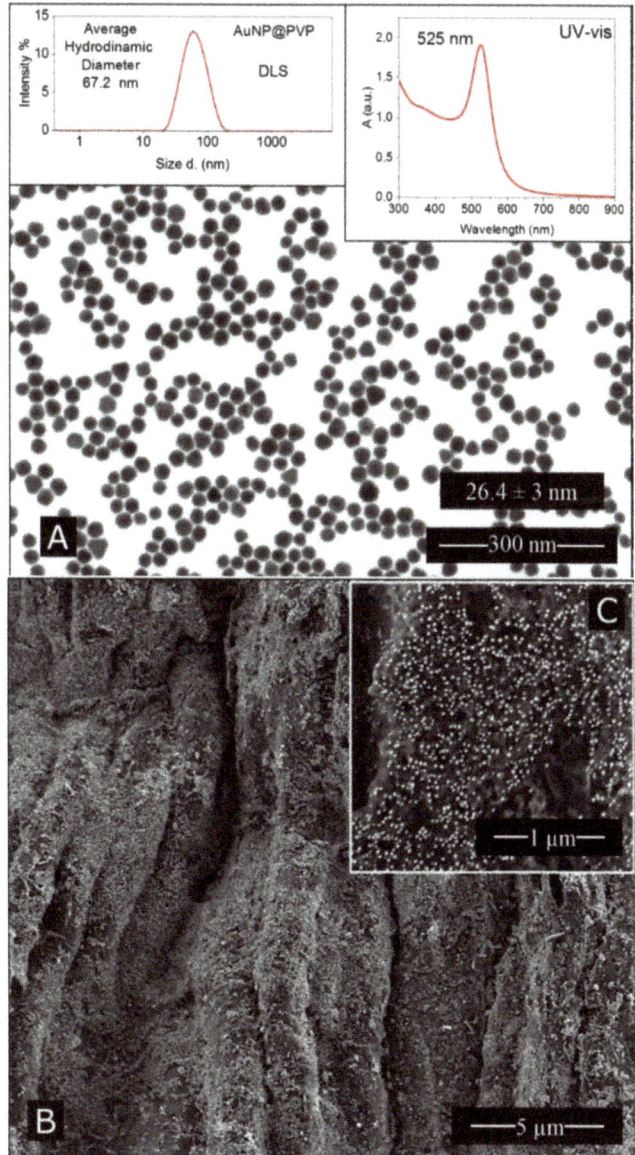

Figure A1. Polyvinylpyrrolidone coated Au NP physicochemical characterisation. (**A**) Bright field—scanning transmission electron microscopy (STEM); dynamic light scattering measurement of the Au NPs (Top left); UV–Vis spectra (Top right). (**B**,**C**) Scanning electron microscopy (SEM) of dried leaves covered with PVP Au NPs.

Table A2. Details regarding the number of animals used in the injection experiment and the stages of the investigation. *, pooled from 4–5 animals; **, pooled from 1–3 animals.

Treatment (Injected)		Biological Repeats (Number of Animals Used)		
		Haemocyte Count	Nitric Oxide *	Phenoloxidase-Like Activity **
Control	Total	22	7 (31)	23 (47)
		22		5 (8)
				6 (13)
			7 (31)	5 (13)
				4 (8)
				3 (5)
LPS	Total	22	7 (35)	23 (61)
		22		
				6 (17)
				5 (14)
			3 (15)	6 (14)
				6 (16)
			4 (20)	
Cerium NPs	Total	17	8 (38)	12 (26)
		17	2 (9)	9 (19)
			2 (10)	
			4 (19)	
				3 (7)
Gold NPs	Total	10	5 (24)	12 (22)
		10		5 (9)
			1 (5)	
			4 (19)	7 (13)

References

1. Usharauli, D.; Kamala, T. An identical mechanism governs self-nonself discrimination and effector class regulation. *PeerJ Prepr.* **2017**. [CrossRef]
2. Schultz, K.T.; Grieder, F. Structure and Function of the Immune System. *Toxicol. Pathol.* **1987**, *15*, 262–264. [CrossRef]
3. Boraschi, D.; Alijagic, A.; Auguste, M.; Barbero, F.; Ferrari, E.; Hernadi, S.; Mayall, C.; Michelini, S.; Navarro Pacheco, N.I.; Prinelli, A.; et al. Addressing Nanomaterial Immunosafety by Evaluating Innate Immunity across Living Species. *Small* **2020**, *16*, 2000598. [CrossRef]
4. Tassanakajon, A.; Rimphanitchayakit, V.; Visetnan, S.; Amparyup, P.; Somboonwiwat, K.; Charoensapsri, W.; Tang, S. Shrimp humoral responses against pathogens: antimicrobial peptides and melanization. *Dev. Comp. Immunol.* **2018**, *80*, 81–93. [CrossRef]
5. Dolar, A.; Kostanjšek, R.; Mayall, C.; Drobne, D.; Kokalj, A.J. Modulations of immune parameters caused by bacterial and viral infections in the terrestrial crustacean *Porcellio scaber*: Implications for potential markers in environmental research. *Dev. Comp. Immunol.* **2020**, *113*. [CrossRef]
6. Gopalakrishnan, S.; Chen, F.Y.; Thilagam, H.; Qiao, K.; Xu, W.F.; Wang, K.J. Modulation and interaction of immune-associated parameters with antioxidant in the immunocytes of crab *Scylla paramamosain* challenged with lipopolysaccharides. *Evidence-based Complement. Altern. Med.* **2011**, *2011*. [CrossRef]
7. Kostanjšek, R.; Pirc Marolt, T. Pathogenesis, tissue distribution and host response to *Rhabdochlamydia porcellionis* infection in rough woodlouse *Porcellio scaber*. *J. Invertebr. Pathol.* **2015**, *125*, 56–67. [CrossRef]
8. Chevalier, F.; Herbinière-Gaboreau, J.; Bertaux, J.; Raimond, M.; Morel, F.; Bouchon, D.; Grève, P.; Braquart-Varnier, C. The immune cellular effectors of terrestrial isopod *armadillidium vulgare*: Meeting with their invaders, wolbachia. *PLoS ONE* **2011**, *6*, e18531. [CrossRef] [PubMed]
9. Chevalier, F.; Herbinière-Gaboreau, J.; Charif, D.; Mitta, G.; Gavory, F.; Wincker, P.; Grève, P.; Braquart-Varnier, C.; Bouchon, D. Feminizing *Wolbachia*: A transcriptomics approach with insights on the immune response genes in *Armadillidium vulgare*. *BMC Microbiol.* **2012**, *12*, S1. [CrossRef] [PubMed]
10. Jin, X.; Li, W.; Xu, M.; Zhu, Y.; Zhou, Y.; Wang, Q. Transcriptome-wide analysis of immune responses in *Eriocheir sinensis* hemocytes after challenge with different microbial derivatives. *Dev. Comp. Immunol.* **2019**, *101*. [CrossRef] [PubMed]
11. Snyman, R.G.; Odendaal, J.P. Effect of cadmium on haemocyte viability of the woodlouse *Porcellio laevis* (Isopoda, Crustacea). *Bull. Environ. Contam. Toxicol.* **2009**, *83*, 525–529. [CrossRef] [PubMed]

12. Hornung, E. Evolutionary adaptation of oniscidean isopods to terrestrial life: Structure, physiology and behavior. *Terr. Arthropod Rev.* **2011**, *4*, 95–130. [CrossRef]
13. Moret, Y.; Moreau, J. The immune role of the arthropod exoskeleton. *Invertebr. Surviv. J.* **2012**, *9*, 200–206.
14. Mount, A.S.; Wheeler, A.P.; Paradkar, R.P.; Snider, D. Hemocyte-Mediated Shell Mineralization in the Eastern Oyster. *Science* **2004**, *304*, 297–300. [CrossRef] [PubMed]
15. Li, S.; Liu, Y.; Liu, C.; Huang, J.; Zheng, G.; Xie, L.; Zhang, R. Hemocytes participate in calcium carbonate crystal formation, transportation and shell regeneration in the pearl oyster *Pinctada fucata*. *Fish Shellfish Immunol.* **2016**, *51*, 263–270. [CrossRef] [PubMed]
16. de Freitas Rebelo, M.; de Souza Figueiredo, E.; Mariante, R.M.; Nóbrega, A.; de Barros, C.M.; Allodi, S. New Insights from the Oyster *Crassostrea rhizophorae* on Bivalve Circulating Hemocytes. *PLoS ONE* **2013**, *8*, e57384. [CrossRef]
17. Da Silva, P.G.C.; De Abreu, I.S.; Cavalcante, L.A.; De Barros, C.M.; Allodi, S. Role of hemocytes in invertebrate adult neurogenesis and brain repair. *Invertebr. Surviv. J.* **2015**, *12*, 142–154.
18. Russo, J.; Bréhelin, M.; Carton, Y. Haemocyte changes in resistant and susceptible strains of *D. melanogaster* caused by virulent and avirulent strains of the parasitic wasp *Leptopilina boulardi*. *J. Insect Physiol.* **2001**, *47*, 167–172. [CrossRef]
19. Du, M.H.; Yan, Z.W.; Hao, Y.J.; Yan, Z.T.; Si, F.L.; Chen, B.; Qiao, L. Suppression of Laccase 2 severely impairs cuticle tanning and pathogen resistance during the pupal metamorphosis of *Anopheles sinensis* (Diptera: Culicidae). *Parasites Vectors* **2017**, *10*, 171. [CrossRef]
20. Jussila, J.; Jago, J.; Tsvetnenko, E.; Dunstan, B.; Evans, L.H. Total and differential haemocyte counts in western rock lobsters (*Panulirus cygnus* George) under post-harvest stress. *Mar. Freshw. Res.* **1997**, *48*, 863–867. [CrossRef]
21. Le Moullac, G.; Haffner, P. Environmental factors affecting immune responses in Crustacea. *Aquaculture* **2000**, *191*, 121–131. [CrossRef]
22. Qin, Q.; Qin, S.; Wang, L.; Lei, W. Immune responses and ultrastructural changes of hemocytes in freshwater crab *Sinopotamon henanense* exposed to elevated cadmium. *Aquat. Toxicol.* **2012**, *106–107*, 140–146. [CrossRef] [PubMed]
23. Cheng, W.; Chen, J.C. Effects of intrinsic and extrinsic factors on the haemocyte profile of the prawn, *Macrobrachium rosenbergii*. *Fish Shellfish Immunol.* **2001**, *11*, 53–63. [CrossRef] [PubMed]
24. Johansson, M.W.; Keyser, P.; Sritunyalucksana, K.; Söderhäll, K. Crustacean haemocytes and haematopoiesis. *Aquaculture* **2000**, *191*, 45–52. [CrossRef]
25. Alikhan, M.A.; Naich, M. Changes in counts of haemocytes and in their physicochemical properties during the moult cycle in *Porcellio spinicornis* Say (Porcellionidae, Isopoda). *Can. J. Zool.* **1987**, *65*, 1685–1688. [CrossRef]
26. Jiang, H.; Kanost, M.R. The clip-domain family of serine proteinases in arthropods. *Insect Biochem. Mol. Biol.* **2000**, *30*, 95–105. [CrossRef]
27. Stevenson, J.R.; Murphy, J.C. Mucopolysaccharide glands in the isopod crustacean *Armadillidium vulgare*. *Trans. Am. Microsc. Soc.* **1967**, *86*, 50–57. [CrossRef] [PubMed]
28. Andersen, S.O. Insect cuticular sclerotization: A review. *Insect Biochem. Mol. Biol.* **2010**, *40*, 166–178. [CrossRef]
29. Rodriguez-Andres, J.; Rani, S.; Varjak, M.; Chase-Topping, M.E.; Beck, M.H.; Ferguson, M.C.; Schnettler, E.; Fragkoudis, R.; Barry, G.; Merits, A.; et al. Phenoloxidase Activity Acts as a Mosquito Innate Immune Response against Infection with Semliki Forest Virus. *PLoS Pathog.* **2012**, *8*, e1002977. [CrossRef]
30. Solano, F. Melanins: Skin Pigments and Much More—Types, Structural Models, Biological Functions, and Formation Routes. *New J. Sci.* **2014**, *2014*, 1–28. [CrossRef]
31. Jiravanichpaisal, P.; Lee, B.L.; Söderhäll, K. Cell-mediated immunity in arthropods: Hematopoiesis, coagulation, melanization and opsonization. *Immunobiology* **2006**, *211*, 213–236. [CrossRef] [PubMed]
32. Santiago, P.B.; De Araújo, C.N.; Motta, F.N.; Praça, Y.R.; Charneau, S.; Bastos, I.M.D.; Santana, J.M. Proteases of haematophagous arthropod vectors are involved in blood-feeding, yolk formation and immunity—A review. *Parasites Vectors* **2017**, *10*, 1–20. [CrossRef] [PubMed]
33. Pan, L.; Zhang, X.; Yang, L.; Pan, S. Effects of *Vibro harveyi* and *Staphyloccocus aureus* infection on hemocyanin synthesis and innate immune responses in white shrimp *Litopenaeus vannamei*. *Fish Shellfish Immunol.* **2019**, *93*, 659–668. [CrossRef] [PubMed]
34. Jaenicke, E.; Fraune, S.; May, S.; Irmak, P.; Augustin, R.; Meesters, C.; Decker, H.; Zimmer, M. Is activated hemocyanin instead of phenoloxidase involved in immune response in woodlice? *Dev. Comp. Immunol.* **2009**, *33*, 1055–1063. [CrossRef] [PubMed]
35. Soderhall, K. Developmental and comparative immunology: Editorial. *Dev. Comp. Immunol.* **1999**, *23*, 263–266.
36. González-Santoyo, I.; Córdoba-Aguilar, A. Phenoloxidase: A key component of the insect immune system. *Entomol. Exp. Appl.* **2012**, *142*, 1–16. [CrossRef]
37. Castillo, J.C.; Robertson, A.E.; Strand, M.R. Characterization of hemocytes from the mosquitoes *Anopheles gambiae* and *Aedes aegypti*. *Insect Biochem. Mol. Biol.* **2006**, *36*, 891–903. [CrossRef]
38. Le Moullac, G.; Le Groumellec, M.; Ansquer, D.; Froissard, S.; Levy, P. Haematological and phenoloxidase activity changes in the shrimp *Penaeus stylirostris* in relation with the moult cycle: Protection against vibriosis. *Fish Shellfish Immunol.* **1997**, *7*, 227–234. [CrossRef]
39. Lai-Fook, J. The repair of wounds in the integument of insects. *J. Insect Physiol.* **1966**, *12*, 195–226. [CrossRef]
40. Nappi, A.J.; Vass, E.; Frey, F.; Carton, Y. Nitric oxide involvement in Drosophila immunity. *Nitric Oxide Biol. Chem.* **2000**, *4*, 423–430. [CrossRef]

41. Radomski, M.W.; Martin, J.F.; Moncada, S. Synthesis of nitric oxide by the haemocytes of the American horseshoe crab (*Limulus polyphemus*). *Philos. Trans. R. Soc. Lond. Ser. B Biol. Sci.* **1991**, *334*, 129–133. [CrossRef]
42. Sharma, J.N.; Al-Omran, A.; Parvathy, S.S. Role of nitric oxide in inflammatory diseases. *Inflammopharmacology* **2007**, *15*, 252–259. [CrossRef] [PubMed]
43. Jia, Z.; Wang, L.; Jiang, S.; Sun, M.; Wang, M.; Yi, Q.; Song, L. Functional characterization of hemocytes from Chinese mitten crab *Eriocheir sinensis* by flow cytometry. *Fish Shellfish Immunol.* **2017**, *69*, 15–25. [CrossRef] [PubMed]
44. Raman, T.; Arumugam, M.; Mullainadhan, P. Agglutinin-mediated phagocytosis-associated generation of superoxide anion and nitric oxide by the hemocytes of the giant freshwater prawn *Macrobrachium rosenbergii*. *Fish Shellfish Immunol.* **2008**, *24*, 337–345. [CrossRef]
45. Davidson, S.K.; Koropatnick, T.A.; Kossmehl, R.; Sycuro, L.; McFall-Ngai, M.J. NO means "yes" in the squid-vibrio symbiosis: Nitric oxide (NO) during the initial stages of a beneficial association. *Cell. Microbiol.* **2004**, *6*, 1139–1151. [CrossRef]
46. Van De Braak, C.B.T.; Botterblom, M.H.A.; Liu, W.; Taverne, N.; Van Der Knaap, W.P.W.; Rombout, J.H.W.M. The role of the haematopoietic tissue in haemocyte production and maturation in the black tiger shrimp (*Penaeus monodon*). *Fish Shellfish Immunol.* **2002**, *12*, 253–272. [CrossRef]
47. Traifalgar, R.F.M.; Corre, V.L.; Serrano, A.E. Efficacy of dietary immunostimulants to enhance the immunological responses and vibriosis resistance of juvenile *Penaeus monodon*. *J. Fish. Aquat. Sci.* **2013**, *8*, 340–354. [CrossRef]
48. Cárdenas, W.; Dankert, J.R.; Jenkins, J.A. Flow cytometric analysis of crayfish haemocytes activated by lipopolysaccharides. *Fish Shellfish Immunol.* **2004**, *17*, 223–233. [CrossRef]
49. Smith, V.J.; Brown, J.H.; Hauton, C. Immunostimulation in crustaceans: Does it really protect against infection? *Fish Shellfish Immunol.* **2003**, *15*, 71–90. [CrossRef]
50. Roach, K.A.; Anderson, S.E.; Stefaniak, A.B.; Shane, H.L.; Boyce, G.R.; Roberts, J.R. Evaluation of the skin-sensitizing potential of gold nanoparticles and the impact of established dermal sensitivity on the pulmonary immune response to various forms of gold. *Nanotoxicology* **2020**, *14*, 1096–1117. [CrossRef]
51. Suchomel, P.; Kvitek, L.; Prucek, R.; Panacek, A.; Halder, A.; Vajda, S.; Zboril, R. Simple size-controlled synthesis of Au nanoparticles and their size-dependent catalytic activity. *Sci. Rep.* **2018**, *8*, 1–11. [CrossRef]
52. Škarková, P.; Romih, T.; Kos, M.; Novak, S.; Kononenko, V.; Jemec, A.; Vávrová, M.; Drobne, D. Gold nanoparticles do not induce adverse effects on terrestrial isopods *Porcellio scaber* after 14-day exposure Nanodelci zlata nimajo negativnih učinkov na kopenske rake vrste *Porcellio scaber* po 14-dnevni izpostavitvi. *Acta Biol. Slov.* **2016**, *59*, 2016.
53. Bourdineaud, J.P.; Štambuk, A.; Šrut, M.; Radić Brkanac, S.; Ivanković, D.; Lisjak, D.; Sauerborn Klobučar, R.; Dragun, Z.; Bačić, N.; Klobučar, G.I.V. Gold and silver nanoparticles effects to the earthworm Eisenia fetida –the importance of tissue over soil concentrations. *Drug Chem. Toxicol.* **2021**, *44*, 12–29. [CrossRef] [PubMed]
54. Hornos Carneiro, M.F.; Barbosa, F. Gold nanoparticles: A critical review of therapeutic applications and toxicological aspects. *J. Toxicol. Environ. Heal. Part B Crit. Rev.* **2016**, *19*, 129–148. [CrossRef] [PubMed]
55. Bednarski, M.; Dudek, M.; Knutelska, J.; Nowiński, L.; Sapa, J.; Zygmunt, M.; Nowak, G.; Luty-Błocho, M.; Wojnicki, M.; Fitzner, K.; et al. The influence of the route of administration of gold nanoparticles on their tissue distribution and basic biochemical parameters: *In vivo* studies. *Pharmacol. Rep.* **2015**, *67*, 405–409. [CrossRef] [PubMed]
56. Paula, M.M.S.; Petronilho, F.; Vuolo, F.; Ferreira, G.K.; De Costa, L.; Santos, G.P.; Effting, P.S.; Dal-Pizzol, F.; Dal-Bō, A.G.; Frizon, T.E.; et al. Gold nanoparticles and/or N-acetylcysteine mediate carrageenan-induced inflammation and oxidative stress in a concentration-dependent manner. *J. Biomed. Mater. Res. Part A* **2015**, *103*, 3323–3330. [CrossRef]
57. Jia, H.; Chen, H.; Wei, M.; Chen, X.; Zhang, Y.; Cao, L.; Yuan, P.; Wang, F.; Yang, G.; Ma, J. Gold nanoparticle-based miR155 antagonist macrophage delivery restores the cardiac function in ovariectomized diabetic mouse model. *Int. J. Nanomed.* **2017**, *12*, 4963–4979. [CrossRef]
58. Sendra, M.; Blasco, J.; Araújo, C.V.M. Is the cell wall of marine phytoplankton a protective barrier or a nanoparticle interaction site? Toxicological responses of *Chlorella autotrophica* and *Dunaliella salina* to Ag and CeO2 nanoparticles. *Ecol. Indic.* **2018**, *95*, 1053–1067. [CrossRef]
59. Malev, O.; Trebše, P.; Piecha, M.; Novak, S.; Budič, B.; Dramićanin, M.D.; Drobne, D. Effects of CeO2 Nanoparticles on Terrestrial Isopod *Porcellio scaber*: Comparison of CeO2 Biological Potential with Other Nanoparticles. *Arch. Environ. Contam. Toxicol.* **2017**, *72*, 303–311. [CrossRef]
60. Nemmar, A.; Yuvaraju, P.; Beegam, S.; Fahim, M.A.; Ali, B.H. Cerium Oxide Nanoparticles in Lung Acutely Induce Oxidative Stress, Inflammation, and DNA Damage in Various Organs of Mice. *Oxid. Med. Cell. Longev.* **2017**, *2017*. [CrossRef]
61. Karakoti, A.S.; Munusamy, P.; Hostetler, K.; Kodali, V.; Kuchibhatla, S.; Orr, G.; Pounds, J.G.; Teeguarden, J.G.; Thrall, B.D.; Baer, D.R. Preparation and characterization challenges to understanding environmental and biological impacts of ceria nanoparticles. *Surf. Interface Anal.* **2012**, *44*, 882–889. [CrossRef] [PubMed]
62. Karakoti, A.S.; Monteiro-Riviere, N.A.; Aggarwal, R.; Davis, J.P.; Narayan, R.J.; Seif, W.T.; McGinnis, J.; Seal, S. Nanoceria as antioxidant: Synthesis and biomedical applications. *JOM* **2008**, *60*, 33–37. [CrossRef] [PubMed]
63. Hauton, C.; Hudspith, M.; Gunton, L. Future prospects for prophylactic immune stimulation in crustacean aquaculture - the need for improved metadata to address immune system complexity. *Dev. Comp. Immunol.* **2015**, *48*, 360–368. [CrossRef] [PubMed]
64. Bastús, N.G.; Comenge, J.; Puntes, V. Kinetically controlled seeded growth synthesis of citrate-stabilized gold nanoparticles of up to 200 nm: Size focusing versus ostwald ripening. *Langmuir* **2011**, *27*, 11098–11105. [CrossRef]

65. Alijagic, A.; Barbero, F.; Gaglio, D.; Napodano, E.; Benada, O.; Kofroňová, O.; Puntes, V.F.; Bastús, N.G.; Pinsino, A. Gold nanoparticles coated with polyvinylpyrrolidone and sea urchin extracellular molecules induce transient immune activation. *J. Hazard. Mater.* **2021**, *402*, 123793. [CrossRef]
66. Kos, M.; Jemec Kokalj, A.; Glavan, G.; Marolt, G.; Zidar, P.; Božič, J.; Novak, S.; Drobne, D. Cerium(IV) oxide nanoparticles induce sublethal changes in honeybees after chronic exposure. *Environ. Sci. Nano* **2017**, *4*, 2297–2310. [CrossRef]
67. Jemec Kokalj, A.; Horvat, P.; Skalar, T.; Kržan, A. Plastic bag and facial cleanser derived microplastic do not affect feeding behaviour and energy reserves of terrestrial isopods. *Sci. Total Environ.* **2018**, *615*, 761–766. [CrossRef]
68. Praetorius, A.; Gundlach-Graham, A.; Goldberg, E.; Fabienke, W.; Navratilova, J.; Gondikas, A.; Kaegi, R.; Günther, D.; Hofmann, T.; Von Der Kammer, F. Single-particle multi-element fingerprinting (spMEF) using inductively-coupled plasma time-of-flight mass spectrometry (ICP-TOFMS) to identify engineered nanoparticles against the elevated natural background in soils. *Environ. Sci. Nano* **2017**, *4*, 307–314. [CrossRef]
69. Mahapatra, I.; Sun, T.Y.; Clark, J.R.A.; Dobson, P.J.; Hungerbuehler, K.; Owen, R.; Nowack, B.; Lead, J. Probabilistic modelling of prospective environmental concentrations of gold nanoparticles from medical applications as a basis for risk assessment. *J. Nanobiotechnology* **2015**, *13*, 93. [CrossRef]
70. Keller, A.A.; Lazareva, A. Predicted Releases of Engineered Nanomaterials: From Global to Regional to Local. *Environ. Sci. Technol. Lett.* **2013**, *1*, 65–70. [CrossRef]
71. Sun, T.Y.; Bornhöft, N.A.; Hungerbühler, K.; Nowack, B. Dynamic Probabilistic Modeling of Environmental Emissions of Engineered Nanomaterials. *Environ. Sci. Technol.* **2016**, *50*, 4701–4711. [CrossRef]
72. Faraldo, A.C.; Sá-Nunes, A.; Del Bel, E.A.; Faccioli, L.H.; Lello, E. Nitric oxide production in blowfly hemolymph after yeast inoculation. *Nitric Oxide Biol. Chem.* **2005**, *13*, 240–246. [CrossRef] [PubMed]
73. Charles, H.M.; Killian, K.A. Response of the insect immune system to three different immune challenges. *J. Insect Physiol.* **2015**, *81*, 97–108. [CrossRef] [PubMed]
74. Setyawan, A.; Isnansetyo, A.; Murwantoko; Indarjulianto, S.; Handayani, C.R. Comparative immune response of dietary fucoidan from three indonesian brown algae in white shrimp *Litopenaeus vannamei*. *AACL Bioflux* **2018**, *11*, 1707–1723.
75. Contreras-Garduño, J.; Lanz-Mendoza, H.; Córdoba-Aguilar, A. The expression of a sexually selected trait correlates with different immune defense components and survival in males of the American rubyspot. *J. Insect Physiol.* **2007**, *53*, 612–621. [CrossRef]
76. Stewart, J.E.; Cornick, J.W.; Dingle, J.R. An electronic method for counting lobster (*Homarus americanus* Milne-Edwards) hemocytes and the influence of diet on hemocyte numbers and hemolymph proteins. *Can. J. Zool.* **1967**, *45*, 291–304. [CrossRef]
77. Pascual, C.; Zenteno, E.; Cuzon, G.; Sánchez, A.; Gaxiola, G.; Taboada, G.; Suárez, J.; Maldonado, T.; Rosas, C. *Litopenaeus vannamei* juveniles energetic balance and immunological response to dietary protein. *Aquaculture* **2004**, *236*, 431–450. [CrossRef]
78. Rosenberger, C.R.; Jones, J.C. Studies on Total Blood Cell Counts of the Southern Armyworm Larva, *Prodenia Eridania* (Lepidoptera). *Ann. Entomol. Soc. Am.* **1960**, *53*, 351–355. [CrossRef]
79. Shapiro, M. Pathologic changes in the blood of the greater wax moth, *Galleria mellonella*, during the course of nucleopolyhedrosis and starvation. I. Total hemocyte count. *J. Invertebr. Pathol.* **1967**, *9*, 111–113. [CrossRef]
80. Matozzo, V.; Gallo, C.; Marin, M.G. Can starvation influence cellular and biochemical parameters in the crab *Carcinus aestuarii*? *Mar. Environ. Res.* **2011**, *71*, 207–212. [CrossRef] [PubMed]
81. Sequeira, T.; Tavares, D.; Arala-Chaves, M. Evidence for circulating hemocyte proliferation in the shrimp *Penaeus japonicus*. *Dev. Comp. Immunol.* **1996**, *20*, 97–104. [CrossRef]
82. Muralisankar, T.; Bhavan, P.S.; Radhakrishnan, S.; Seenivasan, C.; Manickam, N.; Srinivasan, V. Dietary supplementation of zinc nanoparticles and its influence on biology, physiology and immune responses of the freshwater prawn, *Macrobrachium rosenbergii*. *Biol. Trace Elem. Res.* **2014**, *160*, 56–66. [CrossRef] [PubMed]
83. Durstewitz, G.; Terwilliger, N.B. Developmental changes in hemocyanin expression in the dungeness crab, *Cancer magister*. *J. Biol. Chem.* **1997**, *272*, 4347–4350. [CrossRef] [PubMed]
84. Hall, M.; Wang, R.; Van Antwerpen, R.; Sottrup-Jensen, L.; Söderhäll, K. The crayfish plasma clotting protein: A vitellogenin-related protein responsible for clot formation in crustacean blood. *Proc. Natl. Acad. Sci. USA* **1999**, *96*, 1965–1970. [CrossRef]
85. Nel, A.E.; Mädler, L.; Velegol, D.; Xia, T.; Hoek, E.M.V.; Somasundaran, P.; Klaessig, F.; Castranova, V.; Thompson, M. Understanding biophysicochemical interactions at the nano-bio interface. *Nat. Mater.* **2009**, *8*, 543–557. [CrossRef] [PubMed]
86. Westman, J.; Grinstein, S.; Marques, P.E. Phagocytosis of Necrotic Debris at Sites of Injury and Inflammation. *Front. Immunol.* **2020**, *10*, 3030. [CrossRef]
87. Parle, E.; Dirks, J.H.; Taylor, D. Damage, repair and regeneration in insect cuticle: The story so far, and possibilities for the future. *Arthropod Struct. Dev.* **2017**, *46*, 49–55. [CrossRef]
88. Tümer, C.; Bilgin, H.M.; Obay, B.D.; Diken, H.; Atmaca, M.; Kelle, M. Effect of nitric oxide on phagocytic activity of lipopolysaccharide-induced macrophages: Possible role of exogenous l-arginine. *Cell Biol. Int.* **2007**, *31*, 565–569. [CrossRef]
89. Giese, B.; Klaessig, F.; Park, B.; Kaegi, R.; Steinfeldt, M.; Wigger, H.; Von Gleich, A.; Gottschalk, F. Risks, Release and Concentrations of Engineered Nanomaterial in the Environment. *Sci. Rep.* **2018**, *8*, 1–18. [CrossRef]
90. Victor, B.; Narayanan, M.; Nelson, D.J. Gill pathology and hemocyte response in mercury exposed *Macrobrachium idae heller*. *J. Environ. Biol.* **1990**, *11*, 61–66.
91. Johnson, N.G.; Burnett, L.E.; Burnett, K.G. Properties of bacteria that trigger hemocytopenia in the Atlantic Blue Crab, *Callinectes sapidus*. *Biol. Bull.* **2011**, *221*, 164–175. [CrossRef] [PubMed]

92. Matozzo, V.; Gallo, C.; Marin, M.G. Effects of temperature on cellular and biochemical parameters in the crab *Carcinus aestuarii* (Crustacea, Decapoda). *Mar. Environ. Res.* **2011**, *71*, 351–356. [CrossRef] [PubMed]
93. Burnett, L.E.; Holman, J.D.; Jorgensen, D.D.; Ikerd, J.L.; Burnett, K.G. Immune defense reduces respiratory fitness in *Callinectes sapidus*, the Atlantic blue crab. *Biol. Bull.* **2006**, *211*, 50–57. [CrossRef]
94. Truscott, R.; White, K.N. The Influence of Metal and Temperature Stress on the Immune System of Crabs. *Funct. Ecol.* **1990**, *4*, 455. [CrossRef]
95. Singaram, G.; Harikrishnan, T.; Chen, F.Y.; Bo, J.; Giesy, J.P. Modulation of immune-associated parameters and antioxidant responses in the crab (*Scylla serrata*) exposed to mercury. *Chemosphere* **2013**, *90*, 917–928. [CrossRef] [PubMed]
96. Hauton, C.; Hawkins, L.E.; Williams, J.A. In situ variability in phenoloxidase activity in the shore crab, *Carcinus maenas* (L.). *Comp. Biochem. Physiol. B Biochem. Mol. Biol.* **1997**, *117*, 267–271. [CrossRef]
97. Raduolovic, K.; Mak'Anyengo, R.; Kaya, B.; Steinert, A.; Niess, J.H. Injections of lipopolysaccharide into mice to mimic entrance of microbial-derived products after intestinal barrier breach. *J. Vis. Exp.* **2018**, *2018*, 57610. [CrossRef]
98. Goarant, C.; Boglio, E. Changes in Hemocyte Counts in *Litopenaeus stylirostris* Subjected to Sublethal Infection and to Vaccination. *J. World Aquac. Soc.* **2000**, *31*, 123–129. [CrossRef]
99. Lorenzon, S.; de Guarrini, S.; Smith, V.J.; Ferrero, E.A. Effects of LPS injection on circulating haemocytes in crustaceansin vivo. *Fish Shellfish Immunol.* **1999**, *9*, 31–50. [CrossRef]
100. Chiaramonte, M.; Inguglia, L.; Vazzana, M.; Deidun, A.; Arizza, V. Stress and immune response to bacterial LPS in the sea urchin *Paracentrous lividus* (Lamarck, 1816). *Fish Shellfish Immunol.* **2019**, *92*, 384–394. [CrossRef]
101. Xu, H.-S.; Lyu, S.-J.; Xu, J.-H.; Lu, B.-J.; Zhao, J.; Li, S.; Li, Y.-Q.; Chen, Y.-Y. Effect of lipopolysaccharide on the hemocyte apoptosis of *Eriocheir sinensis*. *J. Zhejiang Univ. Sci. B* **2015**, *16*, 971–979. [CrossRef]
102. Yeh, F.C.; Wu, S.H.; Lai, C.Y.; Lee, C.Y. Demonstration of nitric oxide synthase activity in crustacean hemocytes and anti-microbial activity of hemocyte-derived nitric oxide. *Comp. Biochem. Physiol. B Biochem. Mol. Biol.* **2006**, *144*, 11–17. [CrossRef] [PubMed]
103. Salawu, M.O.; Oloyede, H.O.B.; Oladiji, T.A.; Yakubu, M.T.; Amuzat, A.O. Hemolymph coagulation and phenoloxidase activity in *Uca tangeri* induced by *Escherichia coli* endotoxin. *J. Immunotoxicol.* **2016**, *13*, 355–363. [CrossRef] [PubMed]
104. Yoon, K.W. Dead cell phagocytosis and innate immune checkpoint. *BMB Rep.* **2017**, *50*, 496–503. [CrossRef]
105. Hammond, J.A.; Smith, V.J. Lipopolysaccharide induces DNA-synthesis in a sub-population of hemocytes from the swimming crab, *Liocarcinus depurator*. *Dev. Comp. Immunol.* **2002**, *26*, 227–236. [CrossRef]
106. Smith, V.J.; Swindlehurst, R.J.; Johnston, P.A.; Vethaak, A.D. Disturbance of host defence capability in the common shrimp, *Crangon crangon*, by exposure to harbour dredge spoils. *Aquat. Toxicol.* **1995**, *32*, 43–58. [CrossRef]
107. Le Moullac, G.; Soyez, C.; Saulnier, D.; Ansquer, D.; Avarre, J.C.; Levy, P. Effect of hypoxic stress on the immune response and the resistance to vibriosis of the shrimp *Penaeus stylirostris*. *Fish Shellfish Immunol.* **1998**, *8*, 621–629. [CrossRef]
108. Tello-Olea, M.; Rosales-Mendoza, S.; Campa-Córdova, A.I.; Palestino, G.; Luna-González, A.; Reyes-Becerril, M.; Velazquez, E.; Hernandez-Adame, L.; Angulo, C. Gold nanoparticles (AuNP) exert immunostimulatory and protective effects in shrimp (*Litopenaeus vannamei*) against *Vibrio parahaemolyticus*. *Fish Shellfish Immunol.* **2019**, *84*, 756–767. [CrossRef]

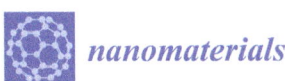

Article

Functional and Morphological Changes Induced in *Mytilus* Hemocytes by Selected Nanoparticles

Manon Auguste [1,*], Craig Mayall [2], Francesco Barbero [3], Matej Hočevar [4], Stefano Alberti [5], Giacomo Grassi [6], Victor F. Puntes [3], Damjana Drobne [2] and Laura Canesi [1]

1. Department of Environmental, Earth, and Life Sciences (DISTAV), University of Genoa, 16136 Genoa, Italy; Laura.Canesi@unige.it
2. Biotechnical Faculty, University of Ljubljana, 1000 Ljubljana, Slovenia; craig_mayall@hotmail.co.uk (C.M.); Damjana.Drobne@bf.uni-lj.si (D.D.)
3. Institut Català de Nanociència i Nanotecnologia (ICN2), CSIC and The Barcelona Institute of Science and Technology (BIST), Campus UAB, Bellaterra, 08193 Barcelona, Spain; fra.barbero@gmail.com (F.B.); victor.puntes@icn2.cat (V.F.P.)
4. Institute of Metals and Technology (IMT), 1000 Ljubljana, Slovenia; matej.hocevar@imt.si
5. Department of Chemistry and Industrial Chemistry, University of Genoa, 16136 Genoa, Italy; stefano.alberti@edu.unige.it
6. Department of Physical, Earth, and Environmental Sciences, University of Siena, 53100 Siena, Italy; giacomograssi6@gmail.com
* Correspondence: manon.auguste@edu.unige.it

Citation: Auguste, M.; Mayall, C.; Barbero, F.; Hočevar, M.; Alberti, S.; Grassi, G.; Puntes, V.F.; Drobne, D.; Canesi, L. Functional and Morphological Changes Induced in *Mytilus* Hemocytes by Selected Nanoparticles. *Nanomaterials* **2021**, *11*, 470. https://doi.org/10.3390/nano11020470

Academic Editor: Diana Boraschi
Received: 18 December 2020
Accepted: 9 February 2021
Published: 12 February 2021

Publisher's Note: MDPI stays neutral with regard to jurisdictional claims in published maps and institutional affiliations.

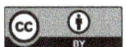

Copyright: © 2021 by the authors. Licensee MDPI, Basel, Switzerland. This article is an open access article distributed under the terms and conditions of the Creative Commons Attribution (CC BY) license (https://creativecommons.org/licenses/by/4.0/).

Abstract: Nanoparticles (NPs) show various properties depending on their composition, size, and surface coating, which shape their interactions with biological systems. In particular, NPs have been shown to interact with immune cells, that represent a sensitive surveillance system of external and internal stimuli. In this light, in vitro models represent useful tools for investigating nano-bio-interactions in immune cells of different organisms, including invertebrates. In this work, the effects of selected types of NPs with different core composition, size and functionalization (custom-made PVP-AuNP and commercial nanopolystyrenes PS-NH$_2$ and PS-COOH) were investigated in the hemocytes of the marine bivalve *Mytilus galloprovincialis*. The role of exposure medium was evaluated using either artificial seawater (ASW) or hemolymph serum (HS). Hemocyte morphology was investigated by scanning electron microscopy (SEM) and different functional parameters (lysosomal membrane stability, phagocytosis, and lysozyme release) were evaluated. The results show distinct morphological and functional changes induced in mussel hemocytes depending on the NP type and exposure medium. Mussel hemocytes may represent a powerful alternative in vitro model for a rapid pre-screening strategy for NPs, whose utilization will contribute to the understanding of the possible impact of environmental exposure to NPs in marine invertebrates.

Keywords: hemocytes; *Mytilus*; in vitro; scanning electron microscopy; immune response

1. Introduction

Due to the rapid expansion of production and use of nanoparticles (NPs) and their consequent release in different ecosystems, there is increasing concern on the utilization of alternative, affordable biological animal models for investigating nanosafety in environmental species. In vitro testing that focuses on specific cellular functions (i.e., immune responses) may provide an ideal starting point for developing a rapid prescreening strategy for NPs [1]. This would apply not only to vertebrate models, but also to invertebrates, which account for over 95% of animal species.

In the aquatic environment, which represents the final sink for all anthropogenic contaminants, including NPs, suspension-feeding invertebrates, due to their filtration ability for nutrition and respiration needs, have been identified as an unique target group for NP ecotoxicity [2–5]. In particular, in bivalve molluscs, abundant cell types involved in digestion or immune responses (digestive cells and hemocytes, respectively), have the capacity to internalize particles from the nano- to the micro-size via endocytic/phagocytic pathways [4–6].

The bivalve immune system relies solely on innate immunity, which mainly involves circulating hemocytes acting in collaboration with other soluble factors present in hemolymph serum [7,8]. This system responds very fast upon its encounter with foreign particles, making it a suitable tool for studying the effects of NPs using in vitro methods [9–13]. In particular, in the hemocytes of the marine mussel *Mytilus galloprovincialis*, the utilization of a battery of immune-related biomarkers has proven useful in the evaluation of the effects of a number of NPs, that can modulate responses with consequent immunotoxic effects or stimulation of immune parameters, leading to inflammation, depending on the NP type and on the conditions of exposure [12,14]. These studies underlined how mussel hemocytes represent a sensitive target for different NPs and their potential application as a starting point to more accurately design further studies that are relevant at the whole animal level.

The utilization of primary cells or cell lines is already established for vertebrates but these existing protocols need to be adapted and/or improved for bivalve in vitro assays [1,15,16]. Hemocytes freshly isolated from adult mussels (*M. galloprovincialis*) can be maintained in different media (artificial seawater, salt-enriched culture medium or hemolymph serum) for some hours, without impacting cell survival and biochemical/functional features [9,12,17,18]. All these media, characterized by a high ionic strength, will however affect NP behavior in terms of agglomeration and surface charge [19] as in the natural marine environment. Moreover, the behavior of NPs in mussel biological fluids (i.e., hemolymph serum) has been shown to be distinct for different types of NPs and important in determining interactions with hemocytes. In mussels, some types of NPs have been shown to associate with serum soluble components, organized into a "hard protein corona", providing a specific biological identity for immune recognition and subsequent cellular responses [20,21]. All these factors are important to consider in the evaluation of the possible biological impact of NPs on the cells of marine invertebrates, to properly utilize these cellular in vitro models as a suitable alternative strategy for testing the immunosafety of NPs in environmental organisms.

In the present study, we investigated the in vitro responses of mussel hemocytes to different types of NPs in different exposure media with the aim of:

(a) investigating the sensitivity of hemocytes to NPs with different surface characteristics and which characteristic of NPs are most potent to provoke the hemocyte response in physiological medium;
(b) defining optimal experimental conditions for a sensitive, alternative, and affordable biological in vitro model for a rapid prescreening strategy for NPs.

Selected NPs were chosen on the basis of two criteria: first, the need to utilize a reference NP that is generally considered biologically inert as in mammalian model systems (i.e., AuNPs) [22,23]. To this aim, custom-made polyvinylpyrrolidone-PVP coated gold NPs (PVP-AuNPs), were designed to be stable in seawater medium and provide baseline information for further NPs testing. Second, the utilization of commercially available surface-modified NPs that could be utilized as model NPs of environmental interests (e.g., nanoplastics). Commercial surface modified polystyrene nanoplastics (amino- and carboxy-modified nanopolystyrene, PS-NH$_2$ and PS-COOH) were utilized to provide an estimate of the role of different surface characteristics in hemocyte nano-bio-interactions.

The short-term in vitro effects of these selected NPs at different concentrations were compared in freshly isolated hemocytes from *M. galloprovincialis* exposed in either artificial seawater (ASW) or filtered hemolymph serum (HS). Upon exposure, the morphological changes induced in different experimental conditions were investigated by scanning electron microscopy (SEM). Complementary experiments were performed to measure different functional immune markers, from functional integrity of lysosomes (lysosomal membrane stability) and phagocytic ability to extracellular defense mechanisms (e.g., lysozyme release and the production of ROS-reactive oxygen species).

2. Materials and Methods

2.1. Nanoparticle Synthesis and Characterization

Custom-made PVP-AuNPs were synthesized by the Catalan Institute of Nanoscience and Nanotechnology (ICN2) (Barcelona, Spain), according to the previously reported seeded-growth methods. Detailed synthetic procedure can be found in Bastús et al. (2011) [24]. Tetrachloroauric (III) acid trihydrate (99.9% purity), sodium citrate tribasic dihydrate (≥99%), and polyvinylpyrrolidone (55 KDa) were purchased from Sigma-Aldrich (Madrid, Spain). Artificial seawater (ASW) was prepared at 35 ppt salinity, pH 7.9–8.1 [25,26]. In brief, AuNPs were synthesized using a sodium citrate aqueous solution, and different synthesis, postproduction, and characterization steps are reported in more detail in Figure S1. The AuNP seeds (~10 nm) were grown to obtain the desired size (~30 nm) and measured by scanning electron microscopy in transmission mode (STEM) (FEI Magellan 400 XHR, Hillsboro, OR, USA) (Figure S1A,B). AuNPs were further coated with PVP, followed by several washing steps. UV-vis analyses using a Carry 4000 spectrophotometer (Agilent, Santa Clara, CA, USA) were performed to verify the AuNP aggregation state and sample concentration (Figure S1C). The final hydrodynamic diameter (Figure S1D) and ζ-potential were determined by dynamic light scattering (DLS) and laser Doppler velocimetry using a Zetasizer Nano ZS instrument (Malvern Panalytical, Malvern, UK).

Commercial surface-modified nanopolystyrenes were from Bangs Laboratories, Inc. (Fishers, IN, USA). Amino-modified nanopolystyrene (PS-NH$_2$), nominal size 50 nm, were previously characterized in different media (milliQ-MQ water, ASW, and HS) as described in Canesi et al. (2015, 2016) [11,12]. Carboxylated nanopolystyrene (PS-COOH), nominal size 60 nm, kindly provided by Ilaria Corsi's lab (Univ. Siena, It), were from the same batch previously characterized in MQ water by DLS analysis [27]. In addition, in the present study, particle behavior was evaluated in suspensions of both ASW and *Mytilus* hemolymph serum (HS). The results on particle characterization are summarized in Table 1.

Table 1. Physicochemical characterization of NPs tested in vitro, PVP-AuNP, nanopolystyrenes (PS-NH$_2$ and PS-COOH) behavior in exposure medium.

NPs	Medium	Z-Average (nm)	PDI	ζ-Potential (mV)
PVP-AuNP	ASW	58.3 ± 0.16	0.12 ± 0.01	−4.1 ± 0.6
PS-NH$_2$	MQ [1]	57 ± 2	0.07 ± 0.02	+42.8 ± 1
	ASW [1]	200 ± 6	0.3 ± 0.02	+14.2 ± 2
	HS [2]	178 ± 2	0.34 ± 0.05	+14.2 ± 1
PS-COOH	MQ [3]	64.5 ± 0.6	0.06 ± 0.02	−59.7 ± 2.6
	ASW	1822 ± 373.6	0.228	−26.9 ± 1.9
	HS	189.1 ± 48.6	0.288	−11.6 ± 1.5

PDI = polydispersity index; ζ = zeta potential; MQ = MilliQ water; ASW= artificial seawater; HS = *Mytilus* hemolymph serum; [1] from [11]; [2] from [12]; [3] from [27].

Possible contamination of NPs by lipopolysaccharides (LPS) was not of first concern, as mussels have shown to be resistant to LPS effects, due to their filtering ability and vicinity with human activities. In particular, mussel hemocytes in vitro show no sensitivity to LPS up to 10 μg/mL [28]. These concentrations are much higher than those of NP-associated LPS [29,30].

2.2. Mussels, Hemolymph Collection, Preparation of Hemolymph Serum and Hemocyte Monolayers and Exposure Conditions

Mussels (*Mytilus galloprovincialis* Lam.) were purchased from an aquaculture farm (Chioggia, IT), transferred to the laboratory, and acclimatized in static tanks containing aerated ASW (1 L/animal), 35 ppt, at $16 \pm 1\ °C$ for 24 h. For each sample, hemolymph was extracted from the adductor muscle of 4–5 animals, using a syringe via a noninvasive method, filtered with gauze, and pooled in Falcon tubes. To obtain hemolymph serum-HS (i.e., hemolymph free of cells), whole hemolymph was centrifuged at $900 \times g$ for 10 min, and the supernatant was passed through a 0.22 µm filter. All procedures were performed as previously described [11,12].

Hemocytes were incubated at 16 °C with different concentrations of NPs in ASW or HS, for 30 min to 1 h (depending on the functional parameter measured) as previously described [9–11,13]. Untreated (control in ASW or HS) hemocyte samples were run in parallel. The in vitro short-term exposure of mussel hemocytes has long been successfully applied to screen the effects of different types of NPs on immune function (see [9–11,13]). The underlying reason is that in these cells, induction of functional responses, as well as of stress responses and apoptotic processes, are particularly rapid, occurring within 1 h of exposure, in line with the physiological role of bivalve hemocytes as the first line of defense against non-self-material (see also [4]).

2.3. Hemocyte Morphology Using Scanning Electron Microscopy (SEM)

Hemocyte monolayers prepared on membrane filters (hydrophilic mixed cellulose esters membrane, Millipore©) of 3 µm pore size were incubated for 30 min with NP suspensions in ASW or HS. Control cells were run in parallel in ASW or HS medium. Cells were fixed for 2 h in 2.5% glutaraldehyde, 0.4% paraformaldehyde in modified PBS (100 mM phosphate-buffered saline adjusted to 450 mM osmolarity by addition of NaCl). Fixed cells were rinsed with the same buffer, postfixed in 1% osmium tetroxide in buffer for 1 h, and then stained with TOTO (thiocarbohydrazide/osmiumtetroxide/thiocarbohydrazide/osmiumtetroxide) conductive stain (adapted from [31,32]). Samples were then dehydrated by graded ethanol solutions and dried with hexamethyldisilizane (HMDS).

The dried samples were mounted on aluminum holders and sputter-coated with gold/palladium using precision etching coating system (Gatan 682, Pleasanton, CA, USA). Hemocytes were then examined with a field emission scanning electron microscope (SEM) (SEM, JEOL JSM-6500F, Tokyo, Japan) equipped with an energy dispersive X-ray spectroscopy (EDX) system. Samples exposed to AuNPs were sputter-coated with carbon in order to detect Au by EDX.

2.4. Hemocyte Functional Assays

Hemocyte functional parameters (lysosomal membrane stability, phagocytosis, lysosomal enzyme release, and extracellular ROS production) were evaluated essentially as previously described [9,11,13].

Lysosomal membrane stability (LMS) was evaluated by the NRR (neutral-red retention time) assay. Hemocyte monolayers (in triplicates) on glass slides were incubated with NP suspensions in filtered ASW or HS for 30 min and then incubated with a neutral-red (NR) solution (final concentration 40 µg/mL). Controls (unexposed samples) were run in parallel. The slides were examined under an optical microscope every 15 min until 50% of the cells showed sign of lysosomal leaking and the results are reported as percentage of control cells.

The percentage of phagocytic cell was evaluated by the uptake of neutral-red-stained zymosan on hemocyte monolayers. After 30 min of NP exposure, the neutral-red-stained zymosan in 0.05 M TrisHCl buffer (TBS) was added to the monolayers and left to incubate for 60 min. Monolayers were then washed three times with ASW, fixed with Baker's formol calcium, and mounted in Kaiser's glycerol gelatine medium for microscopical examination with an optical microscope. For each slide, the percentage of phagocytic hemocytes was calculated from a minimum of 200 cells in triplicates.

Extracellular ROS production was measured by the reduction of cytochrome c. The aliquots of hemolymph (in triplicates) were incubated with 500 µL of cytochrome c solution (75 mM ferricytochrome c in TBS buffer) in presence or not of NPs. The samples were read at 550 nm at different times (0, 30, and 60 min), and the results are expressed as changes in OD per mg of protein.

Lysozyme activity in the extracellular medium was measured in aliquots of serum. Whole hemolymph samples were incubated with or without NPs for 30 to 60 min. Lysozyme activity was determined spectrophotometrically at 450 nm utilizing *Micrococcus lysodeikticus* and was expressed as percentage of controls.

Total protein content was determined according to the Bradford method using bovine serum albumin (BSA) as a standard.

2.5. Statistics

Data are the mean ± SD of four independent experiments (n = 4), with each assay performed in triplicate. Data of functional parameters and hemocyte diameters were analyzed by one-way ANOVA followed by Tukey's test at 95% confidence intervals ($p \leq 0.05$). All statistical calculations were performed using the GraphPad Prism version 7.03 for Windows, GraphPad Software, San Diego, CA, USA.

3. Results

3.1. NP Characterization

Data on NP characteristics and behavior in exposure media are reported in Table 1.

Custom-made PVP-coated gold nanoparticles (PVP-AuNPs) in ASW were characterized by STEM to measure the size of the gold core and by DLS to obtain the hydrodynamic diameter. AuNPs had a gold core of 28.7 ± 3.2 nm (Figure S1B) and a PVP (55 KDa) coating leading to a final hydrodynamic diameter of 58.3 ± 0.16 nm (Figure S1D). PVP-AuNPs ζ-potential in ASW was −4.1 ± 0.6 mV.

For both nanopolystyrenes, in MQ the Z-average were in the same range as reported by the manufacturer, 57 ± 2 and 64.5 ± 0.6 nm for PS-NH$_2$ and PS-COOH, respectively. The ζ-potential was positive (+42.8 ± 1 mV) for PS-NH$_2$ and negative (−59.7 ± 2.6 mV) for PS-COOH [11,27]. In both ASW and HS, PS-NH$_2$ showed a similar behavior, with formation of small agglomerates (~200 nm) and a lower ζ-potential (+14 mV) [11,12]. A distinct behavior was observed for PS-COOH, that in ASW formed large agglomerates (1822 ± 373.6 nm) and a less negative charge value (−26.9 mV). In HS, the size of the agglomerates was greatly reduced (189.1 ± 48.6 nm), and the ζ-potential showed even fewer negative values (−11.6 ± 1.5 mV).

For all NPs, PDI values were smaller in MQ that in ASW and HS, indicating a more homogenous dispersion in the absence of salts.

3.2. Effects of NPs on Hemocyte Morphology: SEM

The effects of different NPs on hemocyte morphology were investigated by SEM. For all NP types, the hemocytes were exposed for 30 min at a concentration of 10 µg/mL in ASW or HS suspension. Control hemocytes (in absence of NPs) were run in parallel in both media.

Control hemocytes in ASW showed a characteristic extremely flat shape, with cells fully spread onto the filter support, with diameters ranging from 20 to 40 µm and showing a rather smooth surface, several short cell-surface extensions and absence of filopodia (Figure 1A,B). Due to the extreme flatness of the cells, fractures were often observed between the periphery and the center of the cells, which was thicker and contained granular structures presumably in the perinuclear region.

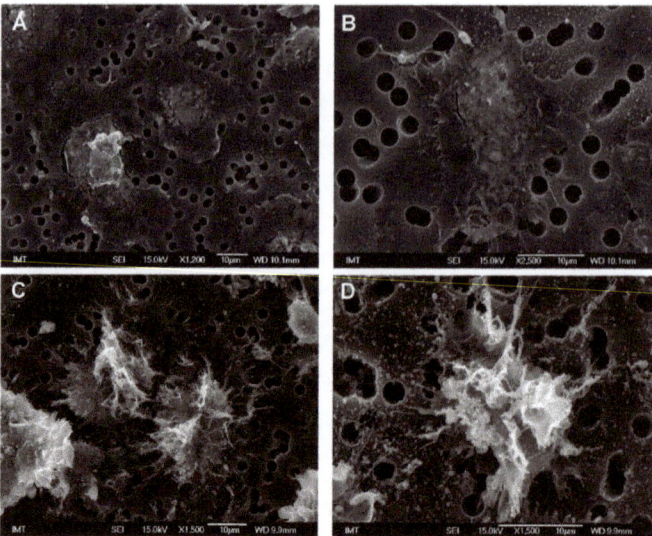

Figure 1. Scanning electron microscopy (SEM) images of control hemocytes from *M. galloprovincialis* in different media. (**A**,**B**) in artificial seawater (ASW); (**C**,**D**) in hemolymph serum (HS). Hemocytes were attached to a paper filter support with pore size of 3 µm.

A different shape was observed in control hemocytes maintained in HS medium. They were not fully spread on the support and therefore thicker with smaller diameters (~20–28 µm). Their surface was irregular with several membrane ruffles and filopodia of variable shapes (Figure 1C,D).

After the addition of PVP-AuNP in ASW, cell morphology was similar to that of controls, even though some cells showed the presence of vesicles of micro-/submicrometric size (≤ 1 µm diameter) on the edge of the plasma membrane (Figure 2). When the presence of Au was investigated by EDX, no gold was detected either inside the cells or in the surrounding environment (Figure S2). Similar observations were made in HS (not shown).

In contrast, PS-NH$_2$ induced changes in hemocyte shape in both media (Figure 3). In ASW, some cells were still spread on the substrate, but they were not fully attached to the support, showing variable shapes (Figure 3A). Other hemocytes were smaller and thicker, showing the typical morphology of activated cells (Figure 3B). Such changes in shape were more evident in HS, where a large number of filopodia was observed (Figure 3D,E). Moreover, in both conditions, the edge of the cells often showed a complex lace-like pattern, due to a network of short filopodia (Figure 3C,F).

Exposure to PS-COOH in ASW did not affect gross morphology of cells with respect to control hemocytes (Figure 4A). Large particle agglomerates were observed around some cells (arrowheads), appearing very white in contrast with the rest of the biological material (Figure 4B and Figure S3 for details of PS-COOH). Moreover, short membrane protrusions could be observed along the border of some cells, as well small extracellular vesicles (Figure 4C). The presence of small PS-COOH agglomerates on the cell surface was observed near vesicles with apparent concave shapes (Figure 4D).

In hemocytes exposed to PS-COOH in HS, cell morphology was apparently similar to those of control cells in HS; however, the formation of thin filopodia of about 3–8 µm in length was observed, apparently enabling communication between adjacent cells (Figure 5A,B). Among these, some longer (>15 µm) filopodia were observed (Figure 5C, arrow), sometimes apparently making contact with apoptotic cells/cell bodies. When observed in more detail (Figure 5D), these filaments appeared thicker (300–400 nm) and containing vesicles (asterisk). Moreover, other shorter filopodia appeared to be formed by a chain of vesicles connected by very thin necks, as in a necklace-like structure (arrowheads). In HS, no particle agglomerates were observed.

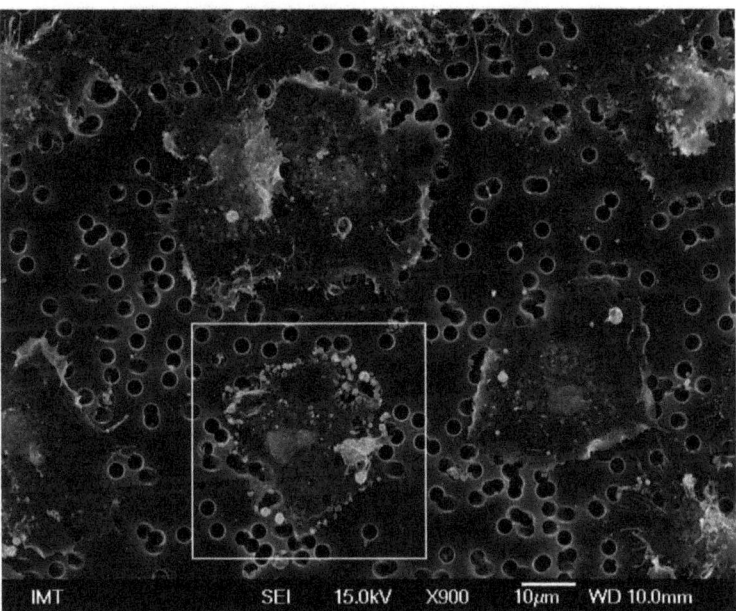

Figure 2. SEM images of hemocytes of *M. galloprovincialis* incubated for 30 min with PVP-AuNPs (10 µg/mL) in ASW suspension. In the framed cell, the presence of PVP-AuNPs was investigated using Energy-dispersive X-ray (EDX) analysis, and the details are presented in Figure S2.

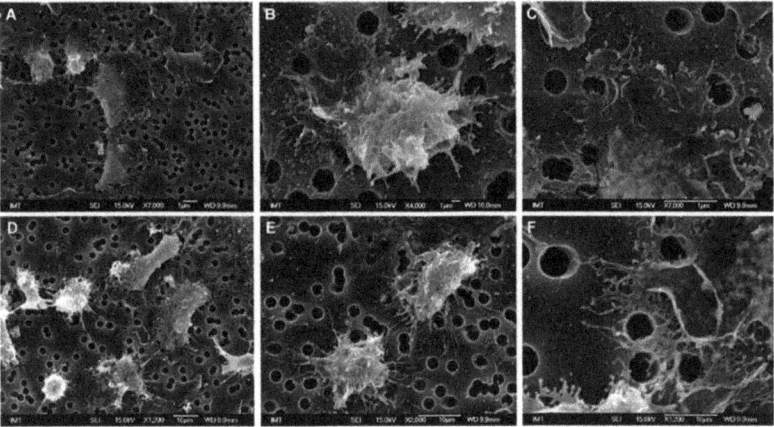

Figure 3. SEM images of hemocytes of *M. galloprovincialis* incubated for 30 min with PS-NH$_2$ in ASW suspension (**A**,**B**) and in HS suspension (**D**,**E**). Details of membrane structures observed in ASW (**C**) and HS (**F**).

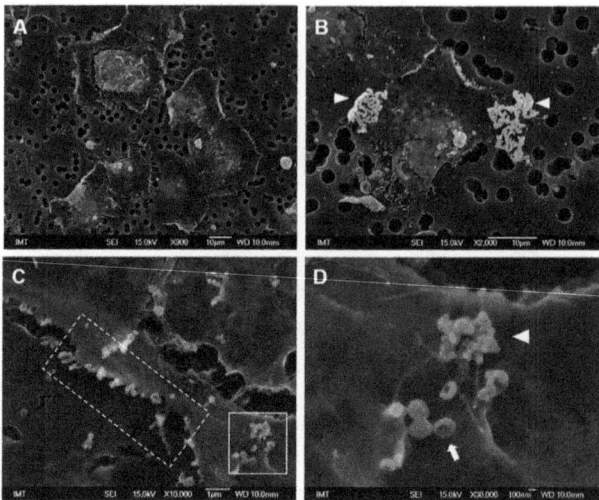

Figure 4. SEM images of *M. galloprovincialis* hemocytes incubated for 30 min with PS-COOH suspensions (10 µg/mL) in ASW (**A**). Arrowheads in (**B**) indicate large agglomerates of PS-COOH; (**C**) short extensions and vesicles along the plasma membrane (dotted frame); (**D**) Enlargement of the white frame in (**C**) indicating the presence of PS-COOH small agglomerates on the cell surface (arrowhead) as well as of concave vesicles (arrow).

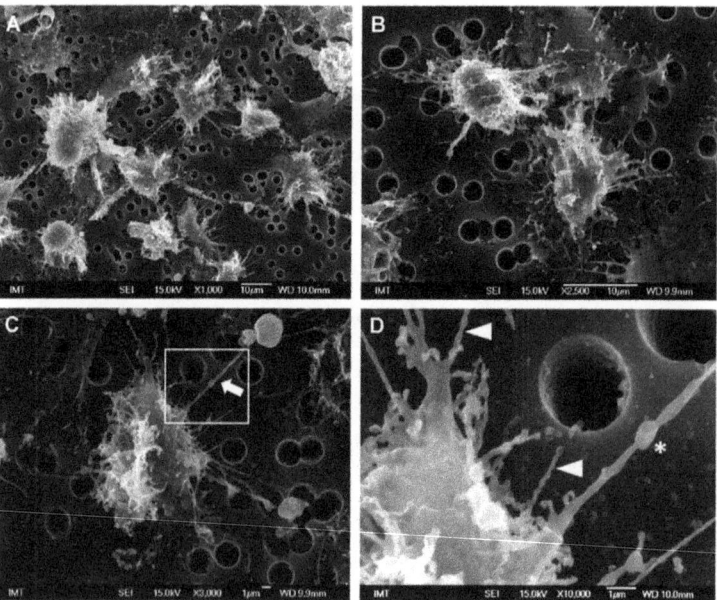

Figure 5. SEM images of *M. galloprovincialis* hemocytes incubated for 30 min with PS-COOH suspensions (10 µg/mL) in HS (**A,B,D**) Detail of cytoplasmic extensions observed in (**C**), indicating thicker filaments containing vesicles (asterisk), and filopodia with necklace-like structure (arrowheads).

3.3. Hemocyte Functional Parameters

3.3.1. PVP-AuNP

PVP-AuNP exposure in ASW did not affect hemocyte LMS and phagocytosis (Figure 6A,B) at any concentration tested up to 100 µg/mL (Figure 6A,B). Moreover, PVP-AuNPs did not affect extracellular ROS production up to 50 µg/mL (Figure 6C). Similarly, no effects were observed using HS as suspension medium (data not shown).

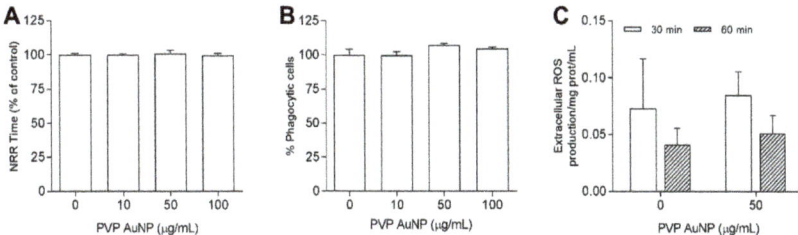

Figure 6. Effects of PVP-AuNPs in ASW on hemocyte: lysosomal membrane stability (LMS) (**A**), phagocytosis (**B**) and extracellular ROS production (**C**).

3.3.2. Amino-Modified Nanopolystyrene—PS-NH$_2$

The effects of PS-NH$_2$ on *Mytilus* hemocytes in different exposure media were previously reported in [11,12]. However, to mirror the effects observed for the changes in cell morphology, in this work further experiments were performed at the same concentration, 10 µg/mL in both media, and the results are reported in Figure 7.

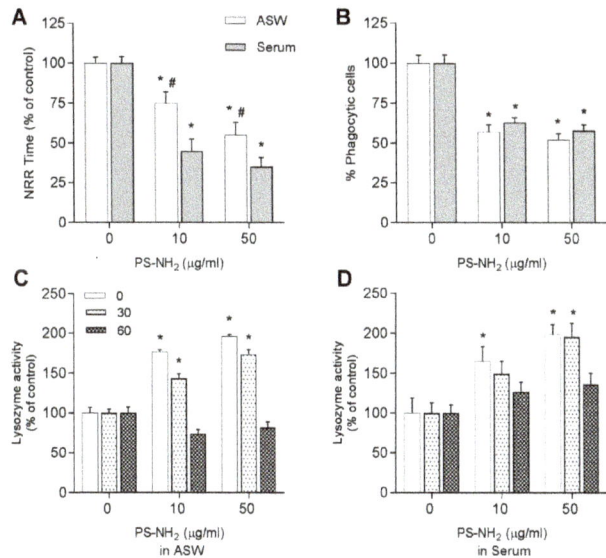

Figure 7. Effects of PS-NH$_2$ in different suspension media in ASW (white bars) or hemolymph serum (HS) (grey bars) on mussel *M. galloprovincialis* hemocytes. (**A**) LMS; (**B**) phagocytosis; and lysozyme activity at time 0, after 30 and 60 min in ASW (**C**) and HS (**D**). Data, representing the mean ± SD of four experiments in triplicate, were analyzed by ANOVA followed by Tukey's post hoc test, ($p < 0.05$): * = all treatments vs. controls; # = ASW vs. serum.

A dose-dependent decrease in LMS was observed from 10 µg/mL in ASW, down to −50% at 50 µg/mL; a significantly stronger effect was observed in HS, at both concentrations (Figure 7A). The phagocytic activity showed a similar decrease (about −40% with respect to controls) at 10 and 50 µg/mL and in both media (Figure 7B). PS-NH$_2$ also stimulated increase in lysozyme activity: the effect was transient in both media with highest values recorded directly immediately after NP addition and after 30 min exposure (Figure 7C,D).

3.3.3. Carboxy-Modified Nanopolystyrene—PS-COOH

The effects of PS-COOH are reported in Figure 8. In ASW suspensions, LMS was decreased from −10 to −45% with respect to controls, at concentrations ranging from 10 to 100 µg/mL, whereas no effects were observed in HS (Figure 8A). Phagocytic activity was unaffected in all experimental conditions (Figure 8B). Addition of PS-COOH immediately triggered lysozyme release by hemocytes in both media although only at 50 µg/mL. Interestingly, in ASW this rise in lysozyme activity was persistent up to 60 min exposure, whereas in HS a rapid decrease over time was observed (Figure 8C,D).

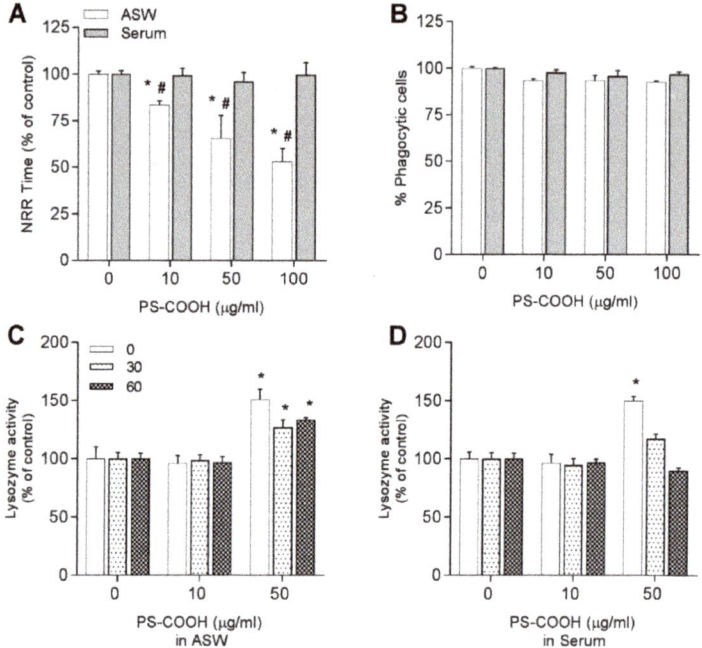

Figure 8. Effects of PS-COOH in different suspension media in ASW (white bars) or hemolymph serum-HS (grey bars) on mussel *M. galloprovincialis* hemocytes. LMS (**A**), phagocytosis (**B**), and lysozyme activity at time 0, after 30 and 60 min in ASW (**C**) and HS (**D**). Data representing the mean ± SD of four experiments in triplicate, were analyzed by ANOVA followed by Tukey's post hoc test, ($p < 0.05$); * = all treatments vs. controls; # = ASW vs. serum.

Because PS-COOH in HS showed distinct agglomeration and effects on hemocyte morphology, lysosomal membrane stability and time course of lysozyme release, its possible interactions with soluble serum components (i.e., the formation of a protein corona) were investigated. PS-COOH was incubated with hemocytes HS and isolation of the corona proteins was performed by centrifugation and 1D-gel electrophoresis as previously described for PS-NH$_2$ and other NPs ([12,20] and Figure S4 for details). When samples were analyzed by gel electrophoresis (Figure S5), no detectable protein bands specific of the corona sample obtained with PS-COOH were observed, indicating the absence of proteins stably bound to the NPs (hard protein corona).

4. Discussion

In the present work, the in vitro interactions and effects of NPs in different media were investigated in the hemocytes of the marine mussel *M. galloprovincialis*. Custom-made PVP-AuNPs stable in ASW were first used as a reference material, and the results were compared with those obtained with two types of nanopolystyrene bearing distinct surface properties (PS-NH$_2$ and PS-COOH). The results highlight distinct morphological and functional responses of mussel hemocytes depending on the core composition and chemicophysical properties of the NPs used and on exposure medium. To our knowledge, these are the first data on the effects of different NPs on detailed cell morphology evaluated by SEM coupled to evaluation of functional parameters in the immune cells of marine invertebrates.

Gold NPs represent a valuable tool for biomedical applications, i.e., diagnosis or targeted drug delivery, due to the peculiar properties of this material [33,34]. AuNPs appear generally inert toward biological systems, since they have been reported to poorly affect natural cell functions [22]. In particular, in mammalian systems, AuNPs have been shown to be relevant to meet the need for immunosafe particles for clinical purposes [23]. In this light, AuNPs can be utilized as a model to compare the interactions of NPs with innate immunity across different species. However, for a proper comparison, the main characteristics and behavior of NPs should be maintained in different experimental settings. Various NPs have been shown to strongly agglomerate in ASW, due to the high salt concentration which reduces the electrostatic repulsion of the particles [35]. To circumvent this problem, custom-made AuNPs, coated with PVP to maintain their dispersion in ASW, were successfully synthesized to allow for exposure of marine invertebrate cells in vitro.

Previous in vitro studies on *M. galloprovincialis* hemocytes exposed to citrate-coated AuNPs of different sizes (5, 15, 40 nm) for 24 h reported a slight decrease in cell viability at concentrations >50 µg/mL, with stronger effects caused by smaller-size AuNPs; however, the citrate coating used appeared to play a major role in the toxicity observed [16]. In gill explants of the clam *Ruditapes philippinarum*, the utilization of an optimized STEM-in-SEM methodology allowed for detection of AuNPs (24 nm) inside the gill cells, attached to the outer membrane of the mitochondria and to the nuclear envelope [36]. In the present work, no internalization of AuNPs was observed by *Mytilus* hemocytes; however, differences in phagocytic activity may be due to the cell type, the incubation time, or the AuNP characteristics. Moreover, the results here obtained show that short-term exposure to PVP-AuNPs did not affect the morphology or main functional parameters of mussel hemocytes. When the presence of Au was investigated by EDX, no gold was detected either inside the cells or in the surrounding environment. However, in some AuNP-exposed cells, small vesicles on the edge of the plasma membrane were observed, resembling ectosomes. Ectosomes are vesicles generated by the direct outward budding of the plasma membrane, which produces microvesicles, microparticles, and large vesicles in the size range of ~50 nm to 1 mm in diameter [37]. Human polymorphonuclear neutrophils (PMNs) upon activation release ectosomes which are characterized by the expression of phosphatidylserine and show anti-inflammatory/immunosuppressive activities toward macrophages [38]. In mussel hemocytes, the production of ectosomes and exchange of signaling molecules might represent an additional component of intercellular communication among different cell subpopulations, contributing to down-regulation of responses to AuNP exposure and immunoregulation as in human PMNs. However, this possibility requires further investigation.

Overall, these data indicate that AuNPs did not strongly interact with hemocytes and/or were lost during the fixing procedure. The data obtained in the present work confirm the suitability of the newly synthetized AuNP to be utilized as a negative control for testing the effects of NP exposure on *Mytilus* hemocytes, as well as any other marine invertebrate cell types. These data reinforce the concept of the importance of the choice of NPs and suitability of the protocols for handling marine invertebrate cells for in vitro testing of NP safety. Many parameters can influence the biological activity of NPs, including core composition, surface charge, and agglomeration state. To evaluate the effects of NP functionalization on *Mytilus* hemocytes, polystyrene NPs (PSNPs) of similar size (50–60 nm) but carrying different surface modifications (–NH_2 and –COOH) were compared in vitro. PS-NH_2 showed little agglomeration (~200 nm) in ASW, and slightly smaller (~178 nm) in HS medium, while retaining a similar positive surface charge (+14.2 mV) in both media [12]. PS-NH_2 induced significant changes in functional parameters in both ASW and HS, with stronger effects observed in HS as previously described [11,12]. These results are supported by the present data here obtained by SEM on cell morphology in HS with respect to ASW.

The difference observed between the two media is in line with the reported formation of a stable biomolecular corona recorded for PS-NH_2 in HS [12], whose unique protein component was identified as the extrapallial protein precursor (EPp) (also called MgC1q6). EPp is the most abundant serum protein encountered in *Mytilus* HS, and it is known to play a key role in the specific recognition of both selected bacterial strains and NP types [39,40]. The presence of a protein corona on PS-NH_2 would likely increase the stability of NPs and contribute to reducing agglomeration, as well as to regulate nano-bio-interactions with hemocytes and the consequent outcome of the cellular response.

Distinct observations were made with PS-COOH, in terms of both particle behavior in exposure media and morphological and functional responses of hemocytes. In ASW, PS-COOH showed the formation of large agglomerates (>1500 nm) and retained a negative surface charge (−26 mV). Such a high agglomeration in ASW is likely to occur due to the interactions between the negative surface charge (-COO^-) retained at pH $\geq$ 5 and high concentrations of divalent cations (e.g., Ca^{2+} and Mg^{2+}) naturally present in seawater [41,42]. The results of SEM analysis indicate the absence of gross morphological changes in hemocytes exposed to PS-COOH at 10 μg/mL in ASW; accordingly, in these conditions, only a slight decrease in LMS was observed, whereas lysozyme release and phagocytosis were unaffected. This confirms that large NP agglomerates show little interactions with hemocytes.

When suspended in HS, PS-COOH formed smaller agglomerates (~180 nm) that were not detectable around the cells by SEM; in addition, under these experimental conditions, gross cell morphology and functional parameters were not significantly affected. However, SEM allowed for the detection of some subtle morphological changes, like formation of multiple filopodial extensions of variable length and shape that were not observed in all the other experimental conditions tested. The roles of filopodia can be various, from sensing or communication with the surrounding environment [43], to mobility, particle engulfment, and the production and release of molecules [44]. In mussel hemocytes exposed to PS-COOH in HS, we observed thicker filopodia containing vesicles, and/or shorter and thinner filopodia apparently formed by a chain of spherical vesicles connected by ultrathin necks. Some of them seemed to connect with the neighboring cell or with apoptotic bodies/vesicles. Drab et al. (2019) recently reported several mechanisms that could explain the presence and formation of these necklace-like structures, which can represent an intermediary stage in the formation of structures known as tunneling nanotubes (TNTs). TNTs are a new emerging cell-to-cell communication tool, that allows for the selective transfer of cellular components, signaling molecules, and pathogens between cells [45]. The presence and roles of TNTs have been mainly described in mammalian cells, including immune cells, where they play several roles in responding to stress, including the transport of nanomaterials [46,47]. Interestingly, we have recently reported the presence of similar structures exchanging lysosomal vesicles and mitochondria in live *M. galloprovincialis* hemocytes [48]. The results here obtained suggest that, under certain experimental conditions, NPs may induce TNT formation in invertebrate immune cells, thus probably allowing for an intercellular communication system that may participate in the protection against NP toxicity. Further work will be needed to confirm and define the presence of these peculiar structures in *Mytilus* hemocytes and appreciate their role in the effects that different NPs have on their immune function.

The results obtained with PS-COOH are the first data on the effects of negatively charged nanoplastics in the cells of marine bivalves. Data obtained in the presence of HS suggest that the observed effects may be due to the formation of a NP-protein corona, in analogy with previous data obtained with other NPs, including PS-NH$_2$ and nano-oxides [20]. However, we could not identify any protein stably bound to PS-COOH (hard corona). These data do not exclude the possible interactions with other hemolymph proteins loosely bound to PS-COOH (soft corona) that may participate in modulating the responses of hemocytes and that cannot be detected with the method utilized. Grassi et al. (2019) studied the corona formation and composition in sea urchin coelomic fluid for PS-NH$_2$ and PS-COOH and reported a similar hard-corona proteomic pattern for both PS-NP types [27]. The discrepancies with this work not only may be due to the profound differences in protein composition between biological fluids of sea urchins and mussels but also to the methodological approach using different protein separation (2D-electrophoresis). Finally, in mussel hemocytes, in contrast with data obtained with PS-NH$_2$, where the presence of a stable protein corona elicited stronger effects/damages, the presence of proteins more loosely interacting with PS-COOH (soft corona) would participate in protective mechanisms, contributing to the biological response, as indicated by the results obtained measuring functional parameters.

Overall, the results further underline the importance of the surface charge, rather than the core material, in determining NP behaviour in exposure medium and consequent specificity of the nano-bio-interactions with mussel hemocytes leading to biological responses in vitro.

The application of SEM revealed for the first time the detailed morphology of hemocytes from *M. galloprovincialis* kept in different media and allowed for the evaluation of the morphological changes induced by different NPs in different experimental conditions. The results obtained on cell morphology are in line with those of determination of functional parameters, because the experimental conditions that elicited more evident morphological changes were always accompanied by the activation of stronger functional responses. The morphological and functional approach thus provides a better understanding of the results obtained when testing different types of NPs in vitro. This basal information will contribute to developing more standardized protocols for the in vitro screening of nanosafety in marine invertebrate cell models. This knowledge will also help better define protocols for in vivo exposure to NPs at environmentally realistic exposure concentrations.

In conclusion, the experimental system used in our study represents a suitable approach for fast evaluation of the biological activity of engineered nanomaterials in mussel immune cells. The most important characteristic of a prescreening tests is its capacity to discriminate among particles with different characteristics and what responses are biologically relevant. Our results confirm the specificity of the responses of mussel hemocytes (morphology and functional parameters) to different NPs.

Supplementary Materials: The following are available online at https://www.mdpi.com/2079-4991/11/2/470/s1, Figure S1: Characterization of synthesis and postproduction steps of synthesized PVP-AuNPs; Figure S2: Energy-dispersive X-ray (EDX) analysis of a SEM sample of a hemocyte exposed to PVP-AuNPs in ASW; Figure S3: SEM images showing in more details PS-COOH suspensions in ASW; Figure S4: Schematic overview of the protocol utilized to identify the mussel PS-COOH corona (C) from *Mytilus galloprovincialis* hemolymph serum (HS); Figure S5: Separation of PS-COOH protein complexes from HS of *M. galloprovincialis* proteins by SDS-PAGE and staining with Coomassie Brilliant Blue.

Author Contributions: Conceptualization, M.A. and L.C.; methodology, C.M. and D.D.; formal analysis, M.H. and S.A.; investigation, resources, F.B., G.G., and V.P.; writing—original draft preparation, M.A.; writing—review and editing, M.A. and L.C.; supervision, D.D. and L.C. All authors have read and agreed to the published version of the manuscript.

Funding: This research has received funding from the European Union's Horizon 2020 research and innovation program under the Marie Skłodowska-Curie grant agreement PANDORA N° 671881 (Probing safety of nano-objects by defining immune responses of environmental organisms). Partial support was given by the Italian Antarctic Project NANOPANTA Nano-Polymers in the Antarctic marine environment and biota PNRA16_00075 B.

Institutional Review Board Statement: The Mediterranean mussel, *M. galloprovincialis*, is not considered an endangered or protected species in any international species catalog, including the CITES list (www.cites.org), and not included in the list of species regulated by EC Directive 2010/63/EU. Therefore, no specific authorization is required to work on mussel samples.

Informed Consent Statement: Not applicable.

Acknowledgments: We would like to thank I. Corsi (Univ. Siena, IT) for providing the PS-COOH used in the present work.

Conflicts of Interest: The authors declare no conflict of interest. The funders had no role in the design of the study; in the collection, analyses, or interpretation of data; in the writing of the manuscript, or in the decision to publish the results.

References

1. Barrick, A.; Guillet, C.; Mouneyrac, C.; Châtel, A. Investigating the Establishment of Primary Cultures of Hemocytes from Mytilus Edulis. *Cytotechnology* **2018**, *70*, 1205–1220. [CrossRef] [PubMed]
2. Canesi, L.; Ciacci, C.; Fabbri, R.; Marcomini, A.; Pojana, G.; Gallo, G. Bivalve Molluscs as a Unique Target Group for Nanoparticle Toxicity. *Mar. Environ. Res.* **2012**, *76*, 16–21. [CrossRef] [PubMed]
3. Rocha, T.L.; Gomes, T.; Sousa, V.S.; Mestre, N.C.; Bebianno, M.J. Ecotoxicological Impact of Engineered Nanomaterials in Bivalve Molluscs: An Overview. *Mar. Environ. Res.* **2015**, *111*, 74–88. [CrossRef]
4. Canesi, L.; Corsi, I. Effects of Nanomaterials on Marine Invertebrates. *Sci. Total Environ.* **2016**, *565*, 933–940. [CrossRef]
5. Canesi, L.; Auguste, M.; Bebianno, M.J. Sublethal effects of nanoparticles on aquatic invertebrates, from molecular to organism level. In *Ecotoxicology of Nanoparticles in Aquatic Systems*; CRC Press: Boca Raton, FL, USA, 2019; pp. 38–61.
6. Moore, M.N. Do Nanoparticles Present Ecotoxicological Risks for the Health of the Aquatic Environment? *Environ. Int.* **2006**, *32*, 967–976. [CrossRef]
7. Allam, B.; Raftos, D. Immune Responses to Infectious Diseases in Bivalves. *J. Invertebr. Pathol.* **2015**, *131*, 121–136. [CrossRef] [PubMed]
8. Gerdol, M.; Gomez-Chiari, M.; Castillo, M.G.; Figueras, A.; Fiorito, G.; Moreira, R.; Novoa, B.; Pallavicini, A.; Ponte, G.; Roumbedakis, K.; et al. Immunity in molluscs: Recognition and effector mechanisms, with a focus on bivalvia. In *Advances in Comparative Immunology*; Springer: Berlin, Germany, 2018; pp. 225–342.
9. Ciacci, C.; Canonico, B.; Bilaničová, D.; Fabbri, R.; Cortese, K.; Gallo, G.; Marcomini, A.; Pojana, G.; Canesi, L. Immunomodulation by Different Types of N-Oxides in the Hemocytes of the Marine Bivalve Mytilus Galloprovincialis. *PLoS ONE* **2012**, *7*, e36937. [CrossRef]
10. Canesi, L.; Ciacci, C.; Vallotto, D.; Gallo, G.; Marcomini, A.; Pojana, G. In Vitro Effects of Suspensions of Selected Nanoparticles (C60 Fullerene, TiO_2, SiO_2) on Mytilus Hemocytes. *Aquat. Toxicol.* **2010**, *96*, 151–158. [CrossRef]
11. Canesi, L.; Ciacci, C.; Bergami, E.; Monopoli, M.P.; Dawson, K.A.; Papa, S.; Canonico, B.; Corsi, I. Evidence for Immunomodulation and Apoptotic Processes Induced by Cationic Polystyrene Nanoparticles in the Hemocytes of the Marine Bivalve Mytilus. *Mar. Environ. Res.* **2015**, *111*, 34–40. [CrossRef]
12. Canesi, L.; Ciacci, C.; Fabbri, R.; Balbi, T.; Salis, A.; Damonte, G.; Cortese, K.; Caratto, V.; Monopoli, M.P.; Dawson, K.; et al. Interactions of Cationic Polystyrene Nanoparticles with Marine Bivalve Hemocytes in a Physiological Environment: Role of Soluble Hemolymph Proteins. *Environ. Res.* **2016**, *150*, 73–81. [CrossRef]
13. Auguste, M.; Ciacci, C.; Balbi, T.; Brunelli, A.; Caratto, V.; Marcomini, A.; Cuppini, R.; Canesi, L. Effects of Nanosilver on Mytilus Galloprovincialis Hemocytes and Early Embryo Development. *Aquat. Toxicol.* **2018**, *203*, 107–116. [CrossRef] [PubMed]
14. Katsumiti, A.; Gilliland, D.; Arostegui, I.; Cajaraville, M.P. Mechanisms of Toxicity of Ag Nanoparticles in Comparison to Bulk and Ionic Ag on Mussel Hemocytes and Gill Cells. *PLoS ONE* **2015**, *10*, e0129039. [CrossRef]
15. Canesi, L.; Ciacci, C.; Balbi, T. Invertebrate Models for Investigating the Impact of Nanomaterials on Innate Immunity: The Example of the Marine Mussel Mytilus Spp. *Curr. Bionanotechnol.* **2016**, *2*, 77–83. [CrossRef]
16. Katsumiti, A.; Arostegui, I.; Oron, M.; Gilliland, D.; Valsami-Jones, E.; Cajaraville, M.P. Cytotoxicity of Au, ZnO and SiO_2 NPs Using In Vitro Assays with Mussel Hemocytes and Gill Cells: Relevance of Size, Shape and Additives. *Nanotoxicology* **2015**, 1–9. [CrossRef]
17. Canesi, L.; Frenzilli, G.; Balbi, T.; Bernardeschi, M.; Ciacci, C.; Corsolini, S.; Della Torre, C.; Fabbri, R.; Faleri, C.; Focardi, S.; et al. Interactive Effects of N-TiO2 and 2,3,7,8-TCDD on the Marine Bivalve Mytilus Galloprovincialis. *Aquat. Toxicol.* **2014**, *153*, 53–65. [CrossRef] [PubMed]

18. Katsumiti, A.; Thorley, A.J.; Arostegui, I.; Reip, P.; Valsami-Jones, E.; Tetley, T.D.; Cajaraville, M.P. Cytotoxicity and Cellular Mechanisms of Toxicity of CuO NPs in Mussel Cells in Vitro and Comparative Sensitivity with Human Cells. *Toxicol. Vitr.* **2018**, *48*, 146–158. [CrossRef]
19. Bruinink, A.; Wang, J.; Wick, P. Effect of Particle Agglomeration in Nanotoxicology. *Arch. Toxicol* **2015**, *89*, 659–675. [CrossRef] [PubMed]
20. Canesi, L.; Balbi, T.; Fabbri, R.; Salis, A.; Damonte, G.; Volland, M.; Blasco, J. Biomolecular Coronas in Invertebrate Species: Implications in the Environmental Impact of Nanoparticles. *NanoImpact* **2017**, *8*, 89–98. [CrossRef]
21. Barbero, F.; Russo, L.; Vitali, M.; Piella, J.; Salvo, I.; Borrajo, M.L.; Busquets-Fité, M.; Grandori, R.; Bastús, N.G.; Casals, E.; et al. Formation of the Protein Corona: The Interface between Nanoparticles and the Immune System. *Semin. Immunol.* **2017**, *34*, 52–60. [CrossRef]
22. Connor, E.E.; Mwamuka, J.; Gole, A.; Murphy, C.J.; Wyatt, M.D. Gold Nanoparticles Are Taken Up by Human Cells but Do Not Cause Acute Cytotoxicity. *Small* **2005**, *1*, 325–327. [CrossRef]
23. Sperling, R.A.; Rivera Gil, P.; Zhang, F.; Zanella, M.; Parak, W.J. Biological Applications of Gold Nanoparticles. *Chem. Soc. Rev.* **2008**, *37*, 1896. [CrossRef]
24. Bastús, N.G.; Comenge, J.; Puntes, V. Kinetically Controlled Seeded Growth Synthesis of Citrate-Stabilized Gold Nanoparticles of up to 200 Nm: Size Focusing versus Ostwald Ripening. *Langmuir* **2011**, *27*, 11098–11105. [CrossRef]
25. La Roche, G.; Eisler, R.; Tarzwell, C. Bioassay Procedure for Oil and Oil Dispersant Toxicity Evaluation. *J. Water Pollut Control. Fed* **1970**, 1982–1989.
26. *ASTM D1141-98 Standard Practice for the Preparation of Substitute Ocean Water*; American Society for Testing and Materials: West Conshohocken, PA, USA, 2013.
27. Grassi, G.; Landi, C.; Della Torre, C.; Bergami, E.; Bini, L.; Corsi, I. Proteomic Profile of the Hard Corona of Charged Polystyrene Nanoparticles Exposed to Sea Urchin *Paracentrotus Lividus* Coelomic Fluid Highlights Potential Drivers of Toxicity. *Environ. Sci. Nano* **2019**, *6*, 2937–2947. [CrossRef]
28. Hernroth, B. The Influence of Temperature and Dose on Antibacterial Peptide Response against Lipopolysaccharide in the Blue Mussel, Mytilus Edulis. *Fish. Shellfish Immunol.* **2003**, *14*, 25–37. [CrossRef]
29. Li, Y.; Boraschi, D. Endotoxin Contamination: A Key Element in the Interpretation of Nanosafety Studies. *Nanomedicine* **2016**, *11*, 269–287. [CrossRef] [PubMed]
30. Li, Y.; Shi, Z.; Radauer-Preiml, I.; Andosch, A.; Casals, E.; Luetz-Meindl, U.; Cobaleda, M.; Lin, Z.; Jaberi-Douraki, M.; Italiani, P.; et al. Bacterial Endotoxin (Lipopolysaccharide) Binds to the Surface of Gold Nanoparticles, Interferes with Biocorona Formation and Induces Human Monocyte Inflammatory Activation. *Nanotoxicology* **2017**, *11*, 1157–1175. [CrossRef] [PubMed]
31. Drobne, D. 3D Imaging of Cells and Tissues by Focused Ion Beam/Scanning Electron Microscopy (FIB/SEM). In *Nanoimaging*; Sousa, A.A., Kruhlak, M.J., Eds.; Humana Press: Totowa, NJ, USA, 2013; pp. 275–292. ISBN 978-1-62703-136-3.
32. Millaku, A.; Drobne, D.; Torkar, M.; Novak, S.; Remškar, M.; Pipan-Tkalec, Ž. Use of Scanning Electron Microscopy to Monitor Nanofibre/Cell Interaction in Digestive Epithelial Cells. *J. Hazard. Mater.* **2013**, *260*, 47–52. [CrossRef] [PubMed]
33. Tiwari, P.; Vig, K.; Dennis, V.; Singh, S. Functionalized Gold Nanoparticles and Their Biomedical Applications. *Nanomaterials* **2011**, *1*, 31–63. [CrossRef]
34. Yeh, Y.-C.; Creran, B.; Rotello, V.M. Gold Nanoparticles: Preparation, Properties, and Applications in Bionanotechnology. *Nanoscale* **2012**, *4*, 1871–1880. [CrossRef]
35. Bundschuh, M.; Filser, J.; Lüderwald, S.; McKee, M.S.; Metreveli, G.; Schaumann, G.E.; Schulz, R.; Wagner, S. Nanoparticles in the Environment: Where Do We Come from, Where Do We Go To? *Environ. Sci. Eur.* **2018**, *30*, 6. [CrossRef] [PubMed]
36. García-Negrete, C.A.; Jiménez de Haro, M.C.; Blasco, J.; Soto, M.; Fernández, A. STEM-in-SEM High Resolution Imaging of Gold Nanoparticles and Bivalve Tissues in Bioaccumulation Experiments. *Analyst* **2015**, *140*, 3082–3089. [CrossRef] [PubMed]
37. Kalluri, R.; LeBleu, V.S. The Biology, Function, and Biomedical Applications of Exosomes. *Science* **2020**, *367*, eaau6977. [CrossRef]
38. Eken, C.; Sadallah, S.; Martin, P.J.; Treves, S.; Schifferli, J.A. Ectosomes of Polymorphonuclear Neutrophils Activate Multiple Signaling Pathways in Macrophages. *Immunobiology* **2013**, *218*, 382–392. [CrossRef]
39. Oliveri, C.; Peric, L.; Sforzini, S.; Banni, M.; Viarengo, A.; Cavaletto, M.; Marsano, F. Biochemical and Proteomic Characterisation of Haemolymph Serum Reveals the Origin of the Alkali-Labile Phosphate (ALP) in Mussel (Mytilus Galloprovincialis). *Comp. Biochem. Physiol. Part. D: Genom. Proteom.* **2014**, *11*, 29–36. [CrossRef] [PubMed]
40. Pezzati, E.; Canesi, L.; Damonte, G.; Salis, A.; Marsano, F.; Grande, C.; Vezzulli, L.; Pruzzo, C. Susceptibility of *V Ibrio Aestuarianus* s 01/032 to the Antibacterial Activity of *M Ytilus* Haemolymph: Identification of a Serum Opsonin Involved in Mannose-Sensitive Interactions: *Vibrio Aestuarianus* and Bivalve Haemocytes. *Environ. Microbiol* **2015**, *17*, 4271–4279. [CrossRef] [PubMed]
41. Tallec, K.; Blard, O.; González-Fernández, C.; Brotons, G.; Berchel, M.; Soudant, P.; Huvet, A.; Paul-Pont, I. Surface Functionalization Determines Behavior of Nanoplastic Solutions in Model Aquatic Environments. *Chemosphere* **2019**, *225*, 639–646. [CrossRef] [PubMed]
42. Zhang, F.; Wang, Z.; Wang, S.; Fang, H.; Wang, D. Aquatic Behavior and Toxicity of Polystyrene Nanoplastic Particles with Different Functional Groups: Complex Roles of PH, Dissolved Organic Carbon and Divalent Cations. *Chemosphere* **2019**, *228*, 195–203. [CrossRef] [PubMed]
43. Heckman, C.A.; Plummer, H.K. Filopodia as Sensors. *Cell. Signal.* **2013**, *25*, 2298–2311. [CrossRef]

44. Gauthier, N.C.; Masters, T.A.; Sheetz, M.P. Mechanical Feedback between Membrane Tension and Dynamics. *Trends Cell Biol.* **2012**, *22*, 527–535. [CrossRef]
45. Drab, M.; Stopar, D.; Kralj-Iglič, V.; Iglič, A. Inception Mechanisms of Tunneling Nanotubes. *Cells* **2019**, *8*, 626. [CrossRef] [PubMed]
46. Sisakhtnezhad, S.; Khosravi, L. Emerging Physiological and Pathological Implications of Tunneling Nanotubes Formation between Cells. *Eur. J. Cell Biol.* **2015**, *94*, 429–443. [CrossRef]
47. Korenkova, O.; Pepe, A.; Zurzolo, C. Fine Intercellular Connections in Development: TNTs, Cytonemes, or Intercellular Bridges? *CST* **2020**, *4*, 30–43. [CrossRef] [PubMed]
48. Auguste, M.; Balbi, T.; Ciacci, C.; Canesi, L. Conservation of Cell Communication Systems in Invertebrate Host–Defence Mechanisms: Possible Role in Immunity and Disease. *Biology* **2020**, *9*, 234. [CrossRef] [PubMed]

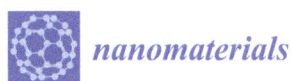

Article

Safety Evaluation of TiO$_2$ Nanoparticle-Based Sunscreen UV Filters on the Development and the Immunological State of the Sea Urchin *Paracentrotus lividus*

Riccardo Catalano [1], Jérôme Labille [1,†], Daniela Gaglio [2,3], Andi Alijagic [4], Elisabetta Napodano [3], Danielle Slomberg [1], Andrea Campos [5] and Annalisa Pinsino [4,*,†]

[1] Aix Marseille University, CNRS, IRD, INRAE, Coll France, CEREGE, 13545 Aix-en-Provence, France; catalano@cerege.fr (R.C.); labille@cerege.fr (J.L.); Slomberg@cerege.fr (D.S.)
[2] Consiglio Nazionale delle Ricerche, Istituto di Bioimmagini e Fisiologia Molecolare (IBFM), 20090 Segrate, MI, Italy; daniela.gaglio@ibfm.cnr.it
[3] SYSBIO.IT, Centre of Systems Biology, University of Milano-Bicocca, 20126 Milano, Italy; elisabetta.napodano@unimib.it
[4] Consiglio Nazionale delle Ricerche, Istituto per la Ricerca e l'Innovazione Biomedica (IRIB), 90146 Palermo, Italy; andialijagic@gmail.com
[5] Aix Marseille Université, CNRS, Centrale Marseille, FSCM, CP2M, 13397 Marseille, France; andrea.campos@univ-amu.fr
* Correspondence: annalisa.pinsino@irib.cnr.it or annalisa.pinsino@cnr.it
† These authors share senior authorship.

Received: 9 September 2020; Accepted: 20 October 2020; Published: 23 October 2020

Abstract: Sunscreens are emulsions of water and oil that contain filters capable of protecting against the detrimental effects of ultraviolet radiation (UV). The widespread use of cosmetic products based on nanoparticulate UV filters has increased concerns regarding their safety and compatibility with both the environment and human health. In the present work, we evaluated the effects of titanium dioxide nanoparticle (TiO$_2$ NP)-based UV filters with three different surface coatings on the development and immunity of the sea urchin, *Paracentrotus lividus*. A wide range of NP concentrations was analyzed, corresponding to different levels of dilution starting from the original cosmetic dispersion. Variations in surface coating, concentration, particle shape, and pre-dispersant medium (i.e., water or oil) influenced the embryonic development without producing a relevant developmental impairment. The most common embryonic abnormalities were related to the skeletal growth and the presence of a few cells, which were presumably involved in the particle uptake. Adult *P. lividus* immune cells exposed to silica-coated TiO$_2$ NP-based filters showed a broad metabolic plasticity based on the biosynthesis of metabolites that mediate inflammation, phagocytosis, and antioxidant response. The results presented here highlight the biosafety of the TiO$_2$ NP-based UV filters toward sea urchin, and the importance of developing safer-by-design sunscreens.

Keywords: cosmetic formulation; cosmetic lifecycle; hydrophobic compound; nano-TiO$_2$; nano safety; marine invertebrate; metabolomics

---

1. Introduction

Ultraviolet (UV) radiation is a main risk factor for skin disorders such as erythema, photoaging, and keratinocyte cancer. As a consequence, effective photoprotection is of utmost importance to humans. Several approaches for skin protection have recently been developed, including organic (e.g., benzophenone, octocrylene) and inorganic UV filters (e.g., zinc oxide, titanium dioxide), topically applied antioxidants, DNA repair enzymes, and oral photoprotective strategies based on nutritional supplements [1]. Sunscreens are emulsions of water and oil that contain UV filters capable of protecting human skin from the detrimental effects of UV radiation [2].

The widespread use of these products has increased concerns regarding their safety and compatibility with both the environment and human health [3]. Thus, sunscreen product-related environmental health risk assessment and management are important issues that need to be carefully considered. Some biological models have shown harmful effects in the presence of organic filters (e.g., benzophenones, camphor) used in sunscreen formulations [4–6]. Moreover, most organic UV filters are able to pass through the skin barrier after one single topical application, raising new concerns regarding consumer safety [7]. Thus, inorganic UV filters are becoming even more promising candidates for photoprotection [8]. They consist of either zinc oxide (ZnO) or titanium dioxide (TiO_2) mineral particles. However, to date, knowledge on the potential health risks associated with sunscreens containing such inorganic UV filters remains limited. ZnO-based UV filters are often less preferred because of their high solubility in water. The dissolved Zn species are more bioavailable than ZnO particles, which increases the potential risk, notably in seawater ecosystems [9–11]. On the other hand, TiO_2-based UV filters are generally considered to be more safe because they are weakly soluble in aqueous media [4,11]. The nanoparticulate form of ZnO and TiO_2 (size < 100 nm) is generally used in sunscreens because their small size leads to a more transparent film on the skin after application, which enhances user acceptance. Moreover, these metal oxides are also more efficient UV blockers when finely dispersed in the sunscreen product [12,13], which also contributes to the considerable use of nanoparticles (NPs).

However, using NPs also implies specific safety concerns due to their well-known higher surface reactivity and bioavailability [14]. Nanoparticle risk assessment must, therefore, be developed in the context of the sunscreen lifecycle. Although nano-TiO_2 is one of the most studied nanomaterials in nanosafety research, few of the studied NPs were relevant to the nanoparticulate TiO_2 UV filters used in sunscreens. In a review of more than 200 scientific articles, Minetto et al. [15] revealed that almost all the safety investigations on TiO_2 NPs were performed with bare anatase or with the highly photocatalytic P25 (mixture of anatase:rutile, 4:1), whereas the TiO_2 NPs used as UV filters in sunscreen consist of pure rutile generally coated with a surface passivation layer [16,17]. The aging, transformation, and environmental fate of TiO_2 NP-based UV filters have scarcely been studied to date [18]. While the important role of the NP coating in controlling fate in the suspension and surface reactivity has already been pointed out, questions as to how its nature and lifetime may influence both exposure and hazard in aquatic systems remain. These are key questions regarding the risk assessment of inorganic UV filters, which cannot be evaluated with the widely studied bare TiO_2 NPs.

Moreover, the dispersing medium carrying the NPs in the original cosmetic formulation may also play an important role on the environmental fate. Either an oil or water phase can be used at the product fabrication stage to disperse the hydrophobic or hydrophilic TiO_2 NP-based UV filters, respectively. While the hydrophilic filters pre-dispersed in the water phase can readily be dispersed, diluted, and transported in the aqueous environment, the hydrophobic filters pre-dispersed in the cosmetic oil may have a different environmental fate [19,20]. Once the sunscreen is washed off the skin, the hydrophobic compounds tend to remain in the oil phase of the cosmetic emulsion and float at the water surface. We can reasonably assume that before NP aging takes place, the local NP concentration in the oil droplet floating at the surface should correspond to that in the original cosmetic oil formulation [19]. This is a NP concentration leveling at 5–10 wt%, much higher than any predicted environmental concentration at the ng or µg/L level [21,22]. Nevertheless, organisms living in coastal zones at low water depths could be exposed to these higher NP concentrations. In such an exposure scenario, the oil droplet may act as a vector, transporting the concentrated NP UV filters between the seawater and living organisms, and significantly impacting the biological effects. Currently, there is no reported environmental threshold for TiO_2 NP-based UV filters inducing a biological effect. It is, thus, mandatory to address the impacts they may have both in the environment and in the organisms.

In the present work, we explored the biosafety of three TiO_2 NP-based UV filters on the sea urchin (*Paracentrotus lividus*) model both in the embryonic and adult life-cycle stages. Sea urchins, found in almost all the marine environments [23], are an effective sentinel of environmental stress, notably in coastal areas that are potentially more impacted by recreational bathing activity. The sea urchin embryonic development and the immunological state of adult sea urchin immune cells were investigated in culture conditions. A wide range of TiO_2 NP concentrations was explored, corresponding to different levels of dilution or aging, starting from the original cosmetic dispersion. Considering the contrasted exposure scenarios expected, with an oil phase carrying hydrophobic UV filters and a water phase carrying hydrophilic UV filters, we varied the nature of the TiO_2 NP coating (hydrophobic: Polydimethylsiloxane and stearic acid; hydrophilic: Silica) and of the cosmetic dispersing medium (water, oil) that were injected into the culture medium. The TiO_2 NP-based UV filters appear safe, as they did not significantly compromise the growth of the sea urchin embryos at the pluteus stage (from 0.001 to 1 mg/L). The hydrophilic silica-coated TiO_2 NPs did not affect immune cell viability or produce toxicity at concentrations representative of the cosmetic lifecycle, and the cells showed a broad metabolic plasticity based on the biosynthesis of metabolites promoting an increase in antioxidant activity and phagocytosis.

2. Materials and Methods

2.1. Commercial TiO_2 NP-Based UV Filters and Sunscreen Oil Phase

Four different types of TiO_2 NPs were used in this work. Three of them were commercial nanoparticulate UV filters commonly used in sunscreen formulations, namely, T-S (Titanium Dioxide and Alumina and Stearic Acid), T-Lite (Titanium Dioxide and Aluminum Hydroxide and Dimethicone/Methicone Copolymer), and T-AVO (Titanium Dioxide and Silica). Both T-S and T-Lite UV filters have a primary mineral layer of aluminium oxide and an outermost organic and hydrophobic layer composed of stearic acid or polydimethylsiloxane, respectively. In contrast, the T-AVO UV filter has one single mineral, hydrophilic silica (SiO_2) coating. In addition, P25 TiO_2, was used as an uncoated nano-TiO_2 reference.

These NPs were directly purchased from the suppliers as dry powders. The respective trade names together with the chemical compositions and primary particle size provided by the manufacturers (when available) are reported in Table 1.

Table 1. TiO_2 NP powder commercial names, supplier name, chemical composition, and primary particle size declared by the suppliers.

Powder Name	Powder Supplier	Chemical Composition	Primary Particle Size
Eusolex® T-S	Merck	TiO_2 (73–79%)/Al_2O_3/stearic acid	ND
T-Lite™ SF	BASF	TiO_2 (79–89%)/$Al(OH)_3$/polydimethylsiloxane	14–16 nm
Eusolex® T-AVO	Merck	TiO_2 (79.6%)/SiO_2	ND
P25 TiO_2	Evonik Degussa	TiO_2 (Anatase/Rutile 4:1)	~21 nm

* ND = not declared.

Two different dispersing media were used to mimic the release of these NPs and their respective life cycles in the environment. The hydrophobic UV filters (T-S and T-Lite) were pre-dispersed in a typical cosmetic oil, while the hydrophilic NPs (T-AVO and P25) were pre-dispersed in pure water. Further dilution was then completed to reach the desired concentrations, as detailed below.

The cosmetic oil was prepared by mixing together two emollient oils and an emulsifying agent provided by the respective suppliers (see Table 2), in a 2:2:1 ratio. The mixture was gently homogenized by magnetic stirring for 10 min. The emulsifying agent contained two surfactant molecules (Octyldodecyl xyloside and PEG30 dipolyhydroxystearate) known to play a role in the exposure route of the hydrophobic NPs via the creation of oil droplets containing the NPs that are stable in pure water [13].

Table 2. Components constituting the typical sunscreen oil phase used in this work: Product names, supplier names, function of each product, and related chemical composition.

Product Name	Supplier	Function	Chemical Composition
Tegosoft P	Evonik	Emollient oil	Isopropyl palmitate
Cetiol LC	BASF	Emollient oil	Coco-Caprylate/Caprate
Easynov	SEPPIC	Emulsifying agent	Octydodecanol; Octyldodecyl xyloside; PEG-30 Dipolyhydroxystearate

2.2. Sea Urchin Paracentrotus Lividus Embryo Exposure during Development

Six males and six females were induced to spawn by injecting 1–2 mL of 0.1 M KCl into the sea urchin body cavity, through the peristomal membrane surrounding the mouth. Eggs were collected by placing spawning females on 100 mL beakers with 0.45 µm filtered artificial seawater (ASW). Egg quality and sperm motility were inspected by observing the gametes under an optical microscope (OLYMPUS CKX31, Olympus, Tokyo, Japan); 10 µL seminal fluid was added to the egg suspension (sperm/egg ratio 50:1) and fertilization success was verified under the microscope (formation of the fertilization membrane with a fertilization rate >95%). After fertilization, the embryonic culture (500 embryos per mL) was transferred into 50-mL disposable, sterile tubes (10 mL in each tube), and embryos were immediately exposed for 48h to increasing NP concentrations (between 0.001 and 1 mg/L). The hydrophilic P25 TiO_2 and T-AVO NPs were pre-dispersed and diluted in water in order to reach the desired exposure concentrations. The hydrophobic T-S and T-Lite NPs were pre-dispersed in the oil phase, as typically done during sunscreen formulation. The oil dispersion was then emulsified by dilution in pure water. An oil/water emulsion with a nominal concentration of 5 mL/L was obtained. This emulsion was then added to the embryo culture medium at nominal concentrations of 0.005, 0.05, and 0.5 mg/L. In preparing the different dispersion concentrations, a constant volume of oil was injected into the culture medium, and only the NP concentration was varied. A pure oil/water emulsion was also prepared as an oil control reference. Tests were accepted if the percentage of control embryos at 48 h of development was ≥80%, as recommended by standard procedure [24].

The degree of toxicity per treatment was calculated using the standard criteria of evaluation based on the calculation of the percentage of normal versus abnormal embryos for a sample of 100 embryos (in triplicate) by optical microscopy (48 h of development endpoint). Embryonic development was also kept under observation to evaluate the occurrence and timing of several morphological events related to the endoderm, ectoderm, and mesoderm (germ layers) development and differentiation, as reported by Pinsino et al. [25].

2.3. Adult Sea Urchin Immune Cell Exposure

Adult sea urchins (*Paracentrotus lividus*) were collected along the northwest coast of Sicily and were acclimated and maintained under controlled conditions of temperature (16 ± 2 °C), pH (8.1 ± 0.1), salinity (38–39‰), and density (1.028–1.030 g/cm^3) in oxygenated ASW (Aqua Ocean Reef Plus Marine Salt, Aquarium Line, Bari, Italy).

Approximately 0.5 mL of coelomic fluid containing freely circulating immune cells were collected from each sea urchin using a 1-mL sterile syringe already containing 0.5 mL of anticoagulant solution, namely Coelomocyte Culture Medium (CCM), composed of 1 M NaCl, 10 mM $MgCl_2$, 40 mM Hepes-4-(2-hydroxyethyl)-1-piperazineethanesulfonic acid- and 2 mM EGTA - ethylene glycol tetra-acetic acid- at pH 7.2. After collection, the immune cells were counted in a Fast-Read chamber (Biosigma, Madison, Wisconsin, USA), and morphological analysis of cells was performed using the optical microscope.

After counting, immune cells were plated at a density of 1×10^5 cells/well in a 96-well white, opaque-walled plate (Thermo Fisher Scientific, Waltham, Massachusetts, USA) and exposed to a final volume of 100 µL T-AVO NPs that had been pre-dispersed in stock solutions of pure water (1 and 100 mg/L nominal concentration), sterilized under UV light, and vortexed for 5 min in order to homogenize the dispersions. The NPs were added to each cell culture medium to achieve five different concentrations (0.1, 1, 10, 100, 500 mg/L final concentration). Culturing was performed in the dark at 16 ± 2 °C. Cell viability and cytotoxicity were measured using the RealTime-Glo MT Cell Viability Assay (Promega, Madison, Wisconsin, USA) and the non-lytic CellTox™ Green Cytotoxicity Assay (Promega, USA), respectively, as previously described [26]. Luminescence and fluorescence were detected using a GloMax Discover high-performance Microplate Reader (Promega). All assays involved at least five biological replicates (specimens).

2.4. Metabolite Renewal Analysis by Mass Spectrometry in Untargeted Liquid Chromatography

Liquid chromatography-mass spectrometry (LC-MS analysis) was performed to analyze the metabolite profile of sea urchin cells exposed to hydrophilic NPs, according to previously established protocols [27]. Metabolites were isolated in 0.5 mL ice-cold 1% acetic acid water–acetonitrile solution (70:30 v/v). Supernatants were recovered in glass inserts for solvent evaporation, dried at 30 °C for approximately 2.5 h (Concentrator plus/Vacufuge® plus, Eppendorf, Juelich, Germany,), re-suspended in 150 µL of H_2O LC-MS grade, and injected into the UHPLC (Ultra high performance liquid chromatography)–MS system for reversed-phase liquid chromatography (RPLC). Data analysis and isotopic natural abundance correction were performed with MassHunter ProFinder and Mass Pro le Professional software (Agilent, Santa Clara, California, USA).

Samples were analyzed using an UHPLC system (Agilent 1290 Infinity UHPLC system) coupled with a quadrupole time-of-flight hybrid mass spectrometer (Agilent 6550 iFunnel Q-TOF) and equipped with an electrospray Dual JetStream source. The LC reversed phase was separated using an InfintyLab Poroshell 120 PFP-pentafluorophenyl-column (2.1 × 100 mm, 2.7 µm; Agilent Technologies) at a volume of 15 µL, a flow rate of 0.2 mL/min, and a temperature of 35 °C. Both the mobile phase A (100% water) and B (100% acetonitrile) contained 0.1% formic acid. The elution gradient was (1) 0 min, 100% A, (2) 2 min, 100% A, (3) 4 min, 99% A, (4) 10 min, 98% A, (5) 11 min, 70% A, (6) 15 min, 70% A, and (7) 16 min, 100% A followed by 5 min of post-run. Mass spectra were recorded in centroid mode in a mass range from m/z 60 to 1050 m/z. The mass spectrometer operated using a capillary voltage of 3.7 kV. Source temperature was set to 285 °C with a 14 L/min drying gas and a nebulizer pressure of 45 psig (pounds per square inch gauge). Fragmentor, skimmer, and octopole voltages were set to 175, 65, and 750 V, respectively.

Active reference mass correction was performed through a second nebulizer using the reference solution (m/z 112.9855 and 1033.9881) dissolved in the mobile phase 2-propanol-acetonitrile-water (70:20:10 v/v).

2.5. Characterization of the NPs by High-Resolution Scanning Electron Microscopy

The primary particle length of the NPs was measured using high-resolution scanning electron microscopy (HR-SEM). Three to four milligrams of the four pristine TiO_2 NP powders (T-S, T-Lite, T-AVO, P25 TiO_2) were dispersed on carbon adhesive tape and analyzed using a Zeiss Gemini500-Field emission SEM. To obtain surface-sensitive imaging at nanoscale resolution, images were recorded at low voltage (1–5 kV) with an in-lens secondary electron detector. Image analysis was then completed in order to distinguish the smallest particulate units constituting the powder grains. The primary particle lengths were obtained from the largest dimension of these smallest units. Fifty particles per sample were measured in order to calculate an average primary particle length.

2.6. Characterization of the NP Dispersions by Dynamic Light Scattering

The size distribution of the studied NPs was measured in their respective original dispersing medium (water or oil) using dynamic light scattering. These dispersions corresponded to the NPs as prepared before injection into the exposure media for the in vivo assay. P25 TiO_2 and T-AVO NPs were each dispersed in pure water at a nominal concentration of 125 mg/L by agitating the appropriate mass of the pristine powders in 5 mL.

The oily dispersions of T-S and T-Lite NPs were prepared by dispersing the UV filters in the commercial cosmetic oil by mechanical agitation at 1000 rpm rotation speed for 10 min, at a nominal NP concentration of 25 g/L using a *Heidolph Hei-Torque* 400 stirrer equipped with a pitcher blade impeller. The hydrophobic UV filters were analyzed in oil at a solid concentration 200 times as high as that for hydrophilic UV filters because in the in vivo assay the oil dispersion was further emulsified by dilution in water but the NP concentration remained locally high in the oil droplets. Moreover, since such complex dispersion/emulsion systems cannot be measured by dynamic light scattering (DLS), only the original oil dispersion was measured here in order to provide insights on the NP aggregation state in the oil droplet.

The size measurements were performed in triplicate at 25 °C with 11 runs per measurement, normal resolution analysis, and 0.01 cumulant fit error tolerance, using a *Zetasizer Nano* (Malvern Instruments, Malvern, UK).

The characterization of the particles and the degree of dispersibility in each pre-dispersant medium are reported in Supplementary Materials.

2.7. Statistical Analysis in Biological Assays

Statistical analyses were performed by GraphPad Prism Software 6.01 (USA). Statistical differences among selected groups were estimated by one-way ANOVA (followed by the multiple comparison tests). The p-value lower than 0.05 was deemed statistically significant. Data were expressed as mean ± standard deviation (SD).

3. Results and Discussion

3.1. Influence of TiO_2 NP-Based UV Filters on the Growth of Sea Urchin Embryos

The TiO_2 NPs used as commercial UV filters in sunscreen consist of the rutile lattice form, which is known to be less photoreactive and less toxic than other forms (i.e., anatase, brookite) [16,17]. They are generally coated with a surface passivation layer aimed at suppressing the rutile photocatalytic activity (e.g., Al_2O_3, SiO_2) and a secondary layer added to enhance particle dispersion in the cosmetic formulation (e.g., hydrophobic polydimethylsiloxane, hydrophilic Na-polyacrylate). Recent field studies of recreational bathing waters have evidenced a distinct fate for the hydrophobic compounds released from sunscreen [19,20]). Notably, measured TiO_2 concentrations were higher (up to 1000x) in the water top surface layer (0.1–0.9 mg/L) than in the water column (0.02–0.05 mg/L).

Here, we investigated the effects of increasing concentrations of three TiO_2 NP-based UV filters on the sea urchin *P. lividus* in the embryonic life-cycle stage. Embryos were classified as normal only when they satisfied all the following morphological criteria: (1) Acceptable schedule in reaching the developmental endpoint; (2) dorso/ventral and left/right embryonic axis symmetry; (3) correct differentiation of oral/aboral endoderm and ectoderm; and (4) correct mesenchyme differentiation, distribution pattern, and shape. At the gastrula stage (24 h of development), embryos exposed from fertilization maintained a regular time schedule and proper sites of spicule elongation at all concentrations tested (not shown). In agreement, at the pluteus stage (48 h) TiO_2 NP-based UV filter-exposed embryos displayed a low number of abnormalities (Figure 1). A slight increase in the incidence of potential morphological abnormalities was observed only in embryos exposed to 1 mg/L of the T-AVO UV filter (hydrophilic) and 0.05 mg/L of the T-Lite UV filter (hydrophobic). Specifically, about 20% of the embryos exhibited problems on arm and skeleton rod development and/or randomly distributed atypical big cells (Figure 2). The most common skeletal malformations observed were: (1) Crossed or separated tips at the hood apex arms (Figure 2, red arrows); (2) asymmetrical arm lengths; and (3) decrease or increase in arm growth and supporting skeletal rods (Figure 2, black arrows, oral and post-oral skeletal rods). Similar skeleton-defective embryos were previously observed in *P. lividus* embryos exposed to other types of NPs, suggesting that skeleton abnormalities could be considered a sensitive target to NP exposure [28,29]. Besides, the formation of big cells or masses (Figure 2, blue arrows) was previously observed in *P. lividus* embryos exposed to PS-NH$_2$ NPs and in *Strongylocentrotus droebachiensis* embryos exposed to Ag NPs [25,30]. These cells could be mesodermal cells involved in NP internalization (immune defense). Others have reported that NP internalization can initiate the immune response responsible for the formation of big mesodermal cells [25], such as those seen in Figure 2. However, this hypothesis remains essentially speculative because NP internalization was not verified here. Notably, other plausible explanations cannot yet be excluded, such as the possibility that the formation of big cells or masses may be caused by other compounds and not by NP internalization. However, similar effects were not observed in embryos exposed to the pure sunscreen oil phase only (Figure 1b), indicating that the oil phase compounds could not be incriminated in the formation of big cells or masses. Further studies are needed to clarify the underlying mechanism.

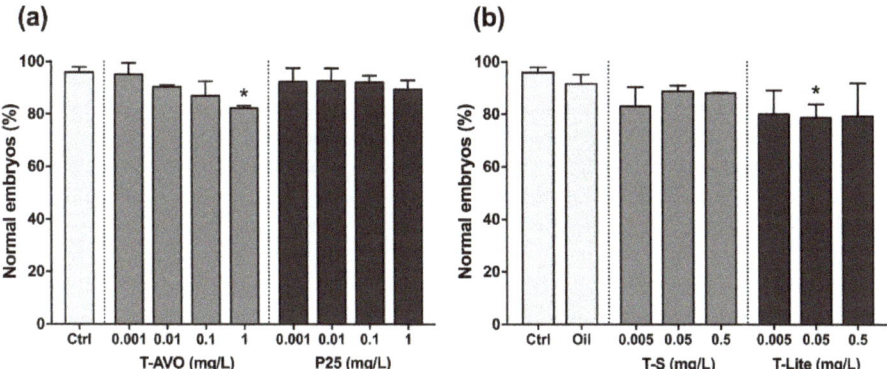

Figure 1. The hydrophilic and hydrophobic TiO$_2$ NP-based UV filters at different concentrations and dispersant phases influence the sea urchin embryonic development without producing a relevant developmental impairment. Histograms represent the results expressed as mean percentage (%) of normal embryos ± standard deviation after 48 h of exposure to the (**a**) hydrophilic (T-AVO and P25) and (**b**) hydrophobic (T-S and T-Lite) TiO$_2$ NP-based UV filters. * $p < 0.05$.

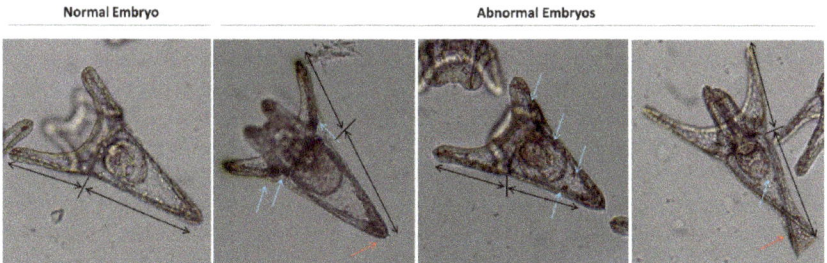

Figure 2. Optical images of representative sea urchin *Paracentrotus lividus* exposed to TiO$_2$ NP-based UV filters. Black arrows indicate decrease or increase in arm growth and supporting skeletal rods. Red arrows indicate crossed or separated tips at the hood apex arms. Blue arrows indicate the atypical big cells found in abnormally developed embryos.

In addition, we would like to point out that the morphological abnormalities observed in the sea urchin embryos exposed to NPs may not even be of ecological significance. Indeed, there was no evidence that these abnormalities reduced larvae survival ability, thus endangering a whole of one population.

Li et al. proposed a model of interaction between NPs and lipid layers of the plasma membrane based on the hydrophobic/hydrophilic nature of particles [31]. Based on the model, they suggested that hydrophobic NPs, which are thermodynamically stable around the core of a bilayer hydrophobic membrane, lead to lipid molecule deformation and distribution, whereas hydrophilic NPs that adsorb on the membrane surface (ready to be phagocytized) enter the hydrophobic core of the membrane, maintaining it intact. The primary particle shape also influences and modulates the particle behavior in a medium and its subsequent biological effect on a living system. Brown et al. argued that rod-shaped NPs could interact more strongly with biological systems than round-shaped NPs because the van der Waals interaction forces in lengthwise-oriented NPs increase proportionally to their length, typically reaching values several orders of magnitude above that of spheres [32]. Based on this theory, the elongated shape of T-AVO NPs compared to the P25 TiO_2 NPs (Figure S1, Supplementary Materials) would facilitate the interaction of particles with the membranes.

It is unclear how the dispersion states of the different UV filters measured here in the aqueous or oil cosmetic medium (Table S1, Supplementary Materials) are altered after dispersion and dilution in the aqueous culture medium. Aggregation and sedimentation will surely occur in artificial seawater for the hydrophilic UV filters pre-dispersed in water because salt-induced aggregation is a well-known effect in such a system [33]. On the contrary, further aggregation is not expected for the hydrophobic UV filters, as they should remain in the oil phase during the exposure. It is important to mention that hydrophobic filters trapped in the surface microlayer may not be bioavailable to the organisms living in suspension because the oil phase does not naturally mix with water. However, the surfactant molecules used in the cosmetic formulation may favor the mixing of the aqueous and oil phases and might play a determining role here (Table 2). For example, it is known that the octyldodecyl xyloside has high affinity for T-Lite NP surface [13]. Thus, we can reasonably assume that once washed of the consumer's skin, these molecules can modify the NP fate in the aquatic environment and their subsequent bioavailability for the marine organisms.

Overall, our results confirmed that the tested hydrophilic and hydrophobic TiO_2 NP-based sunscreen filters do not elicit significant harmful effects on sea urchin embryonic development. Of note, we were not fully satisfied with the efficacy of our evaluation assay with the hydrophobic UV filters pre-dispersed in the oil. Increasing the NP concentration in the oil implies an increase in viscosity. This makes the approach difficult to apply at high concentrations, as well as in tests under static conditions (e.g., primary immune cell culture). For this reason, only the hydrophilic TiO_2 NPs were used in subsequent immune cell-based assays.

3.2. Sea Urchin Adult Immune Cells: Health State and Metabolic Typing under Hydrophilic TiO_2 NPs

An ideal sunscreen active agent should remain localized close to the skin surface without penetrating into the deeper layers because by entering in the systemic circulation it could stimulate immune reactions. The sea urchin *P. lividus* can function as a proxy for humans for in vitro immunological studies [34]. Thus, to focus on the sea urchin immunological tolerance to the silica-coated TiO_2 NP-based UV filters we assessed the viability and cytotoxicity of the exposed immune cells to the hydrophilic T-AVO NPs for 48 h and we characterized their metabolic profile after 72 h of exposure. Cell viability and cytotoxicity were monitored and measured in real time for cells exposed to increasing concentrations of T-AVO NPs (0.1, 1, 10, 100, 500 mg/L). Only the measurements at 48 h are shown (Figure 3). The highest concentrations (100, 500 mg/L) were used as positive controls to demonstrate the appropriateness of the procedures.

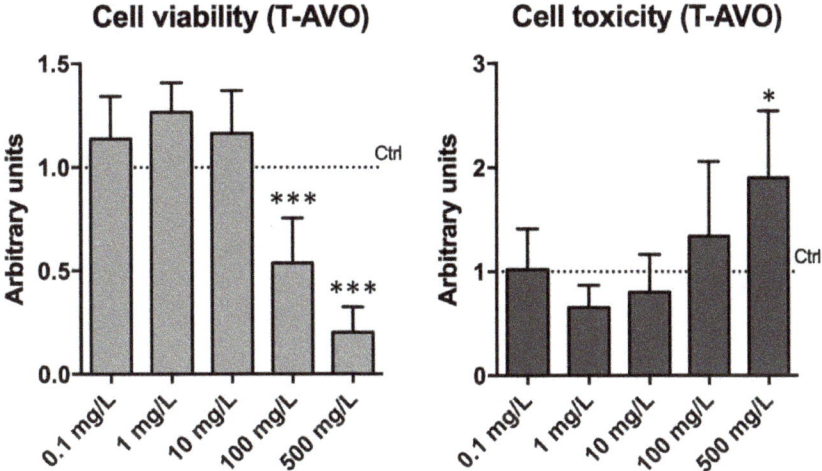

Figure 3. Impact of T-AVO UV filters on the sea urchin immune cell viability and toxicity. Real-time viability over two days of continuous monitoring, of which one measurement point (48) is shown (0.1, 1, 10, 100, 500 mg/L final concentration). The highest doses (100 and 500 mg/L) provoked decreases in cell viability and increase in cell toxicity. Levels are expressed in arbitrary units as fold increase or decrease compared to controls assumed as 1 (dot line). Data are reported as the mean ± SD; stars (*) indicate significant differences among groups (* $p < 0.05$; *** $p < 0.001$).

Our results confirmed those obtained from the sea urchin embryonic development assay, where no significant toxic effects were found at concentrations from 0.1 to 10 mg/L. At the two highest concentrations of exposure (100 and 500 mg/L), a significant decrease in viability and a high cell toxicity were measured, as expected. At these concentrations, faster NP aggregation likely led to particle destabilization and sedimentation, which, in turn, affected cellular viability due to the aggregate–cell physical contact. For samples exposed to 0.1–10 mg/L T-AVO, the RealTime-Glo MT cell viability assay indicated an increase (not statistically significant) in cell viability/metabolic activity compared to unexposed controls. Notably, the chemistry assay is based on the reducing potential of the cell, which is a known metabolic marker of cell viability. This result may be due to a hysteresis response usually observed under drug administration, in which the effect of a drug declines despite its continued presence (drug tolerance) [35]. Studies elucidating metabolic profiles of immune cells exposed to T-AVO were, therefore, carried out to confirm this increased metabolic activity, as reported below.

Immune functions are bio-energetically expensive, requiring accurate management of metabolites coordinated by intracellular and extracellular signals, which direct the uptake, storage, and utilization of substrates (e.g., glucose, amino acids, fatty acids). In turn, metabolites renew and control immune responses [36]. In order to obtain integrated data on the sea urchin immune metabolic state during exposure to hydrophilic TiO_2 NP-based UV filters and their related tolerance state, we characterized the metabolic profile of cells exposed to T-AVO and compared it with the profiles of cells exposed to P25 and unexposed cells (72 h in culture) (Figure 4). To this purpose we used an initial higher dose of particles (2 mg/L, loading dose) to achieve a lower maintenance dose (1 mg/L).

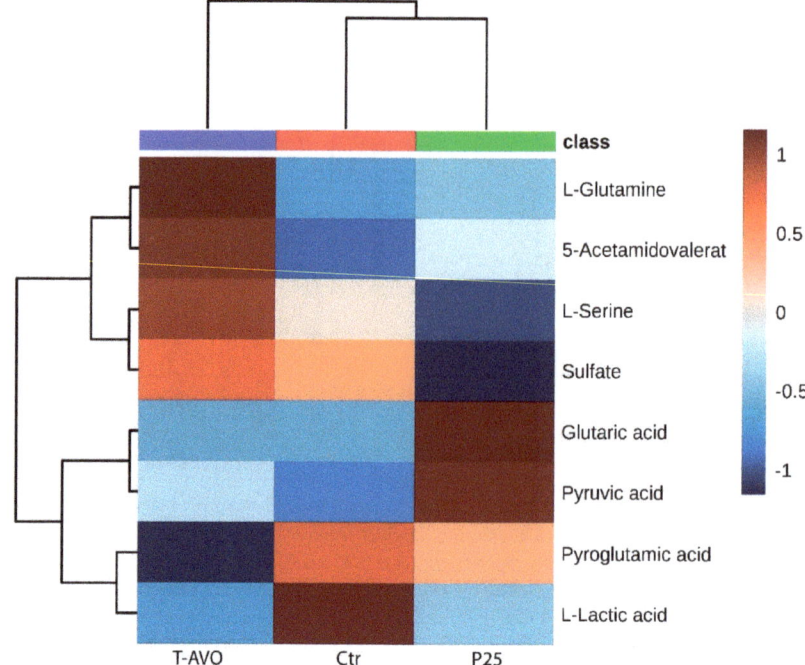

Figure 4. Sea urchin immune cell metabolic profile under hydrophilic nano-TiO$_2$-based UV filters. Untargeted metabolic profiling of T-AVO and P25 exposed for one day at 2 mg/L and for two days at 1 mg/L and unexposed immune cells (Ctr) for 72 h. Hierarchical clustering heatmaps display significantly ($p \leq 0.05$) different intracellular metabolites by LC-MS. Metabolic typing was performed on *P. lividus* primary immune cell cultures obtained from five individual donors.

Metabolite profiling identified level changes of only eight metabolites among groups (Group 1: T-AVO 1-day exposure at 2 mg L^{-1} followed by 2-days exposure at 1 mg L^{-1}; Group 2: Control, 3 days; Group 3: P25 1-day exposure at 2 mg/L followed by 2-days exposure at 1 mg/L), including proteinogenic amino acids (serine, glutamine), amino acid derivatives (L-pyroglutamic acid), organic acids (L-lactic acid, glutaric acid, pyruvic acid), sulfate metabolites (sulfate), and acetamides (acetamidovalerate). Sea urchin T-AVO-responsive metabolites predominantly involved in mediating inflammatory signals and phagocytosis were found. Specifically, glutamine and acetamidovalerate were significantly increased compared to unexposed controls, while L-pyroglutamic acid and L-lactic acid were significantly decreased. It is well known that to re-establish normal cellular and molecular function, immune cells have higher glutamine needs during inflammatory states [37]. Notably, acetamides are known to relieve inflammatory events; in fact, they are used as chemotherapeutic agents for inflammation-associated cancers [38].

Lactic acid is produced in high amounts by innate immune cells during inflammatory activation (anaerobic glycolysis product). A reduction in its amount may be translated into a negative feedback signal to silence or attenuate inflammatory responses [39].

Increased levels of pyroglutamic acid (also called 5-oxoproline) are able to promote lipid and protein oxidation and to enhance hydrogen peroxide content, thus promoting oxidative stress [40]. Consequently, the significantly decreased pyroglutamic acid levels observed under T-AVO exposure may be considered a signal of an increased antioxidant metabolic activity. Although slight, L-serine and pyruvic acid levels were also increased compared to those in unexposed cells. Serine racemase enzyme catalyzes the α, β elimination of water from L-serine to produce pyruvate and ammonia [41].

Notably, L-serine metabolism is required for fueling one-carbon metabolism and nucleotide biosynthesis, and it is known to lower the inflammatory responses in mice during infection [42].

The P25 TiO_2 bare NPs were used here as a negative control for the silica-functionalized T-AVO. In our recent studies we demonstrated that under TiO_2 NP exposure (1 mg/L TiO_2 NPs, 24 h endpoint) the innate sea urchin immune system is able to control inflammatory signaling, excite antioxidant metabolic activity, and acquire immunological tolerance [27,43]. Notably, sea urchin immune system metabolic typing under P25 exposure for 72 h (one day of exposure at 2 mg/L followed by two days of exposure at 1 mg/L) highlighted a different scenario compared to the respective T-AVO and control groups. L-glutamine, acetamidovalerate, and pyriglutamic acid levels all presented a trend similar to controls, while lactic acid levels were similar to T-AVO-exposed cells and pyruvic acid levels were considerably increased. Interestingly, L-serine, sulfate, and glutaric acid levels presented a trend completely different to both T-AVO and control groups. Specifically, L-serine and sulfate were reduced compared to controls, while glutaric acid levels increased, highlighting an ongoing inflammatory state. These findings show the superior immune compatibility of T-AVO compared to P25 when particles stay in contact with the sea urchin immune cells for 72 h (one day of exposure at 2 mg/L, and two days of exposure at the half dose). Based on the notion that the silica coating of commercial TiO_2 NP-based UV filters undergoes a fast degradation once released into aquatic media (88–98% silica removal within 96 h) [44], we speculated that the T-AVO in contact with cells after 72 h of exposure consisted of mainly pure rutile. Worth noting is the fact that not only the shape but also the crystal composition of TiO_2 particles (e.g., T-AVO: Pure rutile; P25: Anatase:Rutile) makes their use more or less safe, as documented in the literature [45].

Overall, our results demonstrate that the commercial TiO_2 NP-based UV filters tested in this work do not show any significant harmful impact toward the development or immunity of the sea urchin (*P. lividus*) at NP concentrations expected near the seashore during summer recreational activities. A summary view of the experimental setup and the results is schematized in Figure 5.

These results are in accordance with the majority of risk assessment studies on different marine organisms using pure rutile or anatase NPs that are summarized in the most relevant reviews [3,46]. The different coatings on the commercial UV filters, together with particle shape and the original dispersant phase, slightly modulate the effects toward embryo development but without causing a relevant developmental impairment. In this context, the particle shape of hydrophilic NPs pre-dispersed in water, predominantly influences the interaction with sea urchin embryos compared with other physical features such as primary particle size or aggregation state. Particularly, the elongated, rod-shaped T-AVO NPs slightly impacted the development compared to the more spherical P25 NPs. The effects of hydrophobic UV filters are, instead, in line with their respective dispersion capacity in the former sunscreen oily dispersant medium, which is directly related to their different particle external coatings. The more finely dispersed T-Lite NPs showed a few visible effects compared to the T-S NPs, probably because of specific interactions with the octyldodecyl xyloside surfactant present in the sunscreen oily medium, which would likely ease its transportation inside the embryonic culture medium.

Viability and toxicity tests on immune cells showed no toxicity of T-AVO NPs at concentrations consistent with that of the cosmetic life cycle. Furthermore, metabolic profile characterization performed on P25 and T-AVO NPs showed that the T-AVO NPs have a superior immune compatibility to that of the P25 after 72 h of interaction with sea urchin immune cells, ultimately supporting the safety of this type of commercial TiO_2-based UV filter on the immunological state of the sea urchin.

Notably, the application of metabolomics in the environmental field is relatively new, but the technique is actively attracting the attention of the scientific community because results obtained successfully describe a "picture" of the biochemistry of an organism, cell, or tissue at any one time [47].

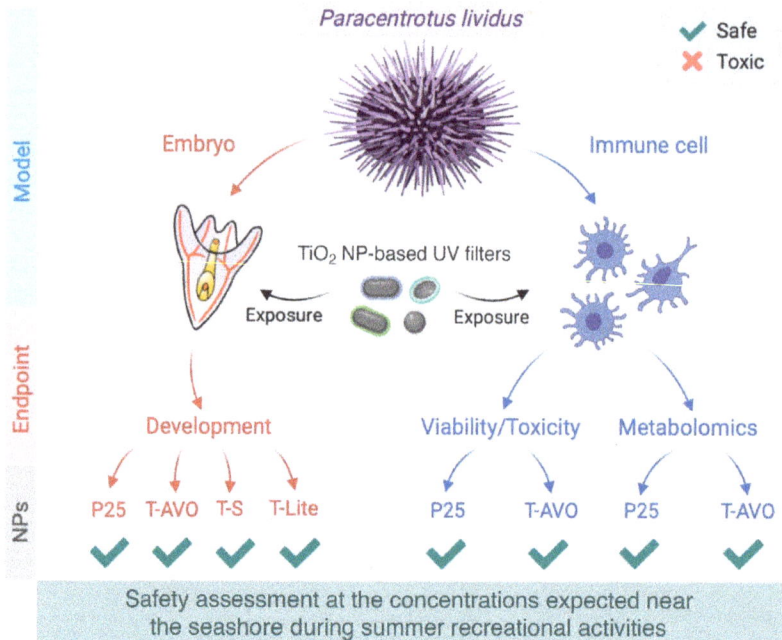

Figure 5. Schematic illustration of the results obtained from the evaluation of the TiO_2 NP-based sunscreen UV filters on the development and the immunological state of the sea urchin *Paracentrotus lividus*. Models: Sea urchin embryos and adult *P. lividus* immune cells in vitro. Endpoints: Sea urchin embryos at the pluteus stage (48 h), immune cell viability/toxicity (48 h), and metabolomics (72 h). Commercial nanoparticulate UV filters with three surface coatings: T-S, T-Lite, and T-AVO tested on embryonic development and T-AVO on immune cells. P25 was used as an uncoated nano-TiO_2 reference. The results presented here highlight the biosafety of TiO_2 NP-based UV filters on sea urchin, and the importance of developing safer-by-design sunscreens and evaluating the associated risk. Created by Andi Alijagic using BioRender.com.

4. Conclusions

Our findings underline the importance of developing sustainable sunscreen formulations based on nanoparticulate UV filters, rather than the bare NP counterpart, to minimize the environmental risk posed by sunscreen products. Further studies with a similar approach need to be performed in the future, on different biological models and with different experimental conditions, in order to fully confirm the safety of these nano-products. Primary cell cultures accurately represent the biological microenvironment in which cells reside in tissues, as cell–cell signaling remains preserved [48]. However, the next step should be to study the immunological state of the sea urchins and other organisms that live in the beaches during recreational activity (field study).

Supplementary Materials: The following are available online at http://www.mdpi.com/2079-4991/10/11/2102/s1, Figure S1: High-resolution scanning electron microscopy (HR-SEM) analysis of the pristine TiO_2-based NPs. Table S1: Comparison of primary particle size and hydrodynamic aggregate size of the TiO_2NPs.

Author Contributions: R.C.: investigation, writing-original draft preparation; J.L.: conceptualisation, data interpretation, writing—review and editing, project administration; D.G., A.A., E.N., and A.C.: methodology and data curation; D.S.: writing—review and editing; A.P.: conceptualisation, supervision, data interpretation, writing—review and editing, project administration. All authors have read and agreed to the published version of the manuscript.

Funding: This project was funded from the European Union's Horizon 2020 research and innovation program under the Marie Skłodowska-Curie grant agreement [No 671881], the Marie Skłodowska-Curie grant agreement [No 713750], and from the Excellence Initiative of Aix-Marseille University—A*MIDEX, a French "Investissements d'Avenir" program, through its associated Labex SERENADE project. This work is also a contribution to the OSU-Institut Pythéas.

Acknowledgments: The authors gratefully acknowledge M. Biondo for his technical support and sea urchin husbandry.

Conflicts of Interest: The authors declare no conflict of interest.

References

1. Schneider, S.L.; Lim, H.W. A Review of Inorganic UV Filters Zinc Oxide and Titanium Dioxide. *Photodermatol. Photoimmunol. Photomed.* **2019**, *35*, 442–446. [CrossRef]
2. Ngoc, L.T.N.; Tran, V.V.; Moon, J.-Y.; Chae, M.; Park, D.; Lee, Y.-C. Recent Trends of Sunscreen Cosmetic: An Update Review. *Cosmetics* **2019**, *6*, 64. [CrossRef]
3. Slijkerman, D.M.E.; Keur, M. *Sunscreen Ecoproducts: Product Claims, Potential Effects and Environmental Risks of Applied UV Filters*; Wageningen Marine Research report C056/18; Wageningen Marine Research: Den Helder, The Netherlands, 2018.
4. Paredes, E.; Perez, S.; Rodil, R.; Quintana, J.B.; Beiras, R. Ecotoxicological Evaluation of Four UV Filters Using Marine Organisms from Different Trophic Levels Isochrysis Galbana, Mytilus Galloprovincialis, Paracentrotus Lividus, and Siriella Armata. *Chemosphere* **2014**, *104*, 44–50. [CrossRef]
5. Fent, K.; Kunz, P.Y.; Zenker, A.; Rapp, M. A Tentative Environmental Risk Assessment of the UV-Filters 3-(4-Methylbenzylidene-Camphor), 2-Ethyl-Hexyl-4-Trimethoxycinnamate, Benzophenone-3, Benzophenone-4 and 3-Benzylidene Camphor. *Mar. Environ. Res.* **2010**, *69*, S4–S6. [CrossRef] [PubMed]
6. Downs, C.A.; Kramarsky-Winter, E.; Segal, R.; Fauth, J.; Knutson, S.; Bronstein, O.; Ciner, F.R.; Jeger, R.; Lichtenfeld, Y.; Woodley, C.M.; et al. Toxicopathological Effects of the Sunscreen UV Filter, Oxybenzone (Benzophenone-3), on Coral Planulae and Cultured Primary Cells and Its Environmental Contamination in Hawaii and the U.S. Virgin Islands. *Arch. Environ. Contam. Toxicol.* **2016**, *70*, 265–288. [CrossRef] [PubMed]
7. Matta, M.K.; Zusterzeel, R.; Pilli, N.R.; Patel, V.; Volpe, D.A.; Florian, J.; Oh, L.; Bashaw, E.; Zineh, I.; Sanabria, C.; et al. Effect of sunscreen application under maximal use conditions on plasma concentration of sunscreen active ingredients: A randomized clinical trial. *JAMA* **2019**, *321*, 2082–2091. [CrossRef]
8. Food and Drug Administration (FDA). FDA Rules Regulations for Sunscreen. 2012. Available online: https://smartshield.com/news/reviews/54-resources/127-new-fda-rules-regulations-for-sunscreen (accessed on 1 March 2020).
9. Yung, M.M.N.; Wong, S.W.Y.; Kwok, K.W.H.; Liu, F.Z.; Leung, Y.H.; Chan, W.T.; Li, X.Y.; Djurišić, A.B.; Leung, K.M.Y. Salinity-Dependent Toxicities of Zinc Oxide Nanoparticles to the Marine Diatom Thalassiosira Pseudonana. *Aquat. Toxicol.* **2015**, *165*, 31–40. [CrossRef]
10. Corinaldesi, C.; Marcellini, F.; Nepote, E.; Damiani, E.; Danovaro, R. Impact of Inorganic UV Filters Contained in Sunscreen Products on Tropical Stony Corals (*Acropora* Spp.). *Sci. Total Environ.* **2018**, *637–638*, 1279–1285. [CrossRef]
11. Miller, R.J.; Lenihan, H.S.; Muller, E.B.; Tseng, N.; Hanna, S.K.; Keller, A.A. Impacts of Metal Oxide Nanoparticles on Marine Phytoplankton. *Environ. Sci. Technol.* **2010**, *44*, 7329–7334. [CrossRef]
12. Cole, C.; Shyr, T.; Ou-Yang, H. Metal Oxide Sunscreens Protect Skin by Absorption, Not by Reflection or Scattering. *Photodermatol. Photoimmunol. Photomed.* **2016**, *32*, 5–10. [CrossRef]
13. Catalano, R.; Masion, A.; Ziarelli, F.; Slomberg, D.; Laisney, J.; Unrine, J.M.; Campos, C.; Labille, J. Optimizing the dispersion of nanoparticulate TiO_2-based UV filters in a non-polar medium used in sunscreen formulations—The roles of surfactants and particle coatings. *Colloid Surface A.* **2020**, *599*, 124792. [CrossRef]
14. Auffan, M.; Rose, J.; Bottero, J.Y.; Lowry, G.V.; Jolivet, J.P.; Wiesner, M.R. Towards a definition of inorganic nanoparticles from an environmental, health and safety perspective. *Nat. Nanotechnol.* **2009**, *4*, 634–641. [CrossRef] [PubMed]
15. Minetto, D.; Libralato, G.; Volpi Ghirardini, A. Ecotoxicity of Engineered TiO_2 Nanoparticles to Saltwater Organisms: An Overview. *Environ. Int.* **2014**, *66*, 18–27. [CrossRef] [PubMed]
16. Gerloff, K.; Fenoglio, I.; Carella, E.; Kolling, J.; Albrecht, C.; Boots, A.W.; Förster, I.; Schins, R.P.F. Distinctive Toxicity of TiO_2 Rutile/Anatase Mixed Phase Nanoparticles on Caco-2 Cells. *Chem. Res. Toxicol.* **2012**, *25*, 646–655. [CrossRef]

17. Botta, C.; Labille, J.; Auffan, M.; Borschneck, D.; Miche, H.; Cabié, M.; Masion, A.; Rose, J.; Bottero, J.-Y. TiO2-Based Nanoparticles Released in Water from Commercialized Sunscreens in a Life-Cycle Perspective: Structures and Quantities. *Environ. Pollut.* **2011**, *159*, 1543–1550. [CrossRef]
18. Labille, J.; Catalano, R.; Slomberg, D.; Motellier, S.; Pinsino, A.; Hennebert, P.; Santaella, C.; Bartolomei, V. Assessing sunscreen lifecycle to minimise environmental risk posed by nanoparticulate UV-filters—A review for safer-by-design products. *Front. Environ. Sci.* **2020**, *8*, 101. [CrossRef]
19. Labille, J.; Slomberg, D.; Catalano, R.; Robert, S.; Apers-Tremelo, M.; Boudenne, J.; Manasfi, T.; Radakovitch, O. Assessing UV filter inputs into beach waters during recreational activity: A field study of three French Mediterranean beaches from consumer survey to water analysis. *Sci. Total Environ.* **2020**, *706*, 136010. [CrossRef]
20. Tovar-Sánchez, A.; Sánchez-Quiles, D.; Basterretxea, G.; Benedé, J.L.; Chisvert, A.; Salvador, A.; Moreno-Garrido, I.; Blasco, J. Sunscreen Products as Emerging Pollutants to Coastal Waters. *PLoS ONE* **2013**, *8*, e65451. [CrossRef]
21. Giese, B.; Klaessig, F.; Park, B.; Kaegi, R.; Steinfeldt, M.; Wigger, H.; von Gleich, A.; Gottschalk, F. Risks, Release and Concentrations of Engineered Nanomaterial in the Environment. *Sci. Rep.* **2018**, *8*, 1565. [CrossRef]
22. Tolaymat, T.; El Badawy, A.; Genaidy, A.; Abdelraheem, W.; Sequeira, R. Analysis of metallic and metal oxide nanomaterial environmental emissions. *J. Clean. Prod.* **2017**, *143*, 401–412. [CrossRef]
23. Pinsino, A.; Matranga, V. Sea Urchin Immune Cells as Sentinels of Environmental Stress. *Dev. Comp. Immunol.* **2015**, *49*, 198–205. [CrossRef] [PubMed]
24. ASTM. Standard Guide for Conducting Static Acute Toxicity Tests with Echinoid Embyos; E 1563-95. In *Annual Book of ASTM Standards*; ASTM: Philadelphia, PA, USA, 1995; Volume 11, pp. 999–1017.
25. Pinsino, A.; Bergami, E.; Della Torre, C.; Vannuccini, M.L.; Addis, P.; Secci, M.; Dawson, K.A.; Matranga, V.; Corsi, I. Amino-modified polystyrene nanoparticles affect signaling pathways of the sea urchin (*Paracentrotus lividus*) embryos. *Nanotoxicology* **2017**, *11*, 201–209. [CrossRef] [PubMed]
26. Pinsino, A.; Alijagic, A. Sea urchin Paracentrotus lividus immune cells in culture: Formulation of the appropriate harvesting and culture media and maintenance conditions. *Biol. Open* **2019**, *8*, bio039289. [CrossRef]
27. Alijagic, A.; Gaglio, D.; Napodano, E.; Russo, R.; Costa, C.; Benada, O.; Kofroňová, O.; Pinsino, A. Titanium Dioxide Nanoparticles Temporarily Influence the Sea Urchin Immunological State Suppressing Inflammatory-Relate Gene Transcription and Boosting Antioxidant Metabolic Activity. *J. Hazard. Mater.* **2020**, *384*, 121389. [CrossRef]
28. Gambardella, C.; Aluigi, M.G.; Ferrando, S.; Gallus, L.; Ramoino, P.; Gatti, A.M.; Rottigni, M.; Falugi, C. Developmental Abnormalities and Changes in Cholinesterase Activity in Sea Urchin Embryos and Larvae from Sperm Exposed to Engineered Nanoparticles. *Aquat. Toxicol.* **2013**, *130–131*, 77–85. [CrossRef] [PubMed]
29. Carballeira, C.; Ramos-Gómez, J.; Martín-Díaz, L.; DelValls, T.A. Identification of Specific Malformations of Sea Urchin Larvae for Toxicity Assessment: Application to Marine Pisciculture Effluents. *Mar. Environ. Res.* **2012**, *77*, 12–22. [CrossRef]
30. Magesky, A.; Pelletier, É. Toxicity Mechanisms of Ionic Silver and Polymer-Coated Silver Nanoparticles with Interactions of Functionalized Carbon Nanotubes on Early Development Stages of Sea Urchin. *Aquat. Toxicol.* **2015**, *167*, 106–123. [CrossRef]
31. Li, Y.; Chen, X.; Gu, N. Computational Investigation of Interaction between Nanoparticles and Membranes: Hydrophobic/Hydrophilic Effect. *J. Phys. Chem. B* **2008**, *112*, 16647–16653. [CrossRef]
32. Brown, S.C.; Kamal, M.; Nasreen, N.; Baumuratov, A.; Sharma, P.; Antony, V.B.; Moudgil, B.M. Influence of Shape, Adhension and Simulated Lung Mechanics on Amorphous Silica Nanoparticle Toxicity. *Adv. Powder Technol.* **2007**, *18*, 69–79. [CrossRef]
33. Labille, J.; Brant, J. Stability of Nanoparticles in Water. *Nanomedicine* **2010**, *5*, 985–998. [CrossRef]
34. Alijagic, A.; Barbero, F.; Gaglio, D.; Napodano, E.; Benada, O.; Kofroňová, O.; Puntes, V.F.; Bastùs, N.G.; Pinsino, A. Gold nanoparticles coated with polyvinylpyrrolidone and sea urchin extracellular molecules induce transient immune activation. *J. Hazard. Mater.* **2021**, *402*, 123793. [CrossRef]
35. Pleuvry, B.J. Hysteresis in Drug Response. *Anaesth. Intensive Care Med.* **2008**, *9*, 372–373. [CrossRef]
36. Ganeshan, K.; Chawla, A. Metabolic Regulation of Immune Responses. *Annu. Rev. Immunol.* **2014**, *32*, 609–634. [CrossRef]

37. De Oliveira, D.C.; da Silva Lima, F.; Sartori, T.; Santos, A.C.A.; Rogero, M.M.; Fock, R.A. Glutamine Metabolism and Its Effects on Immune Response: Molecular Mechanism and Gene Expression. *Nutrire* **2016**, *41*, 14. [CrossRef]
38. Rani, P.; Pal, D.; Hegde, R.R.; Hashim, S.R. Acetamides: Chemotherapeutic Agents for Inflammation-Associated Cancers. *J. Chemother.* **2016**, *28*, 255–265. [CrossRef]
39. Ratter, J.M.; Rooijackers, H.M.M.; Hooiveld, G.J.; Hijmans, A.G.M.; de Galan, B.E.; Tack, C.J.; Stienstra, R. In Vitro and in Vivo Effects of Lactate on Metabolism and Cytokine Production of Human Primary PBMCs and Monocytes. *Front. Immunol.* **2018**, *9*, 2564. [CrossRef]
40. Pederzolli, C.D.; Mescka, C.P.; Zandoná, B.R.; de Moura Coelho, D.; Sgaravatti, Â.M.; Sgarbi, M.B.; de Souza Wyse, A.T.; Duval Wannmacher, C.M.; Wajner, M.; Vargas, C.R.; et al. Acute Administration of 5-Oxoproline Induces Oxidative Damage to Lipids and Proteins and Impairs Antioxidant Defenses in Cerebral Cortex and Cerebellum of Young Rats. *Metab. Brain Dis.* **2010**, *25*, 145–154. [CrossRef]
41. Foltyn, V.N.; Bendikov, I.; De Miranda, J.; Panizzutti, R.; Dumin, E.; Shleper, M.; Li, P.; Toney, M.D.; Kartvelishvily, E.; Wolosker, H. Serine Racemase Modulates Intracellular D-Serine Levels through an α,β-Elimination Activity. *J. Biol. Chem.* **2005**, *280*, 1754–1763. [CrossRef] [PubMed]
42. He, F.; Yin, Z.; Wu, C.; Xia, Y.; Wu, M.; Li, P.; Zhang, H.; Yin, Y.; Li, N.; Zhu, G.; et al. L-Serine Lowers the Inflammatory Responses during *Pasteurella Multocida* Infection. *Infect. Immun.* **2019**, *87*, e00677-19. [CrossRef]
43. Alijagic, A.; Benada, O.; Kofroňová, O.; Cigna, D.; Pinsino, A. Sea Urchin Extracellular Proteins Design a Complex Protein Corona on Titanium Dioxide Nanoparticle Surface Influencing Immune Cell Behavior. *Front. Immunol.* **2019**, *10*, 2261. [CrossRef]
44. Slomberg, D.L.; Catalano, R.; Ziarelli, F.; Viel, S.; Bartolomei, V.; Labille, J.; Masion, A. Aqueous aging of a silica coated TiO2 UV filter used in sunscreens: Investigations at the molecular scale with dynamic nuclear polarization NMR. *RSC Adv.* **2020**, *10*, 8266–8274. [CrossRef]
45. Ziental, D.; Czarczynska-Goslinska, B.; Mlynarczyk, D.T.; Glowacka-Sobotta, A.; Stanisz, B.; Goslinski, T.; Sobotta, L. Titanium Dioxide Nanoparticles: Prospects and Applications in Medicine. *Nanomaterials* **2020**, *10*, 387. [CrossRef] [PubMed]
46. Wang, J.; Wang, W. Significance of Physicochemical and Uptake Kinetics in Controlling the Toxicity of Metallic Nanomaterials to Aquatic Organisms. *J. Zhejiang Univ. Sci. A* **2014**, *15*, 573–592. [CrossRef]
47. Alvarez-Munoz, D.; Farre, M. *Environmental Metabolomics. Applications in Field and Laboratory Studies to Understand from Exposome to Metabolome*, 1st ed.; Elsevier: Amsterdam, The Netherlands, 2020; ISBN 9780128181973.
48. Bols, N.C.; Pham, P.H.; Dayeh, V.R.; Lee, L.E.J. Invitromatics, invitrome, and invitroomics: Introduction of three new terms for in vitro biology and illustration of their use with the cell lines from rainbow trout. *In Vitro Cell. Dev. Biol. Anim.* **2017**, *53*, 383–405. [CrossRef]

Publisher's Note: MDPI stays neutral with regard to jurisdictional claims in published maps and institutional affiliations.

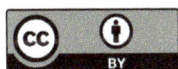 © 2020 by the authors. Licensee MDPI, Basel, Switzerland. This article is an open access article distributed under the terms and conditions of the Creative Commons Attribution (CC BY) license (http://creativecommons.org/licenses/by/4.0/).

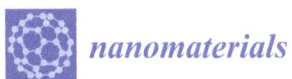

Article

The Effects of In Vivo Exposure to Copper Oxide Nanoparticles on the Gut Microbiome, Host Immunity, and Susceptibility to a Bacterial Infection in Earthworms

Elmer Swart [1,*], Jiri Dvorak [2], Szabolcs Hernádi [3], Tim Goodall [1], Peter Kille [3], David Spurgeon [1], Claus Svendsen [1,*] and Petra Prochazkova [2]

1. UK Centre for Ecology and Hydrology, Maclean Building, Benson Lane, Wallingford OX10 8BB, UK; timgoo@ceh.ac.uk (T.G.); dasp@ceh.ac.uk (D.S.)
2. Laboratory of Cellular and Molecular Immunology, Institute of Microbiology of the Czech Academy of Sciences, Videnska 1083, 142 20 Prague 4, Czech Republic; dvorak@biomed.cas.cz (J.D.); kohler@biomed.cas.cz (P.P.)
3. School of Biosciences, Cardiff University, Sir Martin Evans Building, Museum Avenue, Cardiff CF10 3AX, UK; hernadis1@cardiff.ac.uk (S.H.); kille@cardiff.ac.uk (P.K.)
* Correspondence: elmswa@ceh.ac.uk (E.S.); csv@ceh.ac.uk (C.S.); Tel.: +44-(0)1491-692626 (E.S.); +44-(0)1491-692676 (C.S.)

Received: 9 June 2020; Accepted: 6 July 2020; Published: 9 July 2020

Abstract: Nanomaterials (NMs) can interact with the innate immunity of organisms. It remains, however, unclear whether these interactions can compromise the immune functioning of the host when faced with a disease threat. Co-exposure with pathogens is thus a powerful approach to assess the immuno-safety of NMs. In this paper, we studied the impacts of in vivo exposure to a biocidal NM on the gut microbiome, host immune responses, and susceptibility of the host to a bacterial challenge in an earthworm. *Eisenia fetida* were exposed to CuO-nanoparticles in soil for 28 days, after which the earthworms were challenged with the soil bacterium *Bacillus subtilis*. Immune responses were monitored by measuring mRNA levels of known earthworm immune genes. Effects of treatments on the gut microbiome were also assessed to link microbiome changes to immune responses. Treatments caused a shift in the earthworm gut microbiome. Despite these effects, no impacts of treatment on the expression of earthworm immune markers were recorded. The methodological approach applied in this paper provides a useful framework for improved assessment of immuno-safety of NMs. In addition, we highlight the need to investigate time as a factor in earthworm immune responses to NM exposure.

Keywords: innate immunity; infection; microbiome; survival; nanomaterials; nanoparticles; copper; earthworms; *Eisenia fetida*

1. Introduction

Nanomaterials (NMs) are increasingly used in various applications including surface coatings, biocide pesticides, and electronics [1,2]. The potential risks of NM to human health and the environment have long been identified [3–5]. Over the last decade, research has provided vast amounts of toxicity data that have reduced many of the initial uncertainties around NM risk. There are, however, still some aspects that need further investigation. One of these remaining issues relates to the immuno-safety of NMs [6–8]. Owing to their particulate nature, NMs have an increased potential to interact with the innate immune system of organisms [9–12] and to induce both pro- and anti-inflammatory responses [13]. Most of the current research to investigate such effects has used in vitro models to characterize NM–immune interactions. Although these studies have provided crucial information on how immune systems may interact with NM, it remains unclear how responses in vitro will translate to in vivo effects. Further, immuno-modulation by NM does not necessarily indicate that the immune system is being compromised. In fact, immune reactions are part of a healthy response by the host towards foreign objects. In order to assess whether NMs actually compromise host immunity, co-exposure with infectious pathogens is necessary [7,8].

A major application of NMs is as antimicrobial agents in pesticides and coatings. The effects of biocidal NM on soil microbial communities have been relatively well studied [14–16]. There are, however, uncertainties concerning the impact of NMs on microbes associated with plants and animals (commonly referred to as 'microbiome') [17]. Common roles of the microbiome in host health include the provision of essential nutrients and aiding in digestion, while the role of the microbiome in host immunity is now increasingly being recognized [18–20]. Microbes associated with mucosal surfaces can contribute to immunity by providing resistance against invading pathogens [21–23] and by stimulating the release of antimicrobial peptides by the host [24]. Disruption of the healthy microbiome by, for example, chemical exposure, can lead to reduced immune functioning and reduced survival of bacterial infections [25–27]. Previous studies have shown that, when NMs alter the microbiome of animals, the expression of host immune genes can also change [28–31]. Host immunity and the microbiome are thus a complex and integrally linked system, and it is thus important to include microbiome analysis in the immuno-safety assessment of NM. Invertebrate animals such as earthworms, bivalves, and sea urchins provide suitable models to study in vivo effects of NM on immune functioning under more realistic environmental conditions [31–33].

Earthworms provide crucial ecosystem services in soils through mixing, organic matter degradation of plant material, and nutrient cycling, and thereby contribute to enhanced crop production [34]. Living in soil, earthworms inhabit an environment with high microbial activity. To provide protection from pathogens, cellular immunity in earthworms is provided by immune cells called coelomocytes, which circulate the coelomic cavity. A crucial element of the innate immune system is the recognition of microorganism associated molecular patterns (MAMPs) by host pathogen recognition receptors (PRRs). A well described PRR in earthworms is coelomic cytolytic factor (CCF). This PRR, upon binding to specific MAMPs, induces the prophenoloxidase pathway, which ultimately leads to the production of antimicrobial factors [35–37]. Earthworm pathogens are also controlled by various humoral factors. One of these is lysozyme, an enzyme that can hydrolyse components of the cell wall of Gram-positive bacteria [38]. In the earthworms *Eisenia fetida* and *Eisenia andrei*, immunity is also supported by the humoral factors lysenin [39] and fetidin [40,41], the modes of antibacterial action of which are not fully understood [40,42]. Recent work shows that changes in gene expression of these immune factors can be used as a marker of immune-modulation in earthworms [38,43,44]. In vitro studies have shown that exposure to NM can also alter the expression of earthworm immune genes [45,46]. Effects of in vivo exposure to NM earthworm immune system regulation have not been studied extensively [33] and it remains uncertain whether NM exposure can compromise earthworm immunity by affecting the host susceptibility to infections.

The earthworm gut microbiome has been relatively well described. Gut communities have been identified as being composed of both transient bacteria associated with ingested soil and food [47] and resident bacteria more closely associated to intestinal surfaces [48–50]. Loss of some core earthworm symbionts can lead to reduced host fitness and juvenile development [51,52]. Environmental pollutants can alter the microbiome of earthworms [53–56] and lead to the loss of core symbionts important to host health [57]. An increasing body of literature now indicates that exposure to NMs can also disrupt the microbiome of soil invertebrates [58–60]. In the earthworm *Enchytraeus crypticus*, for example, exposure to CuO-NP can significantly reduce the abundance of core intestinal *Plantomycetes* bacteria [58]. The interplay between microbiome, NMs, and host immunity in earthworms, however, has not been studied. Disruption of host–microbiome interactions can be expected for chemicals that are designed to target microbes (biocides). In agriculture, copper-based NM formulations are being developed for biocidal applications [61]. In widespread application, there is thus the potential for such NMs to negatively affect earthworms through alterations to their microbiome structure.

Because of the integrate link between the microbiome, host immunity, and health status of animals, studies on the immuno-safety assessment of NM require a holistic approach. This paper aims to study whether exposure to copper oxide nanoparticles (NPs) has an effect on the gut microbiome structure, host immunity, and susceptibility to a bacterial infection in earthworms. For this purpose, earthworms were exposed in soil to concentrations of copper forms known to alter the earthworm gut microbiome for a duration of 28 days. The earthworms were subsequently removed from soils and challenged with the bacterium *Bacillus subtilis* for a further four days. The effects of the bacterial challenge were assessed by looking at survival and tissue damage, and by measuring mRNA levels of known immune markers. An analysis of the gut microbiome was concurrently conducted through a metabarcoding approach to link the effects on microbiomes to immune responses. The effects of NP were compared to those of metal salts, to test whether any effects were attributed to particles or ions. We hypothesized that (i) earthworms that have their microbiome changed through exposure to CuO-NP and copper salts are more susceptible to a bacterial infection; and (ii) exposure to CuO-NP, copper salts, and the proceeding bacterial challenge will have an effect on the gene expression of tested immune markers, in line with previous studies [44,62]. The holistic methodological approach applied in this paper provides a useful framework for improved assessment of immuno-safety of NMs.

2. Materials and Methods

2.1. Test Organism, Test Chemicals, and Soil Spiking

Eisenia fetida were reared at 20 °C in a medium consisting of loamy top soil, composted bark, and garden compost in 1:1:1 ratio by volume basis. Earthworms were fed with field collected horse manure from horses grazing on unpolluted pastures and free from recent medical treatment. All earthworms used in the experiment had a stripe patterned outer body characteristic of *E. fetida* with fully developed clitella and were within a weight range between 300 and 600 mg.

Molecular grade $CuCl_2 \cdot 2H_2O$ was supplied by Sigma-Aldrich (Poole, UK). CuO-NPs were manufactured by Promethean Particle Ltd. (Nottingham, UK) and were dispersed in water. Nanoparticles were cuboid in shape, with a stated mean dimension of 20 by 50 nm. Size distributions of NPs were determined with nanoparticle tracking analysis using a Nanosight (Malvern Instruments, Salisbury, UK). Derived mean and modal dimensions were 183 nm (±SE 5.2). Zeta potential of CuO-NPs (33 mV ± SD 0.3 mV) was determined using phase analysis light scattering using a Malvern Zetasize Nano ZS.

All exposures in soil were conducted in LUFA 2.2 natural soil (LUFA-Spreyer, Germany), a sandy loam soil widely used in ecotoxicological testing. Test soils were spiked with a nominal concentration of CuO-NP (160 mg·kg^{-1} d.w. soil) or $CuCl_2$ (160 mg·kg^{-1} d.w. soil) or a negative control (0 mg·kg^{-1} d.w. soil). Test concentrations were based on a previous study that showed changes in the microbiome structure and loss of core symbionts at these copper concentrations [56]. CuO-NP treated soils were spiked one day before the initiation of the exposure. $CuCl_2$ treated soils were spiked five days before the start of the exposure to allow the metal speciation in the soil to reach a quasi-equilibrium [63]. A control consisting of the liquid carrier of the CuO-NP dispersion was not included, as previous work has established that the liquid carrier of this NP dispersion is not toxic to earthworms and does not alter the earthworm microbiome structure [56].

Mixing of the chemicals with the soil was done for each treatment following Waalewijn-Kool et al. [64]. Briefly, the total amounts of CuO-NP and $CuCl_2$ required for all replicates were dissolved in 60 mL of de-ionised water. These stock solutions were then each mixed with 250 g of d.w. LUFA 2.2 soil using a spatula. The mixture was then thoroughly mixed with the remaining soil and subsequently wetted with de-ionised water to reach 55% of the water holding capacity (WHC) before final mixing.

The soil mixtures were divided into replicates each consisting out of a 60 g w.w. aliquot in a 100 mL clear plastic round tub.

2.2. Overview of the Experimental Design

Earthworm were initially exposed to a pre-treatment of either CuO-NP, CuCl$_2$, or a negative control for 28 days, after which time they were removed from soil and challenged with either *Bacillus subtilis* or a negative control for four days (Figure 1). *B. subtilis* was chosen as a model pathogen for the bacterial challenge on the basis of a pilot experiment, which showed that the coelomic fluid of *E. fetida* had inhibiting effects on the growth of this bacterium, possibly indicating an effective immune response by cellular or humoral components (Figure S1). After this bacterial challenge, earthworms were returned to their original soil for recovery for another 28 days, during which time they were periodically sampled for analysis. Details of each of the three experimental steps are described below.

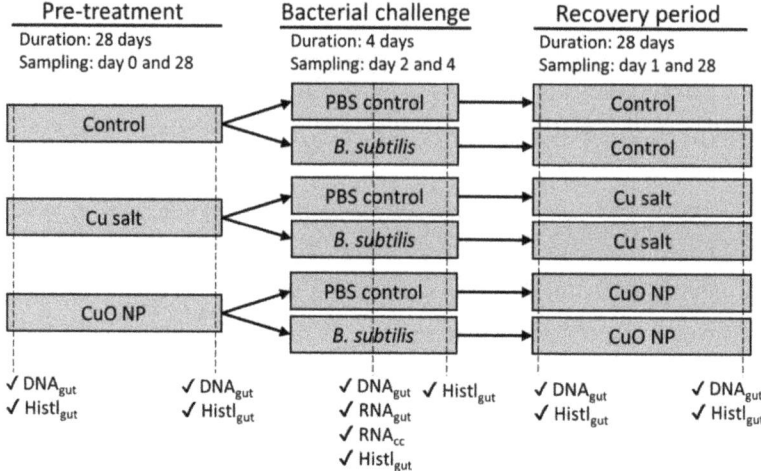

Figure 1. Schematic overview of the study design and collected samples. Dashed lines indicates sampling points. Tick marks indicate the samples collected at the respective sampling point. 'DNA$_{gut}$' indicates sampling of DNA from gut tissue for microbiome analysis; 'RNA$_{gut}$' and 'RNA$_{cc}$' indicate sampling of RNA for gene expression analysis from gut tissue and coelomic fluid, respectively; and 'Histl$_{gut}$' indicates sampling of gut tissue for histological analysis. NP, nanoparticle; PBS, phosphate buffered saline.

2.3. Pre-Treatment Exposure

Prior to the start of the pre-treatment exposure, earthworms were acclimatized to LUFA 2.2 soil for two weeks under the same conditions as the main exposure assay. Before exposure initiation, earthworms were rinsed and weighed. To start the test, one adult *E. fetida* was added to each test replicate. The pre-treatment exposure was conducted at 20 °C for 28 days. Once a week, each replicate received 0.5 g of spiked horse manure on a d.w. basis as food. At the end of the exposure, earthworms from all replicates were removed from soil, rinsed, and weighed. Collected earthworms were subsequently depurated on wetted filter paper to allow egestion of their gut content for two days before bacterial challenge.

2.4. Bacterial Challenge

Following depuration, each earthworm was challenged in a petri dish with either *Bacillus subtilis* (*B. subtilis* subsp. *subtilis*, CCM2217; Czech Collection of Microorganisms, Brno, Czech Republic) or a negative control in a medium consisting of re-wetted paper pellets. The pellets were re-wetted using either 10 mL of phosphate buffered saline (PBS) containing 5×10^8 B. subtilis cells per mL or 10 mL PBS only. B. subtilis cultures used for the challenge were in exponential growth phase at the time of the start of the challenge. Cell concentration was determined by measuring OD_{600}. The bacterial challenge was initiated by placing a depurated earthworm into the prepared Petri dish. The bacterial challenge was conducted at 20 °C in dark conditions for four days. Earthworm survival was monitored at day one, two, and four.

2.5. Recovery Period

After the bacterial challenge, earthworms were rinsed, weighed, and subsequently returned to the original soil exposure replicates to assess responses to exposure after the bacterial challenge. The recovery exposure was conducted at 20 °C and lasted 28 days. Earthworms were fed with 0.5 g of d.w. spiked horse manure every week.

2.6. Sample Points

Six sampling points were used: 'pre-treatment day 0', 'pre-treatment day 28', 'bacterial challenge day 2', 'bacterial challenge day 4', 'recovery period day 1', and 'recovery period day 28' (Figure 1). At every sampling point, except 'bacterial challenge day 4', gut tissue and coelomic fluid from five earthworms were collected (see below). At every sampling point, one additional earthworm was collected for histological analysis (see below). All earthworms collected from soil exposure replicates (i.e., 'pre-treatment day 0', 'pre-treatment day 28', 'recovery period day 1', and 'recovery period day 28') were depurated for two days prior to sampling. Earthworms collected at day two of the bacterial challenge were rinsed in de-ionised water, but not depurated and immediately dissected. At the end of the pre-treatment exposure, 10 g w.w. soil was collected for metal analysis.

2.7. Sampling of Gut Tissue and Coelomic Fluid

Each depurated earthworm was placed in a petri dish containing 500 µL PBS and coelomic fluid was extruded by electrification for 5 s using a 4.5 V battery. The mixture of coelomic fluid and PBS was collected and mixed with 500 µL of 2× RNA/DNA Shield (Zymo Research, Irvine, CA, USA) and placed in a lysis tube. The extruded earthworm was subsequently euthanized in pure ethanol and the midgut (spanning 20 segments posterior to the clitellum) was dissected using sterile equipment. Small incisions were made along the length of the midgut and rinsed in 1 mL PBS for 1 min using a vortex to facilitate removal of any residual soil, and subsequently placed in a lysis tube. All lysis tubes were bead beaten using an MP FastPrep-24™ set at 4.5 m/s for one minute. Lysis tubes were placed at 6 °C overnight and subsequently stored at −20 °C until DNA or RNA extraction.

2.8. Histological Analysis

Earthworms collected for histological analysis were fixed and processed according to Dvorak et al. [44]. Briefly, a whole body sample spanning a 10 segment region posterior to the clitellum was fixed in 4% paraformaldehyde overnight, dehydrated, and embedded in paraffin. For each sample, three 2 µm sections were cut using a microtome, dried overnight, deparaffinised using xylene, rehydrated, and stained using hematoxylin/eosin following Kiernan [65]. Sections were visually inspected for tissue integrity using a light microscope. Damage to the gut epithelium and chloragogen tissue was scored using an ordinal scoring method with four categories ((1) no effects, (2) mild effects, (3) moderate effects, and (4) severe effects), following Gibson-Corley et al. [66].

2.9. Soil Metal Measurements

Soil copper concentrations were measured in 130 mg of d.w. soil, which was mixed with a 4:1 mixture of nitric acid and hydrochloric acid on a volume basis and digested for seven hours at 150 °C. Copper concentration was determined using atomic absorbance spectrometry at the Vrije Universiteit

Amsterdam (The Netherlands). Copper recovery from exposure soils was on average 60.4% and 71.3% for CuO-NP and CuCl$_2$ spiked soils, respectively. The lack of full recovery may be linked to the loss of copper during preparation of stocks solutions and owing to heterogeneity in the distribution of copper forms in soils.

2.10. DNA and RNA Extraction and cDNA Synthesis Procedure

DNA was extracted from gut tissue and soil using a Quick-DNA Fecal/Soil Microbe Miniprep Kit (Zymo Research) according to the protocol supplied by the manufacturer. RNA was extracted from gut tissue and coelomic fluid using Quick-RNA™ Miniprep Kit (Zymo Research) following the protocol supplied by the manufacturer and included a DNA removal step using DNase. Visual inspection through agarose gel electrophoresis under denaturing conditions verified that the RNA in all samples was not degraded. Extracted RNA was subjected to a further clean-up using a Clean and Concentrator™-5 kit (Zymo Research). RNA quantity of the cleaned samples was determined using Qubit™ RNA HS Assay Kit (ThermoFisher Scientific, Waltham, MA, USA). Per sample, 250 ng of RNA was reverse transcribed to cDNA using Reverse Transcription System A3500 (Promega, Madison, WI, USA) following the standard protocol supplied by the manufacturer.

2.11. Earthworm Genotyping

Gene expression analysis relies on accurate binding of primers to target genomic regions. Genetic variation in binding sites between different individuals is likely to reduce the efficacy to elucidate patterns of gene expression. Within species genetic diversity in earthworms is high [67–69]. On the basis of cytochrome c oxidase I (COI) sequence similarities, two distinct genetic *E. fetida* clades have so far been recognised [70]. To screen whether earthworms used in this experiment were part of a single genetic clade, earthworms sampled at day two of the bacterial challenge were genotyped by amplification and sequencing of the mitochondrial COI DNA. PCR reactions were set up using forward primer COI_1490 (5′-GGTCAACAAATCATAAAGATATTGG-3′) and reverse primer HCO_2189 (5′-TAAACTTCAGGGTGACCAAAAAATCA-3′) [71] using One*Taq*® Hot Start polymerase and reaction buffer (New England Biolabs) using the following programme: initial denaturation at 94 °C for 2 min followed by 35 cycles of (1) denaturing at 94 °C for 30 s, (2) annealing at 47 °C for 30 s, and (3) extension at 68 °C for 1 min, followed by a final extension step at 68 °C for 10 min. Amplification of a single fragment was verified through gel electrophoresis. PCR products were cleaned using a QIAquick PCR purification kit (QIAGEN) and DNA quantity was assessed using a Qubit dsDNA HS Assay Kit (ThemoFisher Scientific). Then, 7.5 ng of PCR product was sequenced using Sanger sequencing using 3.2 pg of the forward primer at the University of Birmingham (UK). Sanger sequences were submitted to the National Center for Biotechnology Information (NCBI) BLASTn for taxonomical assignment. Pairwise alignment of sequences was performed using MUSCLE alignment in Geneious 9.1.8. Ambiguous bases and erroneous inserts were manually resolved and low quality ends of sequences were trimmed. The remaining 632 bp alignment was used as input for genetic analysis in MEGA software v7. Gamma-distributed Hasegawa, Kishino, and Yano model was calculated to best fit the data and used to calculate a maximum-likelihood phylogenetic tree using 500 bootstraps. Pairwise between groups genetic distance was calculated in MEGA.

Phylogenetic analysis on the COI gene revealed the existence of three separate genetic clusters. From each cluster, five samples were selected and subjected to further genetic analysis through random amplification of polymorphic DNA (RAPD). The RAPD reactions were conducted using the primer 5′-CAGGCCCTTC-3′ [72] and One*Taq*® polymerase and reaction buffer (New England Biolabs) following the thermal cycling programme: initial denaturation at 94 °C for 2 min followed by 35 cycles of (1) denaturing at 94 °C for 1 min, (2) annealing at 37 °C for 1 min, and (3) extension at 68 °C for 2 min, followed by a final extension step at 68 °C for 10 min. Genomic DNA extracted from the earthworm *Lumbricus rubellus* was used as outgroup. PCR product was run on a 1.5% agarose gel for three hours at 120 V using 1 kb HyperLadder (Bioline, London, UK) as reference. Band patterns were manually scored in a blind manner. Rooted neighbourhood-joining tree was calculated in R 3.5.0 (www.r-project.org) using the package "ape" [73].

2.12. Gut and Soil 16S Sequencing Metagenomics Bioinformatics

The prokaryotic community in genomic DNA extracted from soil and gut tissue was determined by PCR amplification and sequencing following the method outlined by Kozich et al. [74]. Briefly, a ~555 bp fragment spanning the V3–V4 region of the 16S-rRNA gene was amplified using the forward primer 5′-CCTACGGGAGGCAGCAG-3′ and reverse primer 5′-GGACTACHVGGGTWTCTAAT-3′, each modified with the addition of a sequencing primer, an indexing region, and an Illumina flow-cell adaptor such that each sample was uniquely barcoded. PCR amplification was done using Q5® High-Fidelity DNA Polymerase and reaction buffer (New England Biolabs, Ipswich, MA, USA) using the following programme: initial denaturing at 95 °C for 2 min, followed by 30 cycles of (1) denaturing at 95 °C for 30 s, (2) annealing at 55 °C for 15 s, and (3) extension at 72 °C for 40 s, followed by a final extension step at 72 °C for 10 min. Gel electrophoresis was used to verify amplification of a single product. PCR product was normalized using SequalPrep™ Normalization Plate Kit (ThemoFisher Scientific) and samples from each normalization plate were pooled. The pooled samples purified using QIAquick Gel Extraction Kit (QIAGEN, Venlo, The Netherlands). Gel extracted libraries were quantified using Qubit dsDNA HS Assay Kit (ThemoFisher Scientifc) and equimolar pooled and diluted to 7 pM. The pooled library was sequenced with 10% PhiX on a MiSeq using MiSeq Reagent Kit v3—600 cycles (Illumina, Inc., San Diego, CA, USA). The Illumina demultiplexed sequences were processes using the DADA2 bioinformatics pipeline [75] to generate an amplicon sequence table from the forward reads. DADA2 settings were maxEE(2), maxN(0), and truncQ(2). Sequences were trimmed to 290 bases. Sequences were dereplicated and the DADA2 core sequence variant inference algorithm was applied. Chimeric sequences were removed using removeBimeraDenovo default settings. Amplicon sequence variants (ASVs) were subjected to taxonomic assignment using assignTaxonomy at default settings and the Silva database [76]. ASVs assigned to mitochondria, chloroplasts, Archaea, Eukaryotes, and ASVs with unknown kingdom or phylum were removed from the dataset. Nucleotide sequence data have been submitted to NCBI and are available under submission number SUB7500125 as part of BioProject number PRJNA610159.

2.13. Quantitative PCR

Quantitative PCR was used to determine differential levels of mRNA of several earthworm immune genes in gut tissue and coelomic fluid (Table 1). Both tissues were screened for coelomic cytolytic factor (CCF), lysozyme, and lysenin/fetidin. Primer pairs were mapped against reference transcriptomes of both *E. fetida* and *E. andrei* to estimate the binding potential to all known allelic variants. Primer pairs targeting CCF were designed to both *E. fetida* and the *E. andrei* versions of the CCF gene using Primer 3. Amplification efficiency of primer pairs was verified through serial dilution and was between 90% and 110% for all pairs. Amplification of the target fragment was verified by Sanger sequencing of the PCR products. qPCR reactions were conducted using GoTaq® qPCR Master Mix (Promega) in a 20 µL reaction volume using 6.25 ng of cDNA as input. qPCR was performed using a Roche LightCycler® 480II with PCR conditions: initial denaturation at 95 °C for 3 min, followed by 40 cycles of (1) denaturation at 95 °C for 10 s and (2) annealing and extension at 60 °C for 30 s. Melt curve analysis was conducted to verify single PCR product. Changes in gene expression were calculated using the $2^{-\Delta\Delta Ct}$ method [77]. EF1α was used as a reference gene for the normalization of the target immune genes. Log2 fold change was expressed in relation to the negative control (earthworms exposed to control soils in the pre-exposure and PBS in the bacterial challenge).

2.14. Statistical Analysis

All data analysis was done in R (www.r-project.org). Non-metric dimensional scaling (NMDS), distance-based redundancy analysis (db-rda) (using Bray–Curtis distance matrix), permutational analysis of variance (Permanova), and calculation of diversity indices were conducted using the R package 'vegan' [78] using datasets rarefied to 4959 reads per sample with removal of samples below this threshold. Differences between treatments in diversity indices and gene expression values were tested using two-way analysis of variance (2w-ANOVA) and Tukey's post hoc test. Differential abundance analysis of bacterial taxa was done using Kruskal–Wallis Rank Sum Test and Mann–Whitney test using datasets rarefied to 2448 reads. For the differential abundance analysis, rarefaction to this lower read number was done to prevent losing replicates and, therefore, statistical power.

Table 1. Details of primers targeting housekeeping gene (EF1α) and target immune system genes.

Primer Name	Target Gene(s)	F/R	Sequence (5′ → 3′)	Amplicon Length (bp)
EF1α_F	Elongation factor 1 alpha	F	ATCGGTCATGTCGATTCCGG	213
EF1α_R	Elongation factor 1 alpha	R	GGCAGTCTCGAACTTCCACA	
CCF_721F	Coelomic cytolytic factor	F	ACGACAACCGATACTGGCTG	193
CCF_914R	Coelomic cytolytic factor	R	CTCCCAGAAATCCACCCACC	
Lysfet_F	Lysenin/fetidin	F	TGGCCAGCTGCAACTCTT [a]	177
Lysfet_R	Lysenin/fetidin	R	CCAGCGCTGTTTCGGATTAT [a]	
Lysozyme_F	Lysozyme	F	GCCATTCCAAATCAAGGAAC [a]	129
Lysozyme_R	Lysozyme	R	TAGGTACCGTAGCGCTTCAT [a]	

[a] from Dvorak et al. [43].

3. Results

3.1. Earthworm Population Genotypes

Sequencing of the COI gene from earthworms sampled during the bacterial challenge indicated three separate genetic clusters (Figure 2A). Local alignment using NCBI BLASTn indicated that one of those clusters was most similar to *E. andrei* COI, while the COI of the two other clusters aligned best with *E. fetida* COI. The two *E. fetida* COI sub-clusters did not group together in the phylogenetic tree. However, the overall genetic distance between the two *E. fetida* COI clusters was smaller (0.160) than that between the *E. andrei* COI cluster and *E. fetida* COI cluster 1 (0.186) (Figure 2B). RAPD analysis based on 26 polymorphic markers indicated the existence of two genetic clusters (Figure 2C). One of these clusters consisted of individuals carrying an *E. andrei* COI gene copy. The other cluster comprised individuals carrying an *E. fetida* COI copy and one COI assigned *E. andrei* individual.

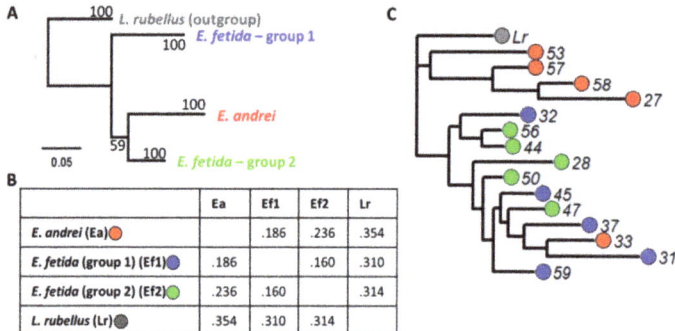

Figure 2. Phylogenetic trees showing relationship between cytochrome c oxidase I (COI) cluster and genetic distances between COI clusters. (**A**) Maximum-likelihood phylogenetic tree of showing phylogenetic relation between the three COI clusters. Samples are collapsed to COI cluster level, see Figure S2 for full tree. Bootstrap values are derived using 500 bootstraps. (**B**) Table with genetic distances between the three COI clusters. (**C**) Rooted neighbourhood-joining tree based on random amplification of polymorphic DNA (RAPD) profiles with *L. rubellus* (Lr) as outgroup. Different number indicate sample number. Colours indicate COI grouping.

3.2. The Effects of Pre-Treatment Exposure and Bacterial Challenge on the Gut Microbiome

The earthworm gut community at the start of the pre-treatment was composed of a consortium of bacteria comparable to that found in previous studies [56,79]. The gut community was dominated by *Verminephrobacter* (*Proteobacteria*), '*Candidatus* Lumbricincola' (*Mollicutes*), a member of the *Spirochaetaceae* family (*Spirochaetes*), and multiple ASVs belonging to the genus *Aeromonas* (*Proteobacteria*) (Figure S3). Transfer of earthworms from culture soil ('pre-treatment day 0') to LUFA control soils ('pre-treatment day 28') did not significantly alter the total community structure in the gut (Permanova: $F(1,8) = 1.059$, $p = 0.356$) (Figure S3) nor Shannon diversity ($F(1,8) = 0.882$, $p = 0.375$) or species richness ($F(1,8) = 0.074$, $p = 0.375$) (Table S1). Average Shannon diversity and richness across all replicates were 3.0 (±SD 1.1) and 239 (±SD 146), respectively.

At the end of the pre-treatment exposure (i.e., 'pre-treatment day 28'), there were no significant differences in overall community structure between the treatment groups (Permanova: $F(2,12) = 1.252$, $p = 0.256$) (Figure 3A). Bacterial diversity was also not affected by pre-treatment exposure (Shannon: $(F(2,12) = 0.176, p = 0.84$; richness: $F(2,12) = 1.695, p = 0.225$) and was on average 2.5 (±0.9) (Shannon) and 189 (±114) (richness) (Table S1). Among the most abundant gut bacteria (ASVs with a relative abundance >1% in any of the samples), three ASVs were significantly negatively affected by exposure to both copper forms (Kruskal–Wallis: $p < 0.05$). These ASVs included '*Candidatus* Lumbricinola' (ASV 4876) and two ASVs belonging to *Luteolibacter* (ASV 4960 and 4963) (Figure 3C–E). These taxa together comprised an average of 8% of the total community in controls, but were at or below the limit of detection in the copper-treated earthworms.

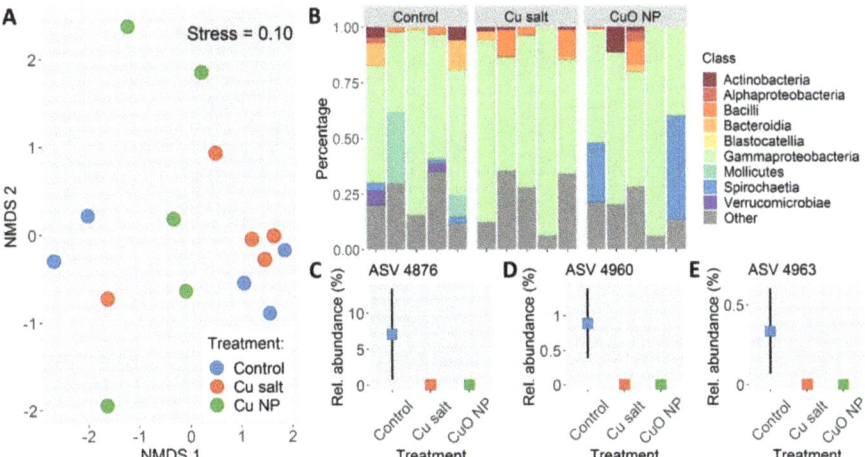

Figure 3. Bacterial community composition and structure of earthworm gut samples at the end of the pre-treatment exposure (i.e., 'pre-treatment day 28'). (**A**) Plot of non-metric dimensional scaling (NMDS) showing ordination of samples at amplicon sequence variant (ASV) level. (**B**) Relative abundance of dominant ASV at class level per sample. All ASVs with a relative abundance <1% of the total community are grouped under "Other". Mean relative abundance (±se) per treatment as percentage of total community of (**C**) '*Candidatus* Lumbricincola' (ASV 4876), (**D**) *Luteolibacter pohnpeiensis* (ASV 4960), and (**E**) *Luetolibacter* (ASV 4963).

In earthworms that were sampled at 'bacterial challenge day 2', treatment (i.e., pre-treatment exposure followed and bacterial challenge combined) had a nearly statistically significant effect on the bacterial community composition in earthworms, with treatment explaining 24% of the total variance (Permanova: $F(5,23) = 1.423$, $p = 0.075$) (Figure S4). Pre-treatment exposure and bacterial challenge treatment alone explained 10% (Permanova: $F(2,26) = 1.453$, $p = 0.108$) and 4% of the total variance (Permanova: $F(2,26) = 1.222$, $p = 0.265$), respectively (Table 2). No significant effect of treatment on diversity indices, which averaged 1.95 (±0.6) (Shannon) and 57 (±22) (richness) across all samples, was found (Table S1). Among the most dominant gut bacteria (ASVs with relative abundance >1%), '*Candidatus* Lumbricincola' (ASV 4876) relative abundance was significantly negatively affected by copper treatment (Figure S4D) (Kruskal–Wallis: $X^2(5) = 12.1$, $p < 0.05$), while *Aeromonas* (ASV 10149) was positively affected (Figure S4D) (Kruskal–Wallis: $X^2(5) = 14.0$, $p < 0.05$).

Table 2. Outcomes of models testing the relationship between bacterial community composition in the gut of earthworms sampled at 'bacterial challenge day 2' and different combinations of explanatory variables. Db-rda: distance based redundancy analysis using Bray–Curtis distance matrix and applying square root transformation and Wisconsin double standardization. Permanova: Permutational multivariate analysis of variance using Bray–Curtis distance matrix and 999 permutations. 'Explained' and 'Unexplained' represent in db-rda models the proportion of inertia either explained or unexplained by explanatory variables. In brackets (in the 'Explained' column), the fraction of the inertia that is conditioned is shown (i.e., removed). In Permanova models, 'Explained' and 'Unexplained' refer to the model R^2 and residual R^2 values.

Model Type	Model	Explanatory Variables	Explained	Un-Explained	F-Value	p-Value
Db-rda	Community~Pre-treatment + Bacterial treatment + Genotype	All	0.202	0.798	1.167	0.008 **
Db-rda	Community~Pre-treatment + Bacterial treatment	All	0.118	0.882	1.114	0.084
Db-rda	Community~Pre-treatment + Bacterial treatment + conditioned (Genotype)	Pre-treatment + Bacterial treatment	0.085 (0.117)	0.798	1.130	0.079
Db-rda	Community~Pre-treatment	Pre-treatment	0.041	0.959	1.159	0.103
Db-rda	Community~Bacterial treatment	Bacterial treatment	0.077	0.924	1.077	0.189
Db-rda	Community~Genotype	Genotype	0.085	0.915	1.205	0.021*
Permanova	Community~Pre-treatment + Bacterial treatment + Genotype	Pre-treatment	0.101	0.899	1.614	0.074
		Bacterial treatment	0.044	0.956	1.428	0.173
		Genotype	0.139	0.861	2.229	0.019 *
Permanova	Community~Pre-treatment + Bacterial treatment	Pre-treatment	0.101	0.899	1.470	0.128
		Bacterial treatment	0.044	0.956	1.300	0.220
Permanova	Community~Pre-treatment	Pre-treatment	0.101	0.899	1.453	0.108
Permanova	Community~Bacterial treatment	Bacterial treatment	0.043	0.957	1.221	0.265
Permanova	Community~Genotype	Genotype	0.167	0.833	2.598	0.004 **

* indicates $p < 0.05$, ** indicates $p < 0.01$.

3.3. Relation between Earthworm Genotype and Bacterial Community Structure

Permanova and db-rda indicated that genotype was a better predictor for the bacterial community composition than either pre-treatment exposure or bacterial challenge treatment (Table 2) with samples clustering primarily by COI genotype (Figure 4). After removal of the variation associated to COI genotype using partial db-rda models, the effect of pre-treatment and bacterial challenge treatment on community composition was still not significant (Table 2).

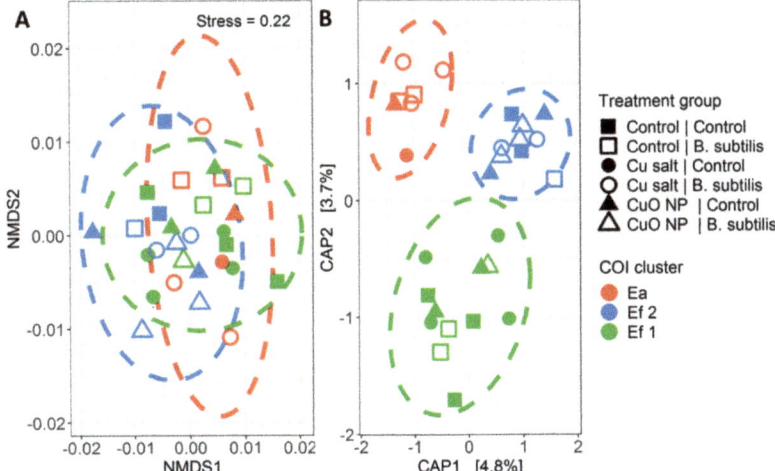

Figure 4. (**A**) NMDS plot showing ordination of 'bacterial challenge day 2' samples. (**B**) First two-axis of distance based redundancy analysis (db-rda) including 'pre-treatment exposure', 'bacterial challenge treatment', and 'genotype' as explanatory variables. Percentage following axis labels in (**B**) indicate percentage of total inertia explained by the respective axis. In both figures, different colours indicate different COI genotypes, while different shapes and filling indicate different treatments. Ellipses indicate 90% confidence interval (CI) of the respective COI cluster. In the legend, the text before the vertical bar indicates 'pre-treatment exposure' and the text following the vertical bar indicates 'bacterial challenge treatment'. 'Ea' (*E. andrei*), 'Ef1' (*E. fetida* 1), and 'Ef2' (*E. fetida* 2) indicate COI genotype.

3.4. Impact of Treatments on Bacillus Subtilis Abundance in Gut Tissue, Earthworm Survival, Tissue Integrity, and Immune Responses

All control earthworms exposed to the PBS control for four days survived. The survival of earthworms exposed to *B. subtilis* was on average 79% at day four, with no statistically significant effects of pre-treatment on the survival rate observed ($X^2(2) = 0.875$, $p = 0.646$) (Figure 5A). Abundance of *Bacillus* in gut tissue from earthworms challenged with *B. subtilis* was significantly higher than in control animals, indicating successful inoculation (Figure 5B). No differences in the abundance of *Bacillus* in gut tissue were observed during the recovery period. Histological analysis indicated a possible effect of pre-treatment exposure with copper (in both forms) on the integrity of the gut epithelium and longitudinal muscle tissue. The average integrity scores in copper treatment were between 0.8 and 1.3 points higher than controls (Table S2). The effects of copper treatment were manifested as the thinning of the gut epithelium tissue lining as well as the thinning of muscle fibres (Figure S5). Gene expression levels were assessed through qPCR analysis, targeting several known earthworm immune genes using EF1α as reference gene (Figure S6). No significant effect of treatments was found on immune gene expression in both tissue types (2w-ANOVA: $p > 0.05$) (Figure 5C–H).

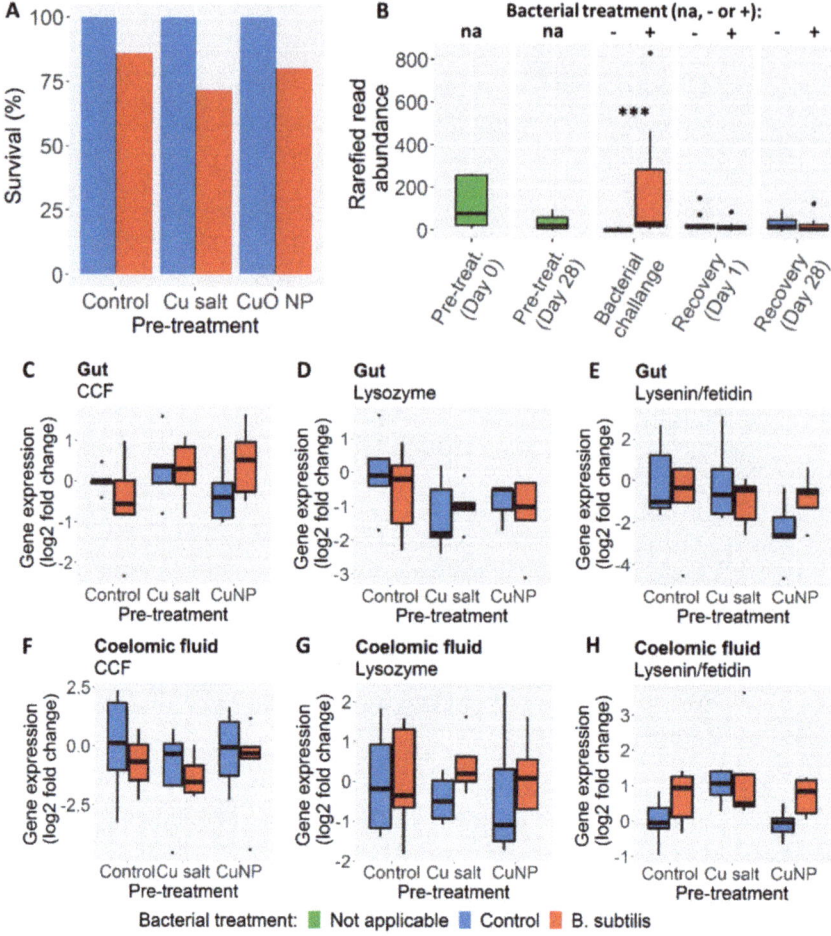

Figure 5. (**A**) Survival at day four of the bacterial challenge. (**B**) Boxplots of rarefied read abundance of *Bacillus* per sample point. Annotation at top of the graph indicates bacterial treatment: na (not applicable), − (PBS control), and + (*B. subtilis* treatment). Triple asterisks indicate statistical significance between bacterial challenge control and bacterial challenge treatment with $p < 0.001$. Relative high abundance of *Bacillus* at 'pre-treatment day 0' is driven by the two samples in that sample group (Figure S2). Boxplots of fold change in gene expression of earthworm immune responses in (**C–E**) gut tissue and (**F–H**) coelomic fluid at 'bacterial challenge day 2'. All gene expression values are log2 fold change values derived through $2^{-\Delta\Delta Ct}$ method. Expression values represent fold changes of treatments compared to control animals (control pre-treatment + control bacterial challenge) and are normalized to the expression of the housekeeping gene EF1α. There were no significant differences in gene expression between groups for all tested genes ($\alpha = 0.05$). Different colours in all panels indicate different bacterial challenge treatments. CCF, coelomic cytolytic factor.

3.5. Relation between Earthworm Genotype and Gene Expression

No significant relation between gene expression and COI genotype was found, with the exception of lysozyme expression in coelomic fluid samples. For this gene, expression in the *E. andrei* COI genotype was marginally, but significantly higher than the *E. fetida* group 2 (2w-ANOVA: $F(2,26) = 4.646$,

$p < 0.05$; Tukey's post hoc test: $p < 0.05$), with the difference in mean fold change of 1.4 indicating a small magnitude effect (data not shown).

4. Discussion

Innate immunity provides a first line of defence against invading pathogens. NMs are known to interact with the immune system of organisms and can induce both pro- and anti-inflammatory responses [8,13]. NMs are developed and applied as antimicrobial agents in personal care products and in an agricultural setting. In many animals, microbial symbionts play an important role in host defence. Therefore, when animals are exposed to biocidal NM, disruption of their microbiome can be expected, which, accordingly, may lead to effects on host immunity. It remains unclear, however, whether NM exposure can compromise host immunity through effects on the microbiome when hosts are infected by pathogens. This paper aimed to study the impact of biocidal CuO-NPs and its ionic counterpart on the gut microbial community, host immune responses, and infection susceptibility in an earthworm.

Previous in vitro studies have shown that NPs can be taken up by earthworm immune cells (coelomocytes) [45,80,81], and can alter the expression of earthworm immune markers [45,46], leading to cellular toxicity [82,83]. In this study, in vivo exposure to metal biocides (in both metal salt and NP form) caused changes to microbiome structure, with several bacterial symbionts being negatively affected by exposure to copper. Following these exposures and microbiome changes, survival rates were unaffected when earthworms were challenged with a high dose of the soil bacterium *B. subtilis*. Histological analysis indicated possible tissue damage owing to copper exposure, although this analysis is based on observations for a limited number of samples, and thus further assessment of this response is needed. Overall, we found no evidence for altered infection susceptibility or altered immune gene regulation at biocide concentrations where the gut microbiome is already affected.

The lack of an immune response after NP exposure contrasts with the results of previous studies [45,46]. Hayashi and colleagues, for example, found that in vitro exposure in earthworm immune cells to Ag-NP significantly alters the temporal expression of immune genes [45]. Studies in other invertebrates, such as mussels and sea urchins, have also shown that both in vivo and in vitro exposure to NMs can modulate the immune system of these animals [30,31,84]. NMs that are released into the environment are likely to undergo transformations [85–87]. Uptake by organisms may further modify the shape, size, and form of NPs [88,89]. Therefore, the NMs that earthworm immune systems are exposed to in vivo may be different to the pristine forms that have often been used in in vitro studies. The discrepancy between the impact of NM on earthworm immune reactivity in vivo and those in vitro may thus be linked to the transformations of NMs in soil media and the resulting change in the immuno-reactivity of NMs.

Previous research has shown that the microbiome of animals can be altered by NM exposure. In rodents, for example, exposure to Ag-NP can negatively affect the abundance of *Firmicutes* and *Lactobacillus* and induce histological damage to intestinal tissue [28,29]. In soil invertebrates such as springtails and earthworms, metal NP exposure was also shown to alter intestinal microbiomes [58–60]. Exposure to Ag-NP in the springtail *Folsomia candida*, for example, negatively affects the abundance of *Firmicutes* and *Actinobacteria* in the gut of these soil invertebrates [59]. Although implications on host functioning were not further studied, other research shows that microbiome dysbiosis induced by environmental pollution can be associated to changes in the isotopic composition of springtails, suggesting an impact on nutrient turnover [90]. In this study, we found that the earthworm symbiont '*Candidatus* Lumbricincola' is negatively affected by an exposure to copper forms. '*Candidatus* Lumbricincola' is a bacterium exclusively associated to earthworms and has a possible role in the degradation of polysaccharides [47,91]. However, the implications of the near loss of this symbiont for the health and functioning of earthworms require further investigation.

Contrary to our hypothesis, a two-day exposure to a high bacterial level did not change the expression of known earthworm immune markers. Successful inoculation with the bacterium was confirmed by the mortality data and the abundance of *Bacillus* in gut tissue. The lack of an immune response at concentrations of bacteria at which 21% of the exposed individuals die is thus unexpected. Earthworms can show large variation in the expression of immune genes over time [45,92]. Timing of the expression of components of the immune system can be gene-specific [44], but can also depend on the specific pathogen to which the earthworm is exposed [92]. For example, in *E. andrei*, lysozyme is expressed within several hours of exposure to *Escherichia coli*, but only after 16 h following exposure to *B. subtilis* [38]. Similarly, in *E. andrei*, lysenin/fetidin has been reported to be upregulated after six hours in response to a *Staphylococcus aureus* exposure, but downregulated when exposed to *E. coli* [93]. The methodology adopted in this study was based on studies by Dvorak and colleagues, who showed that exposure to high levels of *B. subtilis* can induce changes in immune regulation of earthworms [43,44]. Discrepancy between measured immune responses in *E. fetida*, as reported in this study, and those measured in previous studies in a related species under similar condition show that earthworm immune responses are also species-dependent. Investigations into the molecular structure of the earthworm immune gene CCF in eight different species have shown that some earthworm species have a wider recognition capacity than others [37]. Even within closely related *Eisenia* spp., there are differences in the reactivity of immune genes and immunity related enzymatic activity [43]. These differences in immune reactivity between related earthworms may reflect differences in microbial environments, which may require niche-specific immune responses and lead to differing basal immune reactivities. Time as a factor in earthworm immune responses is thus not fully understood [33] and requires further species-specific investigation. Sufficient sampling over a time-course is needed to fully elucidate patterns of immune expression in earthworms under various environmental stressors and, in particular, to identify the specific points of highest upregulation for key genes.

Earthworm coelomocytes are composed of three subpopulations, each with a unique function [94,95] and molecular immune-expression profile [93–96]. This cellular complexity means that it is possible for different cell subpopulations to have different sensitivities to pollutant exposure [82,97]. Exposure to metals and xenobiotics, but also immunostimulants like LPS [98], has been demonstrated to change the ratio between the different coelomocyte cell subpopulations [82,97,99] and to alter the expression of earthworm immune markers [62]. In this study, coelomic fluid was extruded and sampled without separation of different cell subpopulations. Accordingly, the measured immune responses to *B. subtilis* exposure are an average of the expression levels of these genes across these different subpopulations. This, in combination with high variation between individuals in expression of some of the tested genes as previously reported [100], may limit the ability to elucidate differences in the patterns of gene expression within any individual cell subpopulation [82].

In this study, we found that 7 out of the 30 genotyped earthworms carried an *E. andrei* COI copy. Moreover, for the remaining *E. fetida* individuals, two COI clades were recorded. COI genotype, however, did not affect measured immune responses. The finding of clade structure for earthworms from the *E. fetida/E. andrei* complex is in agreement with previous studies [70,101–103]. *E. fetida* are phenotypically characterized by their stripped pigmentation pattern, whereas *E. andrei* are classically more uniformly red coloured. These two species were formally described as two different subspecies (e.g., *E. fetida fetida* and *E. fetida andrei*) [104], but, on the basis of crossbreeding experiments and differences in biochemical markers, were classified as separate species [105]. More recent research has shown that, in laboratory conditions, *E. fetida* and *E. andrei* can hybridize and produce fertile hybrid offspring [101,106]. Field studies also confirm that gene flow between these two species does occur [102]. Earthworms in this study were characterized by typical *E. fetida* pigmentation. Previous studies, however, report that pigmentation is not always a good predictor for COI genotype [101,103]. Here, RAPD profiling suggests that COI genotype does not always predict genomic variability, as indicated by the presence of an individual carrying an *E. andrei* COI copy within a clade consisting of *E. fetida* COI carrying individuals. The COI genotype was shown to be a better predictor for the bacterial community composition than any treatment. Host genetics is one of the components shaping the human gut microbiome [107,108], but similar relationships have also been observed in other animals such as mice [109] and invertebrates. In the water flea *Daphnia manga*, for example, host genotype shapes not only the structure, but also the functionality of the gut microbiome, in particular its ability to respond to toxic cyanobacteria [110]. The gut microbiome of *Eisenia* spp. is dominated by a consortium of bacteria that are vertically transmitted from parental animal to offspring [79,111]. The relation between COI genotype and gut microbiome structure may thus be linked to the concurrent maternal transmission of both mitochondria and bacterial symbionts.

5. Conclusions

We show that the microbiome of earthworms can change when exposed to a copper (in both NP and salt form). However, these biocide-mediated changes of the microbiome do not lead to altered susceptibility to a bacterial infection. Despite mortality when challenged with a bacterium, no effects of treatment on the measured earthworm immune markers were observed. The absence of an effect on immune function needs to be further validated by studies of gene expression using a greater time resolution of immune responses in earthworms and further identification of markers of immunity through, for example, full transcriptomic analysis. The methodological approach applied in this paper may guide future studies to improve the assessment of immuno-safety of NMs.

Supplementary Materials: The following are available online at http://www.mdpi.com/2079-4991/10/7/1337/s1, Figure S1: Growth over time of (**A**) *Bacillus subtilis*, (**B**) *Bacillus thuringiensis*, and (**C**) *Citrobacter rodentium* in LB medium (i.e., 'Control'), filter sterilized culture medium consiting out of 800 µL LB medium and 200 µL 10x diluted coelomic fluid ('Coelomic fluid') or culture medium containing both diluted coelomic fluid and antibiotics ('Antibiotics'); Figure S2: Maximum-likelihood phylogenetic tree of showing phylogenetic relation between all samples; Figure S3: Bacterial community composition and structure of earthworm gut samples from control replicates at start and end of pre-treatment; Figure S4: Bacterial community composition and structure of earthworm gut samples during bacterial challenge (i.e., 'bacterial challenge day 2'); Figure S5: Examples of cross sections of *E. fetida* stained with hematoxylin/eosin representing a range of tissue integrity scores; Figure S6: Boxplots of C_p values of elongation factor 1 alpha (ef1α) per treatment in coelomic fluid and gut tissue; Table S1: Mean Shannon diversity index and bacterial richness (±SD) per sampling point and treatment group; Table S2: Integrity scores of gut epithelium and chloragogen tissue per sample point and treatment. Values are means of the scores of three sections from a single replicate.

Author Contributions: Conceptualization, E.S., D.S., P.P., P.K., and C.S.; Methodology, E.S., D.S., P.P., P.K., and C.S.; Formal analysis, E.S. and J.D.; Investigation, E.S., J.D., S.H., and P.P.; Data curation, E.S.; Data interpretation: E.S., J.D., P.K., D.S., C.S., and P.P.; Resources: P.P., T.G., S.H., and P.K.; Writing—Original draft preparation, E.S.; Writing—Review and editing, J.D., D.S., T.G., and P.P.; Visualization, E.S.; Supervision, D.S., P.K., C.S., and P.P.; Project administration, E.S., D.S., C.S., and P.P.; Funding acquisition, D.S., C.S., P.K., and P.P. All authors have read and agreed to the published version of the manuscript.

Funding: This work has received funding from the European Union's Horizon 2020 research and innovation programme under the Marie Skłodowska-Curie grant agreement No 671881. The contributions by David Spurgeon and Claus Svendsen were supported by the UK Natural Environment Research Council (NERC) UK Centre for Ecology & Hydrology Institute Funding award.

Acknowledgments: The authors would like to thank Denny Rigby (UK CEH), Natividad Isabel Navarro Pacheco (IMIC), and Frantisek Skanta (IMIC) for their help.

Conflicts of Interest: The authors declare no conflict of interest.

References

1. Sun, T.Y.; Bornhöft, N.A.; Hungerbühler, K.; Nowack, B. Dynamic Probabilistic Modeling of Environmental Emissions of Engineered Nanomaterials. *Environ. Sci. Technol.* **2016**, *50*, 4701–4711. [CrossRef] [PubMed]
2. Keller, A.A.; McFerran, S.; Lazareva, A.; Suh, S. Glob al life cycle releases of engineered nanomaterials. *J. Nanopart. Res.* **2013**, *15*. [CrossRef]
3. Colvin, V.L. The potential environmental impact of engineered nanomaterials. *Nat. Biotechnol.* **2003**, *21*, 1166–1170. [CrossRef]
4. Moore, M.N. Do nanoparticles present ecotoxicological risks for the health of the aquatic environment? *Environ. Int.* **2006**, *32*, 967–976. [CrossRef] [PubMed]
5. Handy, R.D.; Owen, R.; Valsami-Jones, E. The ecotoxicology of nanoparticles and nanomaterials: Current status, knowledge gaps, challenges, and future needs. *Ecotoxicology* **2008**, *17*, 315–325. [CrossRef] [PubMed]

6. Dobrovolskaia, M.A.; McNeil, S.E. Immunological properties of engineered nanomaterials. *Nat. Nanotechnol.* **2007**, *2*, 469–478. [CrossRef] [PubMed]
7. Boraschi, D.; Oostingh, G.J.; Casals, E.; Italiani, P.; Nelissen, I.; Puntes, V.F.; Duschl, A. Nano-immunosafety: Issues in assay validation. *J. Phys. Conf. Ser.* **2011**, *304*, 012077. [CrossRef]
8. Boraschi, D.; Alijagic, A.; Auguste, M.; Barbero, F.; Ferrari, E.; Hernadi, S.; Mayall, C.; Michelini, S.; Navarro Pacheco, N.I.; Prinelli, A.; et al. Addressing Nanomaterial Immunosafety by Evaluating Innate Immunity across Living Species. *Small* **2020**, *16*. [CrossRef]
9. Fadeel, B. Hide and seek: Nanomaterial interactions with the immune system. *Front. Immunol.* **2019**, *10*, 133. [CrossRef]
10. Boraschi, D.; Italiani, P.; Palomba, R.; Decuzzi, P.; Duschl, A.; Fadeel, B.; Moghimi, S.M. Nanoparticles and innate immunity: New perspectives on host defence. *Semin. Immunol.* **2017**, *34*, 33–51. [CrossRef]
11. Pallardy, M.J.; Turbica, I.; Biola-Vidamment, A. Why the immune system should be concerned by nanomaterials? *Front. Immunol.* **2017**, *8*, 544. [CrossRef] [PubMed]
12. Alsaleh, N.B.; Brown, J.M. Immune responses to engineered nanomaterials: Current understanding and challenges. *Curr. Opin. Toxicol.* **2018**, *10*, 8–14. [CrossRef]
13. Bhattacharya, K.; Kiliç, G.; Costa, P.M.; Fadeel, B. Cytotoxicity screening and cytokine profiling of nineteen nanomaterials enables hazard ranking and grouping based on inflammogenic potential. *Nanotoxicology* **2017**, *11*, 809–826. [CrossRef]
14. Simonin, M.; Richaume, A. Impact of engineered nanoparticles on the activity, abundance, and diversity of soil microbial communities: A review. *Environ. Sci. Pollut. Res.* **2015**, *22*, 13710–13723. [CrossRef] [PubMed]
15. McKee, M.S.; Filser, J. Impacts of metal-based engineered nanomaterials on soil communities. *Environ. Sci. Nano* **2016**, *3*, 506. [CrossRef]
16. Courtois, P.; Rorat, A.; Lemiere, S.; Guyoneaud, R.; Attard, E.; Levard, C.; Vandenbulcke, F. Ecotoxicology of silver nanoparticles and their derivatives introduced in soil with or without sewage sludge: A review of effects on microorganisms, plants and animals. *Environ. Pollut.* **2019**, *253*, 578–598. [CrossRef]
17. Judy, J.D.; McNear, D.H.; Chen, C.; Lewis, R.W.; Tsyusko, O.V.; Bertsch, P.M.; Rao, W.; Stegemeier, J.; Lowry, G.V.; McGrath, S.P.; et al. Nanomaterials in Biosolids Inhibit Nodulation, Shift Microbial Community Composition, and Result in Increased Metal Uptake Relative to Bulk/Dissolved Metals. *Environ. Sci. Technol.* **2015**, *49*, 8751–8758. [CrossRef]
18. Brestoff, J.R.; Artis, D. Commensal bacteria at the interface of host metabolism and the immune system. *Nat. Immunol.* **2013**, *14*, 676–684. [CrossRef]
19. Buffie, C.G.; Pamer, E.G. Microbiota-mediated colonization resistance against intestinal pathogens. *Nat. Rev. Immunol.* **2013**, *13*, 790–801. [CrossRef]
20. Nyholm, S.V.; Graf, J. Knowing your friends: Invertebrate innate immunity fosters beneficial bacterial symbioses. *Nat. Rev. Microbiol.* **2012**, *10*, 815–827. [CrossRef]
21. Koch, H.; Schmid-Hempel, P. Socially transmitted gut microbiota protect bumble bees against an intestinal parasite. *Proc. Natl. Acad. Sci. USA* **2011**, *108*, 19288–19292. [CrossRef] [PubMed]
22. Dillon, R.J.; Vennard, C.T.; Buckling, A.; Charnley, A.K. Diversity of locust gut bacteria protects against pathogen invasion. *Ecol. Lett.* **2005**, *8*, 1291–1298. [CrossRef]
23. Cirimotich, C.M.; Dong, Y.; Clayton, A.M.; Sandiford, S.L.; Souza-Neto, J.; Mulenga, M.; Dimopoulos, G. Natural microbe-mediated refractoriness to Plasmodium infection in Anopheles gambiae. *Science* **2011**, *332*, 855–858. [CrossRef] [PubMed]
24. Kwong, W.K.; Mancenido, A.L.; Moran, N.A. Immune system stimulation by the native gut microbiota of honey bees. *R. Soc. Open Sci.* **2017**, *4*, 1–9. [CrossRef]
25. Weiss, B.L.; Maltz, M.; Aksoy, S. Obligate symbionts activate immune system development in the tsetse fly. *J. Immunol.* **2012**, *188*, 3395–3403. [CrossRef] [PubMed]
26. Motta, E.V.S.; Raymann, K.; Moran, N.A. Glyphosate perturbs the gut microbiota of honey bees. *Proc. Natl. Acad. Sci. USA* **2018**, *115*, 10305–10310. [CrossRef] [PubMed]
27. Kim, J.K.; Lee, J.B.; Huh, Y.R.; Jang, H.A.; Kim, C.H.; Yoo, J.W.; Lee, B.L. Burkholderia gut symbionts enhance the innate immunity of host Riptortus pedestris. *Dev. Comp. Immunol.* **2015**, *53*, 265–269. [CrossRef]
28. Chen, H.; Zhao, R.; Wang, B.; Cai, C.; Zheng, L.; Wang, H.; Wang, M.; Ouyang, H.; Zhou, X.; Chai, Z.; et al. The effects of orally administered Ag, TiO2 and SiO2 nanoparticles on gut microbiota composition and colitis induction in mice. *NanoImpact* **2017**, *8*, 80–88. [CrossRef]

29. Williams, K.; Milner, J.; Boudreau, M.D.; Gokulan, K.; Cerniglia, C.E.; Khare, S. Effects of subchronic exposure of silver nanoparticles on intestinal microbiota and gut-associated immune responses in the ileum of Sprague-Dawley rats. *Nanotoxicology* **2015**, *9*, 279–289. [CrossRef]
30. Auguste, M.; Balbi, T.; Montagna, M.; Fabbri, R.; Sendra, M.; Blasco, J.; Canesi, L. In vivo immunomodulatory and antioxidant properties of nanoceria (nCeO2) in the marine mussel Mytilus galloprovincialis. *Comp. Biochem. Physiol. Part—C Toxicol. Pharmacol.* **2019**, *219*, 95–102. [CrossRef]
31. Auguste, M.; Lasa, A.; Pallavicini, A.; Gualdi, S.; Vezzulli, L.; Canesi, L. Exposure to TiO2 nanoparticles induces shifts in the microbiota composition of Mytilus galloprovincialis hemolymph. *Sci. Total Environ.* **2019**, *670*, 129–137. [CrossRef] [PubMed]
32. Alijagic, A.; Pinsino, A. Probing safety of nanoparticles by outlining sea urchin sensing and signaling cascades. *Ecotoxicol. Environ. Saf.* **2017**, *144*, 416–421. [CrossRef]
33. Hayashi, Y.; Heckmann, L.H.; Simonsen, V.; Scott-Fordsmand, J.J. Time-course profiling of molecular stress responses to silver nanoparticles in the earthworm *Eisenia fetida*. *Ecotoxicol. Environ. Saf.* **2013**, *98*, 219–226. [CrossRef] [PubMed]
34. Edwards, C.A.; Bohlen, P.J. The role of earthworms in organic matter and nutrient cycles. In *Biology and Ecology of Earthworms*; Chapman & Hall: London, UK, 1996; pp. 155–180.
35. Beschin, A.; Bilej, M.; Hanssens, F.; Raymakers, J.; Van Dyck, E.; Revets, H.; Brys, L.; Gomez, J.; De Baetselier, P.; Timmermans, M. Identification and Cloning of a Glucan- and Lipopolysaccharide-binding Protein from Eisenia foetida Earthworm Involved in the Activation of Prophenoloxidase Cascade. *J. Biol. Chem.* **1998**, *273*, 24948–24954. [CrossRef]
36. Bilej, M.; De Baetselier, P.; Van Dijck, E.; Stijlemans, B.; Colige, A.; Beschin, A. Distinct Carbohydrate Recognition Domains of an Invertebrate Defense Molecule Recognize Gram-negative and Gram-positive Bacteria. *J. Biol. Chem.* **2001**, *276*, 45840–45847. [CrossRef]
37. Šilerová, M.; Procházková, P.; Josková, R.; Josens, G.; Beschin, A.; De Baetselier, P.; Bilej, M. Comparative study of the CCF-like pattern recognition protein in different Lumbricid species. *Dev. Comp. Immunol.* **2006**, *30*, 765–771. [CrossRef]
38. Josková, R.; Šilerová, M.; Procházková, P.; Bilej, M. Identification and cloning of an invertebrate-type lysozyme from Eisenia andrei. *Dev. Comp. Immunol.* **2009**, *33*, 932–938. [CrossRef]
39. Sekizawa, Y.; Hagiwara, K.; Nakajima, T.; Kobayashi, H. A novel protein, lysenin, that causes contraction of the isolated rat aorta: Its purification from the coelomic fluid of the earthworm Eisenia foetida. *Biomed. Res.* **1996**, *17*, 197–203. [CrossRef]
40. Lassegues, M.; Milochau, A.; Doignon, F.; Du Pasquier, L.; Valembois, P. Sequence and expression of an Eisenia-fetida-derived cDNA clone that encodes the 40-kDa fetidin antibacterial protein. *Eur. J. Biochem.* **1997**, *246*, 756–762. [CrossRef]
41. Cooper, E.L.; Roch, P. Earthworm immunity: A model of immune competence. *Pedobiologia* **2003**, *47*, 676–688. [CrossRef]
42. Bruhn, H.; Winkelmann, J.; Andersen, C.; Andrä, J.; Leippe, M. Dissection of the mechanisms of cytolytic and antibacterial activity of lysenin, a defence protein of the annelid Eisenia fetida. *Dev. Comp. Immunol.* **2006**, *30*, 597–606. [CrossRef]
43. Dvořák, J.; Mančíková, V.; Pižl, V.; Elhottová, D.; Šilerová, M.; Roubalová, R.; Škanta, F.; Procházková, P.; Bilej, M. Microbial environment affects innate immunity in two closely related earthworm species Eisenia andrei and Eisenia fetida. *PLoS ONE* **2013**, *8*, e0079257. [CrossRef] [PubMed]
44. Dvořák, J.; Roubalová, R.; Procházková, P.; Rossmann, P.; Škanta, F.; Bilej, M. Sensing microorganisms in the gut triggers the immune response in Eisenia andrei earthworms. *Dev. Comp. Immunol.* **2016**, *57*, 67–74. [CrossRef] [PubMed]
45. Hayashi, Y.; Engelmann, P.; Foldbjerg, R.; Szabó, M.; Somogyi, I.; Pollák, E.; Molnár, L.; Autrup, H.; Sutherland, D.S.; Scott-Fordsmand, J.; et al. Earthworms and humans in vitro: Characterizing evolutionarily conserved stress and immune responses to silver nanoparticles. *Environ. Sci. Technol.* **2012**, *46*, 4166–4173. [CrossRef]
46. Hayashi, Y.; Miclaus, T.; Engelmann, P.; Autrup, H.; Sutherland, D.S.; Scott-Fordsmand, J.J. Nanosilver pathophysiology in earthworms: Transcriptional profiling of secretory proteins and the implication for the protein corona. *Nanotoxicology* **2016**, *10*, 303–311. [CrossRef] [PubMed]

47. Zeibich, L.; Schmidt, O.; Drake, H.L. Fermenters in the earthworm gut: Do transients matter? *FEMS Microbiol. Ecol.* **2019**, *95*, 1–12. [CrossRef]
48. Singleton, D.R.; Hendrix, P.F.; Coleman, D.C.; Whitman, W.B. Identification of uncultured bacteria tightly associated with the intestine of the earthworm *Lumbricus rubellus* (Lumbricidae; Oligochaeta). *Soil Biol. Biochem.* **2003**, *35*, 1547–1555. [CrossRef]
49. Thakuria, D.; Schmidt, O.; Finan, D.; Egan, D.; Doohan, F.M. Gut wall bacteria of earthworms: A natural selection process. *ISME J.* **2010**, *4*, 357–366. [CrossRef]
50. Swart, E.; Newbold, L.; Kille, P.; Spurgeon, D.; Svendsen, C. The midgut of the earthworm Eisenia fetida harbours a resident host specific bacterial community independent from soil. *Environ. Microbiol.* under review.
51. Lund, M.B.; Holmstrup, M.; Lomstein, B.A.; Damgaard, C.; Schramm, A. Beneficial effect of verminephrobacter nephridial symbionts on the fitness of the earthworm aporrectodea tuberculata. *Appl. Environ. Microbiol.* **2010**, *76*, 4738–4743. [CrossRef]
52. Viana, F.; Paz, L.C.; Methling, K.; Damgaard, C.F.; Lalk, M.; Schramm, A.; Lund, M.B. Distinct effects of the nephridial symbionts Verminephrobacter and Candidatus Nephrothrix on reproduction and maturation of its earthworm host Eisenia andrei. *FEMS Microbiol. Ecol.* **2018**, *94*, 1–7. [CrossRef] [PubMed]
53. Šrut, M.; Menke, S.; Höckner, M.; Sommer, S. Earthworms and cadmium—Heavy metal resistant gut bacteria as indicators for heavy metal pollution in soils? *Ecotoxicol. Environ. Saf.* **2019**, *171*, 843–853. [CrossRef] [PubMed]
54. Yausheva, E.; Sizova, E.; Lebedev, S.; Skalny, A.; Miroshnikov, S.; Plotnikov, A.; Khlopko, Y.; Gogoleva, N.; Cherkasov, S. Influence of zinc nanoparticles on survival of worms Eisenia fetida and taxonomic diversity of the gut microflora. *Environ. Sci. Pollut. Res.* **2016**, *23*, 13245–13254. [CrossRef] [PubMed]
55. Ma, L.; Xie, Y.; Han, Z.; Giesy, J.P.; Zhang, X. Responses of earthworms and microbial communities in their guts to Triclosan. *Chemosphere* **2017**, *168*, 1194–1202. [CrossRef]
56. Swart, E.; Goodall, T.; Kille, P.; Spurgeon, D.; Svendsen, C. The earthworm microbiome is resilient to exposure to biocidal metal nanoparticles. *Environ. Pollut.* accepted.
57. Pass, D.A.; Morgan, A.J.; Read, D.S.; Field, D.; Weightman, A.J.; Kille, P. The effect of anthropogenic arsenic contamination on the earthworm microbiome. *Environ. Microbiol.* **2015**, *17*, 1884–1896. [CrossRef]
58. Ma, J.; Chen, Q.-L.; O'Connor, P.; Sheng, G.D. Does soil CuO nanoparticles pollution alter the gut microbiota and resistome of *Enchytraeus crypticus*? *Environ. Pollut.* **2019**, 113467. [CrossRef]
59. Zhu, D.; Zheng, F.; Chen, Q.-L.; Yang, X.-R.; Christie, P.; Ke, X.; Zhu, Y.-G. Exposure of a soil collembolan to Ag nanoparticles and AgNO$_3$ disturbs its associated microbiota and lowers the incidence of antibiotic resistance genes in the gut. *Environ. Sci. Technol.* **2018**, *52*, 12748–12756. [CrossRef]
60. Ma, J.; Sheng, G.D.; Chen, Q.L.; O'Connor, P. Do combined nanoscale polystyrene and tetracycline impact on the incidence of resistance genes and microbial community disturbance in *Enchytraeus crypticus*? *J. Hazard. Mater.* **2020**, *387*, 122012. [CrossRef]
61. Keller, A.A.; Adeleye, A.S.; Conway, J.R.; Garner, K.L.; Zhao, L.; Cherr, G.N.; Hong, J.; Gardea-Torresdey, J.L.; Godwin, H.A.; Hanna, S.; et al. Comparative environmental fate and toxicity of copper nanomaterials. *NanoImpact* **2017**, *7*, 28–40. [CrossRef]
62. Mincarelli, L.; Tiano, L.; Craft, J.; Marcheggiani, F.; Vischetti, C. Evaluation of gene expression of different molecular biomarkers of stress response as an effect of copper exposure on the earthworm Eisenia Andrei. *Ecotoxicology* **2019**, *28*, 938–948. [CrossRef] [PubMed]
63. Smit, C.E.; Van Gestel, C.A.M. Effects of soil type, prepercolation, and ageing on bioaccumulation and toxicity of zinc for the springtail Folsomia candida. *Environ. Toxicol. Chem.* **1998**, *17*, 1132–1141. [CrossRef]
64. Waalewijn-Kool, P.L.; Ortiz, M.D.; Van Gestel, C.A.M. Effect of different spiking procedures on the distribution and toxicity of ZnO nanoparticles in soil. *Ecotoxicology* **2012**, *21*, 1797–1804. [CrossRef] [PubMed]
65. Kiernan, J.A. *Histological and Histochemical Methods: Theory and Practice*, 4th ed.; Scion Publishing Ltd.: Banbury, UK, 2008; ISBN 9781904842422.
66. Gibson-Corley, K.N.; Olivier, A.K.; Meyerholz, D.K. Principles for Valid Histopathologic Scoring in Research. *Vet. Pathol.* **2013**, *50*, 1007–1015. [CrossRef]
67. Novo, M.; Almodóvar, A.; Fernández, R.; Trigo, D.; Díaz Cosín, D.J. Cryptic speciation of hormogastrid earthworms revealed by mitochondrial and nuclear data. *Mol. Phylogenet. Evol.* **2010**, *56*, 507–512. [CrossRef]
68. King, R.A.; Tibble, A.L.; Symondson, W.O.C. Opening a can of worms: Unprecedented sympatric cryptic diversity within British lumbricid earthworms. *Mol. Ecol.* **2008**, *17*, 4684–4698. [CrossRef]

69. Anderson, C.; Cunha, L.; Sechi, P.; Kille, P.; Spurgeon, D. Genetic variation in populations of the earthworm, Lumbricus rubellus, across contaminated mine sites. *BMC Genet.* **2017**, *18*. [CrossRef]
70. Pérez-Losada, M.; Eiroa, J.; Mato, S.; Domínguez, J. Phylogenetic species delimitation of the earthworms Eisenia fetida (Savigny, 1826) and Eisenia andrei Bouché, 1972 (Oligochaeta, Lumbricidae) based on mitochondrial and nuclear DNA sequences. *Pedobiologia* **2005**, *49*, 317–324. [CrossRef]
71. Folmer, O.; Black, M.; Hoeh, W.; Lutz, R.; Vrijenhoek, R. DNA primers for amplification of mitochondrial cytochrome c oxidase subunit I from diverse metazoan invertebrates. *Mol. Mar. Biol. Biotechnol.* **1994**, *3*, 294–299. [CrossRef]
72. Sharma, A.; Sonah, H.; Deshmukh, R.K.; Gupta, N.K.; Singh, N.K.; Sharma, T.R. Analysis of Genetic Diversity in Earthworms using DNA Markers. *Zool. Sci.* **2010**, *28*, 25. [CrossRef]
73. Paradis, E.; Schliep, K. ape 5.0: An environment for modern phylogenetics and evolutionary analyses in R. *Bioinformatics* **2019**, *35*, 526–528. [CrossRef] [PubMed]
74. Kozich, J.J.; Westcott, S.L.; Baxter, N.T.; Highlander, S.K.; Schloss, P.D. Development of a dual-index sequencing strategy and curation pipeline for analyzing amplicon sequence data on the MiSeq Illumina sequencing platform. *Appl. Environ. Microbiol.* **2013**, *79*, 5112–5120. [CrossRef]
75. Callahan, B.J.; McMurdie, P.J.; Rosen, M.J.; Han, A.W.; Johnson, A.J.A.; Holmes, S.P. DADA2: High-resolution sample inference from Illumina amplicon data. *Nat. Methods* **2016**, *13*, 581–583. [CrossRef] [PubMed]
76. Callahan, B. Silva taxonomic training data formatted for DADA2 (Silva version 132) [Data set]. *Zenodo* **2018**.
77. Livak, K.J.; Schmittgen, T.D. Analysis of relative gene expression data using real-time quantitative PCR and the 2-∆∆CT method. *Methods* **2001**, *25*, 402–408. [CrossRef]
78. Oksanen, J.; Blanchet, F.G.; Friendly, M.; Kindt, R.; Legendre, P.; McGlinn, D.; Minchin, P.R.; O'Hara, R.B.; Simpson, G.L.; Solymos, P.; et al. Vegan: Community Ecology Package. R Package Version 2.5-3. 2018. Available online: https://CRAN.R-project.org/package=vegan (accessed on 25 October 2018).
79. Procházková, P.; Hanč, A.; Dvořák, J.; Roubalová, R.; Drešlová, M.; Částková, T.; Šustr, V.; Škanta, F.; Pacheco, N.I.N.; Bilej, M. Contribution of Eisenia andrei earthworms in pathogen reduction during vermicomposting. *Environ. Sci. Pollut. Res.* **2018**, *25*, 26267–26278. [CrossRef]
80. Hayashi, Y.; Miclaus, T.; Scavenius, C.; Kwiatkowska, K.; Sobota, A.; Engelmann, P.; Scott-Fordsmand, J.J.; Enghild, J.J.; Sutherland, D.S. Species differences take shape at nanoparticles: Protein corona made of the native repertoire assists cellular interaction. *Environ. Sci. Technol.* **2013**, *47*, 14367–14375. [CrossRef]
81. Bigorgne, E.; Foucaud, L.; Caillet, C.; Giambérini, L.; Nahmani, J.; Thomas, F.; Rodius, F. Cellular and molecular responses of E. fetida cœlomocytes exposed to TiO 2 nanoparticles. *J. Nanoparticle Res.* **2012**, *14*. [CrossRef]
82. Patricia, C.S.; Nerea, G.V.; Erik, U.; Elena, S.M.; Eider, B.; Darío, D.M.W.; Manu, S. Responses to silver nanoparticles and silver nitrate in a battery of biomarkers measured in coelomocytes and in target tissues of Eisenia fetida earthworms. *Ecotoxicol. Environ. Saf.* **2017**, *141*, 57–63. [CrossRef]
83. Garcia-Velasco, N.; Irizar, A.; Urionabarrenetxea, E.; Scott-Fordsmand, J.J.; Soto, M. Selection of an optimal culture medium and the most responsive viability assay to assess AgNPs toxicity with primary cultures of Eisenia fetida coelomocytes. *Ecotoxicol. Environ. Saf.* **2019**, *183*, 109545. [CrossRef]
84. Alijagic, A.; Gaglio, D.; Napodano, E.; Russo, R.; Costa, C.; Benada, O.; Kofroňová, O.; Pinsino, A. Titanium dioxide nanoparticles temporarily influence the sea urchin immunological state suppressing inflammatory-relate gene transcription and boosting antioxidant metabolic activity. *J. Hazard. Mater.* **2020**, *384*, 121389. [CrossRef]
85. Meier, C.; Voegelin, A.; Pradas Del Real, A.; Sarret, G.; Mueller, C.R.; Kaegi, R. Transformation of Silver Nanoparticles in Sewage Sludge during Incineration. *Environ. Sci. Technol.* **2016**, *50*, 3503–3510. [CrossRef]
86. Sekine, R.; Marzouk, E.R.; Khaksar, M.; Scheckel, K.G.; Stegemeier, J.P.; Lowry, G.V.; Donner, E.; Lombi, E. Aging of dissolved copper and copper-based nanoparticles in five different soils: Short-term kinetics vs. long-term fate. *J. Environ. Qual.* **2017**, *46*, 1198–1205. [CrossRef] [PubMed]
87. Levard, C.; Hotze, E.M.; Lowry, G.V.; Brown, G.E. Environmental Transformations of Silver Nanoparticles: Impact on Stability and Toxicity. *Environ. Sci. Technol.* **2012**, *46*, 6900–6914. [CrossRef]
88. Baccaro, M.; Undas, A.K.; De Vriendt, J.; Van Den Berg, J.H.J.; Peters, R.J.B.; Van Den Brink, N.W. Ageing, dissolution and biogenic formation of nanoparticles: How do these factors affect the uptake kinetics of silver nanoparticles in earthworms? *Environ. Sci. Nano* **2018**, *5*, 1107–1116. [CrossRef]

89. Peng, C.; Duan, D.; Xu, C.; Chen, Y.; Sun, L.; Zhang, H.; Yuan, X.; Zheng, L.; Yang, Y.; Yang, J.; et al. Translocation and biotransformation of CuO nanoparticles in rice (*Oryza sativa* L.) plants. *Environ. Pollut.* **2015**, *197*, 99–107. [CrossRef] [PubMed]
90. Xiang, Q.; Zhu, D.; Chen, Q.L.; O'Connor, P.; Yang, X.R.; Qiao, M.; Zhu, Y.G. Adsorbed Sulfamethoxazole Exacerbates the Effects of Polystyrene (~2 μm) on Gut Microbiota and the Antibiotic Resistome of a Soil Collembolan. *Environ. Sci. Technol.* **2019**, *53*, 12823–12834. [CrossRef]
91. Nechitaylo, T.Y.; Timmis, K.N.; Golyshin, P.N. "Candidatus Lumbricincola", a novel lineage of uncultured Mollicutes from earthworms of family Lumbricidae. *Environ. Microbiol.* **2009**, *11*, 1016–1026. [CrossRef]
92. Tak, E.S.; Cho, S.; Park, S.C. Gene expression profiling of coelomic cells and discovery of immune-related genes in the earthworm, Eisenia andrei, using expressed sequence tags. *Biosci. Biotechnol. Biochem.* **2015**, *8451*, 1–7. [CrossRef]
93. Opper, B.; Bognár, A.; Heidt, D.; Németh, P.; Engelmann, P. Revising lysenin expression of earthworm coelomocytes. *Dev. Comp. Immunol.* **2013**, *39*, 214–218. [CrossRef]
94. Adamowicz, A. Morphology and ultrastructure of the earthworm Dendrobaena veneta (Lumbricidae) coelomocytes. *Tissue Cell* **2005**, *37*, 125–133. [CrossRef] [PubMed]
95. Engelmann, P.; Cooper, E.L.; Opper, B.; Németh, P. Earthworm Innate Immune System. In *Biology of Earthworms*; Karaca, A., Ed.; Soil Biology; Springer: Berlin/Heidelberg, Germany, 2011; Volume 24, pp. 229–245. ISBN 978-3-642-14635-0.
96. Bodó, K.; Ernszt, D.; Németh, P.; Engelmann, P. Distinct immune-and defense-related molecular fingerprints in sepatated coelomocyte subsets of Eisenia andrei earthworms. *Invertebr. Surviv. J.* **2018**, *15*, 338–345.
97. Irizar, A.; Rivas, C.; García-Velasco, N.; de Cerio, F.G.; Etxebarria, J.; Marigómez, I.; Soto, M. Establishment of toxicity thresholds in subpopulations of coelomocytes (amoebocytes vs. eleocytes) of Eisenia fetida exposed in vitro to a variety of metals: Implications for biomarker measurements. *Ecotoxicology* **2015**, *24*, 1004–1013. [CrossRef] [PubMed]
98. Homa, J.; Zorska, A.; Wesolowski, D.; Chadzinska, M. Dermal exposure to immunostimulants induces changes in activity and proliferation of coelomocytes of Eisenia andrei. *J. Comp. Physiol. B.* **2013**, 313–322. [CrossRef] [PubMed]
99. Olchawa, E.; Bzowska, M.; Stürzenbaum, S.R.; Morgan, A.J.; Plytycz, B. Heavy metals affect the coelomocyte-bacteria balance in earthworms: Environmental interactions between abiotic and biotic stressors. *Environ. Pollut.* **2006**, *142*, 373–381. [CrossRef] [PubMed]
100. Procházková, P.; Silerová, M.; Felsberg, J.; Josková, R.; Beschin, A.; De Baetselier, P.; Bilej, M. Relationship between hemolytic molecules in Eisenia fetida earthworms. *Dev. Comp. Immunol.* **2006**, *30*, 381–392. [CrossRef]
101. Plytycz, B.; Bigaj, J.; Osikowski, A.; Hofman, S.; Falniowski, A.; Panz, T.; Grzmil, P.; Vandenbulcke, F. The existence of fertile hybrids of closely related model earthworm species, *Eisenia andrei* and *E. fetida*. *PLoS ONE* **2018**, *13*, e0191711. [CrossRef]
102. Martinsson, S.; Erséus, C. Hybridisation and species delimitation of Scandinavian Eisenia spp. (Clitellata: Lumbricidae). *Eur. J. Soil Biol.* **2018**, *88*, 41–47. [CrossRef]
103. Römbke, J.; Aira, M.; Backeljau, T.; Breugelmans, K.; Domínguez, J.; Funke, E.; Graf, N.; Hajibabaei, M.; Pérez-Losada, M.; Porto, P.G.; et al. DNA barcoding of earthworms (Eisenia fetida/andrei complex) from 28 ecotoxicological test laboratories. *Appl. Soil Ecol.* **2016**, *104*, 3–11. [CrossRef]
104. Bouché, M.B. Lombriciens de France. *Ecol. Syst.* **1972**, *72*, 671.
105. Domínguez, J.; Velando, A.; Ferreiro, A. Are Eisenia fetida (Savigny, 1826) and Eisenia andrei Bouche (1972) (Oligochaeta, Lumbricidae) different biological species? *Pedobiologia* **2005**, *49*, 81–87. [CrossRef]
106. Plytycz, B.; Bigaj, J.; Panz, T.; Grzmil, P. Asymmetrical hybridization and gene flow between Eisenia andrei and E. fetida lumbricid earthworms. *PLoS ONE* **2018**, *13*, e0204469. [CrossRef] [PubMed]
107. Goodrich, J.K.; Davenport, E.R.; Beaumont, M.; Bell, J.T.; Clark, A.G.; Ley, R.E.; Goodrich, J.K.; Davenport, E.R.; Beaumont, M.; Jackson, M.A.; et al. Genetic Determinants of the Gut Microbiome in UK Twins Resource Genetic Determinants of the Gut Microbiome in UK Twins. *Cell Host Microbe* **2016**, 731–743. [CrossRef]
108. Kolde, R.; Franzosa, E.A.; Rahnavard, G.; Hall, A.B.; Vlamakis, H.; Stevens, C.; Daly, M.J.; Xavier, R.J.; Huttenhower, C. Host genetic variation and its microbiome interactions within the Human Microbiome Project. *Genome Med.* **2018**, *10*, 1–13. [CrossRef] [PubMed]
109. Buhnik-Rosenblau, K.; Danin-Poleg, Y.; Kashi, Y. Predominant effect of host genetics on levels of Lactobacillus johnsonii bacteria in the mouse gut. *Appl. Environ. Microbiol.* **2011**, *77*, 6531–6538. [CrossRef]

110. Macke, E.; Callens, M.; De Meester, L.; Decaestecker, E. Host-genotype dependent gut microbiota drives zooplankton tolerance to toxic cyanobacteria. *Nat. Commun.* **2017**, *8*. [CrossRef]
111. Davidson, S.K.; Davidson, S.K.; Stahl, D.A. Transmission of Nephridial Bacteria of the Earthworm Eisenia fetida. *Appl. Environ. Microbiol.* **2006**, *72*, 769–775. [CrossRef]

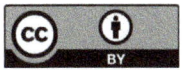

© 2020 by the authors. Licensee MDPI, Basel, Switzerland. This article is an open access article distributed under the terms and conditions of the Creative Commons Attribution (CC BY) license (http://creativecommons.org/licenses/by/4.0/).

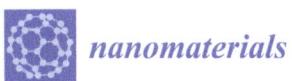

Article

An OMV-Based Nanovaccine Confers Safety and Protection against Pathogenic *Escherichia coli* via Both Humoral and Predominantly Th1 Immune Responses in Poultry

Rujiu Hu [1], Haojing Liu [1], Mimi Wang [1], Jing Li [2], Hua Lin [1], Mingyue Liang [1], Yupeng Gao [1,*] and Mingming Yang [1,*]

1. College of Animal Science and Technology, Northwest A&F University, No.22 Xinong Road, Yangling 712100, Shaanxi, China; hurujiu@nwsuaf.edu.cn (R.H.); lhj1995@nwsuaf.edu.cn (H.L.); wmm@nwsuaf.edu.cn (M.W.); 17208046@nwsuaf.edu.cn (H.L.); lmy20@nwsuaf.edu.cn (M.L.)
2. Department of Animal Engineering, Yangling Vocational and Technical College, No.24 Weihui Road, Yangling 712100, Shaanxi, China; lijing0916@nwafu.edu.cn
* Correspondence: gaoyupeng@nwsuaf.edu.cn (Y.G.); ymm@nwsuaf.edu.cn (M.Y.)

Received: 6 September 2020; Accepted: 16 November 2020; Published: 20 November 2020

Abstract: Avian pathogenic *Escherichia coli* (APEC) infection in poultry causes enormous economic losses and public health risks. Bacterial outer membrane vesicles (OMVs) and nano-sized proteolipids enriched with various immunogenic molecules have gained extensive interest as novel nanovaccines against bacterial infections. In this study, after the preparation of APEC O2-derived OMVs (APEC_OMVs) using the ultracentrifugation method and characterization of them using electron microscopy and nanoparticle tracking analyses, we examined the safety and vaccination effect of APEC_OMVs in broiler chicks and investigated the underlying immunological mechanism of protection. The results showed that APEC_OMVs had membrane-enclosed structures with an average diameter of 89 nm. Vaccination with 50 µg of APEC_OMVs had no side effects and efficiently protected chicks against homologous infection. APEC_OMVs could be effectively taken up by chicken macrophages and activated innate immune responses in macrophages in vitro. APEC_OMV vaccination significantly improved activities of serum non-specific immune factors, enhanced the specific antibody response and promoted the proliferation of splenic and peripheral blood lymphocytes in response to mitogen. Furthermore, APEC_OMVs also elicited a predominantly IFN-γ-mediated Th1 response in splenic lymphocytes. Our data revealed the involvement of both non-specific immune responses and specific antibody and cytokine responses in the APEC_OMV-mediated protection, providing broader knowledge for the development of multivalent APEC_OMV-based nanovaccine with high safety and efficacy in the future.

Keywords: avian pathogenic *Escherichia coli*; nanovaccine; outer membrane vesicles; immune response; broiler

---

1. Introduction

Avian pathogenic *Escherichia coli* (APEC) is one of the major pathogens that have been recognized as serious threats to the global poultry industry [1–3]. APEC causes a variety of local and systemic diseases in many avian species, such as colibacillosis in broiler chickens [2,4]. Chicken colibacillosis is characterized by high morbidity and mortality, leading to substantial economic losses every year in the poultry industry worldwide [5]. In commercial production, antibiotic regimens are used as a common measure to control APEC. However, the prevalence of multidrug-resistant APEC caused by the extensive usage of antibiotics has attracted significant concerns. In many countries, antibiotics have been banned in the animal food industry [6]. Furthermore, drug residues and transfers of resistant genes through poultry products are becoming severe threats to public health [7]. Therefore, it is necessary to explore novel preventive approaches. To date, the use of effective vaccines is recognized as an important way to control APEC infections in today's large-scale poultry industry [8,9].

Many attempts have been made to develop various biological materials as vaccine candidates against APEC infections. Some cell-wall components and virulence factors from APEC strains, such as lipopolysaccharide (LPS), outer membrane proteins, siderophore receptor protein, fimbriae and adhesins, have been shown to induce protective immunity against their corresponding serotypes [8,10,11]. Accordingly, numerous APEC vaccines, mainly inactivated, live-attenuated and subunit vaccines, have been developed for commercial use. Although these vaccines have been proven to be effective, there are still some drawbacks in practical application [8]. Inactivated vaccines are prepared by inactivating the live whole-bacteria with heat or chemicals, which can provide short-term protection against the homologous serogroups only [8]; live-attenuated bacteria vaccines may cause public safety concerns due to their potential risk of bacterial spread [9]. Subunit or recombinant vaccines, mainly including iron regulated outer membrane proteins-based vaccines, fimbriae-based vaccines and increased serum survival protein-based vaccines, could induce better protective immunity against heterologous challenges than inactivated vaccines, but they are rarely used in practice because of their limitations, such as unstable efficacy and the requirement of strong adjuvants [8,9]. Additionally, APEC isolates commonly have a variety of O serogroups (according to the O-antigens); and three main serogroups, including O1, O2 and O78, are frequently associated with disease formation in poultry farms, which can cause over 80% of chicken colibacillosis cases [2,4,8]. It may be difficult to achieve better prevention efficiency for APEC multi-serogroups using these above-mentioned vaccines. Therefore, it is still necessary to develop new vaccine candidates with both higher safety and better efficacy.

Almost all domains of life, including bacteria, archaea and eukaryotes, can secrete nanosized membrane vesicles during their normal growth [12]. These nanovesicles released by Gram-negative bacteria originate from the outer membrane of the cell envelope, and thus are also termed outer membrane vesicles (OMVs) [13]. Biochemical and proteomic analyses have shown that OMVs are naturally enriched with many bioactive molecules of the parental bacteria, including outer membrane proteins and lipids, periplasmic proteins, polysaccharides, nucleic acids (DNA and RNA) and virulence-associated factors [14–17]. Bacterial OMVs have been proven to play important roles in host–bacteria interactions, such as mediating pathogenesis, enhancing bacterial survival under various environmental stress conditions and modulating host immunity [18,19]. Due to the unique structural and immunological properties, such as biocompatible nanometer-scale structure, and the feature of being genetically modified and naturally carrying both adjuvants and multiple antigens, OMVs are generally considered to be emerging candidates for drug delivery platforms and nanovaccines [20–23]. Numerous studies have demonstrated that OMVs secreted by a variety of pathogens, such as *Neisseria meningitidis* [24], *Klebsiella pneumoniae* [25], *Vibrio cholerae* [26] *Bordetella pertussis* [27], *Salmonella* [28] and *Staphylococcus aureus* [29], can elicit protection against the corresponding bacterial infections in mice. Moreover, some studies have shown that immunization with OMVs can provide broad cross-protection against heterologous serogroups [30–32].

Although extensive studies have revealed that OMVs secreted by pathogenic *E. coli* species can induce protective immunity in mouse models, very few investigations have focused on whether OMVs produced by APEC (APEC_OMVs) have the potential to be developed as a novel vaccine candidates in chickens [21,33,34]. Recently, Wang and colleagues have revealed that vaccination with APEC O78-derived OMVs can protect broiler chickens against homologous infection, suggesting the potential of APEC-derived OMVs as APEC vaccine candidates [35]. Wang's report only characterized the specific antibody responses induced by OMVs; however, the safety of APEC_OMVs and the protective mechanisms involving both innate and specific cellular immunity have not been clearly identified.

In this study, we isolated and purified APEC_OMVs from a clinical APEC O2 strain, a major APEC serogroup causing chicken colibacillosis. Compared with Wang's study, the present study investigated the immunogenicity of APEC_OMVs in a broiler chick model using both in vitro and in vivo experiments, including innate immune responses in chicken macrophages; non-specific immune factor activities and specific antibody responses in the serum; and lymphocyte proliferation and cytokine responses in splenic lymphocytes. Moreover, we also evaluated the adverse effects of APEC_OMVs and estimated the window dose between effectiveness and toxicity for APEC_OMVs. Our work reveals the detailed immunologic mechanisms of APEC_OMV-mediated protection, providing the basic information for the development of an effective and multivalent APEC_OMV-based nanovaccine in the future.

2. Materials and Methods

2.1. Bacterial Strain and Preparation of APEC_OMVs

A clinical APEC O2 strain from a chicken with colisepticemia (collection number CVCC1554) was purchased from China Veterinary Culture Collection Center (China Veterinary Drug Supervision Institute, Beijing, China) and used in this study. This APEC isolate was grown in Luria–Bertani (LB) broth at 37 °C. Native OMVs were isolated and purified from bacterial culture supernatant by a series of centrifugal processes, as described in our previous studies [36,37]. Briefly, the bacteria-free supernatant was collected from the culture medium in the logarithmic phase by centrifugation (12,000× g, 15 min, 4 °C), and filtered through a 0.45-μm membrane (Merck Millipore, Tullagreen, Carrigtwohill, Ireland) followed by ultracentrifugation (150,000× g, 2 h, 4 °C). After washing with sterile phosphate buffer saline (PBS; pH 7.4), the obtained APEC_OMV pellet was purified by discontinuous density centrifugation. For purification, APEC_OMVs were covered with 20% (1.127 g/mL) and 35% (1.199 g/mL) OptiPrep (Sigma, catalogue number D1556) and then subjected to ultracentrifugation (16 h, 180,000× g, 4 °C) [38]. The interlayer of the 20% and 35% OptiPrep containing the majority of vesicles was collected, dispersed in sterile PBS and then centrifuged (150,000× g, 2 h, 4 °C) to completely remove OptiPrep. The purified APEC_OMVs were uniformly dispersed in sterile PBS and any bacterial contaminations were removed by filter sterilization with a 0.45-μm membrane. The APEC_OMVs samples were stored at −80 °C for future use. The protein quantification of APEC_OMVs was performed using a TaKaRa BCA Protein Assay Kit (TaKaRa Bio, Beijing, China; catalogue number T9300A) following the manufacturer's instructions.

2.2. Electron Microscopy Analysis

APEC_OMVs were visualized by scanning electron microscopy (SEM) and transmission electron microscopy (TEM). For SEM visualization, 10 μL of the purified APEC_OMVs was dropped on a 5 mm × 5 mm silicon slice, dried at 20 °C and sputter-coated with gold-palladium using an ion-sputtering coater (E-1045; Hitachi, Tokyo, Japan). The prepared nanovesicles were observed using a Field Emission Scanning Electron Microscope (S-4800, Hitachi, Tokyo, Japan). For TEM visualization, 200 μg/mL of the nanovesicles was adhered to 300-mesh copper grids for 10 min followed by negatively staining with 1% phosphotungstic acid (pH 7.2), and then viewed using FEI Tecnai™ G2 Spirit BioTWIN (FEI Company, Hillsboro, OR, USA) at 100 kV.

2.3. Nanoparticle Tracking Analysis

Nanoparticle tracking analysis (NTA) was performed to measure the diameter size and particle number of APEC_OMVs using an NS300 nanoparticle analyzer (Malvern, Worchestershire, UK). These nanovesicle samples were uniformly dispersed in PBS and detected with a camera level of 15. Five 60 s video records were obtained for each sample and analyzed using NTA software version 2.3. The detection threshold was set at 6.

2.4. Animals and Housing

Broiler chicks (Arbor Acres) were hatched from fertilized eggs in an automatic incubator (Beijing LanTianJiao Electronic Technology Co., Ltd., Beijing, China) following routine incubation procedures in a sterilized room with filtered air. All hatching eggs and the incubator were sterilized before incubation. The hatching eggs were sterilized by wiping the surface of the eggshell with 75% alcohol cotton balls before putting them into the incubator. The incubator was placed in an isolation room and the isolation room was disinfected by formaldehyde fumigation. Newly hatched chicks were housed in stainless-steel cages in sterilized rooms with filtered air, strict sanitary conditions and age-appropriate temperatures. All chicks were fed an age-appropriate commercial diet containing no antibiotic additives. Drinking water and diets were offered ad libitum. All procedures of animal experiments were approved by the Ethics Committee of Animal Care and Use at Northwest A&F University with the permit number 2018NWAFU-052.

2.5. Maternal Anti-APEC Antibody Levels in Broiler Chicks

The objective of this experiment was to detect the optimal age for the immunization in young broiler chicks. A total of 30 newly hatched chicks were randomly divided into 6 replicates with 5 birds per replicate. The serum samples were collected at 1, 3, 5, 7, 10, 14, 18 and 21 days of age to determine the natural anti-APEC maternal antibody levels as described below.

2.6. Effect of APEC_OMV Vaccination on the Growth Performance, Immune Organ Index and Blood Cell Counts

This experiment aimed to evaluate the potential adverse effects of APEC_OMVs. For vaccination procedures, a total of 120 seven-day-old broiler chicks were randomly divided into four groups. Each group contained 6 replicates with 5 birds per replicate, which were respectively immunized with 200 µL PBS (as a control) and 10, 50 and 200 µg of APEC_OMVs in 200 µL PBS via intramuscular injection into the right thigh muscle using the disposable syringe at 7 and 14 days of age. The body weight, feed intake and the number of deaths were recorded on a replicate basis and used to calculate average daily weight gain (ADWG), average daily feed intake (ADFI) and feed conversion rate (FCR) from 7 to 21 days of age. At 21 days of age (one week after the secondary vaccination), 6 chicks of each group were chosen and euthanized to collect immune organs (thymus, spleen and bursa of Fabricius) and blood samples for the determination of immune organ index and blood cell counts. The organ index was calculated based on the following formula: organ index = organ weight (g)/body weight (kg). The numbers of red blood cells (RBC) and white blood cells (WBC) were estimated by a manual hemocytometer using Natt–Herrick's stain solution [39].

2.7. Effect of APEC_OMV Vaccination on the Protective Efficacy against Homologous Infection in Broiler Chicks

After the vaccination procedures, the remaining 24 chicks of each group were challenged by the air sac route with 5×10^8 CFU/bird of APEC O2 recommended by the previous study at 21 days of age [10]. The survival rate of chicks in each group was calculated daily for 10 consecutive days. Blood samples were collected from PBS- and APEC_OMV-immunized chicks at 12, 24 and 36 h after bacterial challenge for the determination of bacterial loads. Blood samples were prepared by 10-fold serial dilution in sterile PBS, followed by plating on LB agar plates in triplicate. The counts of bacterial colonies under 37 °C for 12 h were recorded. Serum samples were collected from PBS- and APEC_OMV-immunized chicks at 24 h after bacterial challenge for the determination of proinflammatory cytokines interleukin (IL)-1β and IL-6 using the Chicken Interleukin 1β ELISA Kit (Cloud-Clone Corp., Houston, TX, USA; catalogue number SEA563Ga) and Chicken Interleukin 6 ELISA Kit (Cloud-Clone Corp., Houston, TX, USA; catalogue number SEA079Ga) according to the manufacturer's instructions, respectively.

2.8. In Vitro Chicken Macrophage Assays

HD11 cells, a chicken macrophage cell line derived from bone marrow [40], were used in this study and cultured in the complete PRMI-1640 medium (Gibco, catalogue number 22400089) supplemented with 10% heat-inactivated fetal bovine serum (FBS; Zeta-Life, catalogue number Z7181FBS-500), 100 U/mL penicillin and 100 μg/mL streptomycin (Sigma, catalogue number P4333) in an atmosphere of 5% CO_2 at 37 °C. APEC_OMVs (5 μg/mL) were stained with 1 μM dialkylcarbocyanine iodide (DiI; Sigma, catalogue number 42364) as described previously [41]. The DiI-labeled APEC_OMVs were co-incubated with HD11 cells (5×10^6 cells/well) in a 24-well culture plate. After 4 h-incubation, the cells were collected, washed and then fixed with 4% paraformaldehyde in PBS followed by cell nucleus staining with 10 μg/mL of 4′,6-diamidino-2-phenylindole (DAPI; Sigma, catalogue number D9542). Subsequently, the samples were placed on glass slides and viewed by an Andor Revolution XD spinning-disk confocal microscope (Andor Technology, UK).

To investigate innate immune responses induced by the APEC_OMVs, HD11 cells (5×10^6 cells/well) were stimulated with serial doses of APEC_OMVs (0–1000 ng/mL) in a 24-well culture plate. After a 16 h treatment, the cells were harvested for the measurement of the expression of major histocompatibility complex class II β (MHC IIβ) and cytokines tumor necrosis factor α (TNF-α) and IL-6 by quantitative real-time PCR (qRT-PCR).

2.9. Serum Non-Specific Immune Factor Activities

Serum samples were collected from PBS- and APEC_OMV-immunized chicks at 14 and 21 days of age (one week after the primary and secondary vaccinations, respectively) before APEC_OMV vaccination or bacterial challenge. The activities of lysozyme and superoxide dismutase (SOD) in the serum were measured using commercial assay kits (Nanjing Jiancheng Bioengineering Institute, Jiangsu, China; catalogue number A050-1-1 and A001-3-2). Serum complement 3 level was estimated using a chicken-specific ELISA kit (Cloud-Clone Corp., Houston, TX, USA, catalogue number SEA861Ga). The respiratory burst activity in blood leukocyte was estimated as described previously [42].

2.10. Determination of Specific Antibody Titer and Bactericidal Activity in Serum

The natural antibody levels in nonimmunized serum and the levels of APEC_OMV-reactive IgY and APEC-reactive IgY in PBS- and APEC_OMV-immunized serums were determined by the ELISA method as previously described [35]. Bacterial lysates or APEC_OMVs (200 ng/well) were used as antigens and the diluted serum samples (1:200) were used as the primary antibodies. After incubation with antigens, the primary antibodies were reacted with the secondary horseradish peroxidase-conjugated rabbit anti-chicken IgY (200 ng/mL; abcam, catalogue number ab97140) followed by termination with substrate tetramethylbenzidine (100 μL). The OD_{450} was detected using a BioTek synergy2 microplate reader (Biotek, Winooski, VT, USA).

To further evaluate serum antibody responses induced by APEC_OMVs, the ability of bacteria-killing by PBS- and APEC_OMV-immunized serum samples was estimated according to the previously described method [35]. The bacterial survival rate was calculated by comparing bacterial colony-forming unit (CFU) counts after and before the treatment with the serum. Each sample was detected in triplicate.

2.11. Lymphocyte Proliferation Assays

Splenic and peripheral blood lymphocytes were freshly isolated from PBS- and APEC_OMV-immunized chicks at 21 days of age (one week after the secondary vaccination) using the Chicken Splenic and Peripheral Blood Lymphocyte Isolation Kits (Solarbio, catalogue number P9120 and P8740), respectively, following the manufacturer's instructions. These isolated lymphocytes were maintained in complete PRMI-1640 medium supplemented with 10% FBS, 100 U/mL penicillin and 100 μg/mL streptomycin in an atmosphere of 5% CO_2 at 37 °C. Cell proliferation responses were detected by

3-(4,5-dimethylthiazol-2-yl)-2,5-diphenyl tetrazolium bromide (MTT) assay using an MTT Cell Growth Assay Kit (Sigma, catalogue number CT02) as previously described [43]. The results of the tests were expressed as proliferation index according to the formula: proliferation index = (OD_{570} of test sample-OD_{570} of the negative control)/OD_{570} of the negative control. Each sample was determined in triplicate.

2.12. Re-Stimulation Assay of Splenic Lymphocyte

Splenic lymphocytes were obtained and cultured as described above. These cells were adjusted to a concentration of 5×10^6 cells/well in a 24-well culture plate and then re-stimulated with APEC_OMVs (5 μg/mL) for 12 h. The cells were harvested to measure the gene expressions of IFN-γ, IL-4 and IL-17A.

2.13. Quantitative Real-Time PCR (qRT-PCR) for mRNA Quantification

Total RNA was extracted from the cultured HD11 cells and splenic lymphocytes using a Total RNA Kit (Omega Bio-Tek, catalogue number R1034) following the manufacturer's instructions. After examination of RNA purity and quality with an ND-1000 spectrophotometer (Nano-drop Technologies, Wilmington, Delaware), the qRT-PCR analysis was performed with One Step TB Green® PrimeScript™ PLUS RT-PCR Kit (TaKaRa Bio, Beijing, China; catalogue number RR096A) on an iCycler IQ5™ Real-Time PCR Detection System (Bio-Rad, Hercules, CA, USA) according to the manufacturer's instructions. The primer sequences of the target genes and a housekeeping gene (β-actin) are shown in Supplementary Table S1. Triplicate qRT-PCR reactions for each sample were conducted with the following protocol: 95 °C for 1 min; 40 cycles of 95 °C for 15 s and 60 °C for 30 s, 72 °C for 30 s; 72 °C for 10 min. Relative mRNA expression was calculated using the $2^{-\Delta\Delta Ct}$ method as described previously [44], and expressed as the fold-change relative to the control, which was normalized to 1.

2.14. Statistical Analysis

Experimental data were shown as mean ± standard error (S.E.). Data were analyzed by Graph Pad Prism software 5.0 (San Diego, CA, USA). The analysis of differences between the two groups was performed by Student's *t*-test. The analysis of differences among greater than two groups was performed by one-way ANOVA analysis with the Newman–Keuls post-test. The survival data after bacterial infection were analyzed by the log-rank test. Statistical significance was declared at $P < 0.05$.

3. Results

3.1. Characterization of APEC_OMVs

APEC_OMVs were obtained from the culture supernatant of APEC O2 strain using a series of centrifugation procedures and then purified using the density gradient centrifugation method. The morphology and integrity of APEC_OMVs were detected by SEM (Figure 1A) and TEM (Figure 1B). The results showed that these vesicles were intact nanosized structures with spherical morphology, and the majority of these nanovesicles ranged from 50 to 150 nm in diameter. Typical results characterized by NTA are shown in Figure 1C,D. The diameter of APEC_OMVs peaked at 89 nm, which is in accordance with the results of electron microscopy analyses and the previously determined sizes of bacterial OMVs [34].

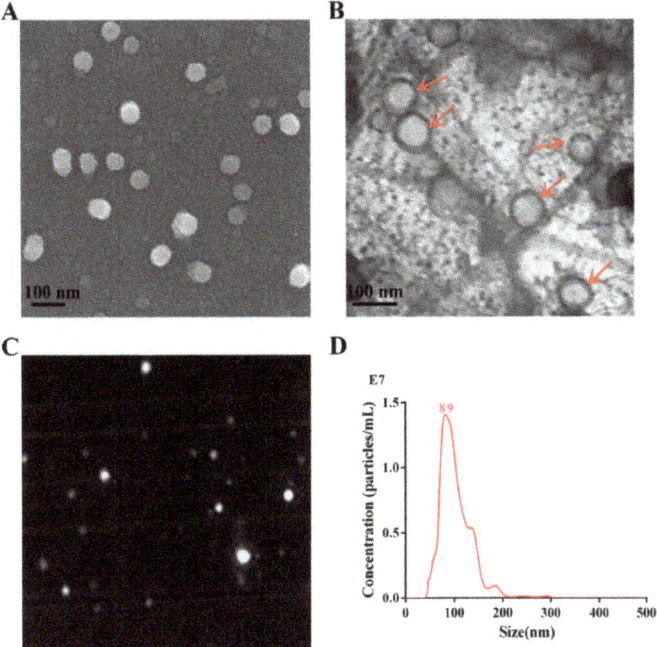

Figure 1. Characterization of outer membrane vesicles secreted by avian pathogenic *E. coli* O2 (APEC_OMVs). (**A**) The purified APEC_OMVs were viewed with a scanning electron microscope. (**B**) After negative staining with 1% phosphotungstic acid, APEC_OMVs were visualized by transmission electron microscopy. The red arrows indicate several visible APEC_OMVs. (**C**) The image from the movie captured using a SCMOS camera of Malven NTA 3.0 when APEC_OMVs were characterized by nanoparticle tracking analysis (NTA). (**D**) Concentration and size distribution of APEC_OMVs determined by NTA.

3.2. Natural Antibody Levels in Nonimmunized Chicks

As shown in Figure 2, a high antibody level was observed in the serum before 5 days of age. The antibody titer dropped to a low level at 7 days of age and remained stable thereafter. These findings suggested that the optimal age of vaccination should not be earlier than 7 days of age.

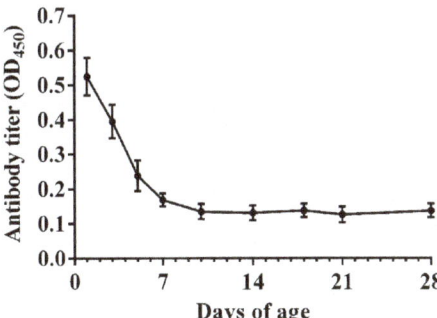

Figure 2. Natural anti-APEC maternal antibody levels in the serum collected from commercial broiler chicks during the 1–28 days of age (n = 5). Data are presented as mean ± SE.

3.3. Effect of APEC_OMVs Vaccination on the Growth Performance, Immune Organ Index and Blood Cell Counts

As shown in Table 1, vaccination with 10 and 50 µg of APEC_OMVs had no significant impacts on ADFI, ADWG, FCR, immune organ index or WBC and RBC counts. However, vaccination with 200 µg of APEC_OMVs significantly reduced ADFI and ADWG, and increased FCR and WBC count, suggesting that this vaccination dose can have adverse effects on chicks. The immune organ indexes were slightly improved in all APEC_OMV-immunized groups compared with the control group, but an increase in the dose of APEC_OMVs to 200 µg had no statistically significant effect on the immune organ indexes. No chicks died in all groups during the vaccination period (data not shown). These results demonstrated that vaccination with an appropriate dose of APEC_OMVs was safe, while high doses of APEC_OMVs could be toxic.

Table 1. Effects of various doses of APEC_OMV vaccination on the growth performance, immune organ index and blood cell counts.

Item [2]	APEC_OMVs [1] (µg/bird)				SE [3]	P-Value
	0	10	50	200		
Growth Performance						
ADFI (g/d)	64.5 [a]	63.9 [a]	62.6 [a]	57.2 [b]	1.35	0.024
ADWG (g/d)	51.3 [a]	49.6 [a]	49.2 [a]	42.4 [b]	1.40	0.003
FCR	1.26 [b]	1.29 [b]	1.27 [b]	1.35 [a]	0.013	0.031
Immune Organ Index (g/kg body weight)						
Thymus index	2.06	2.40	2.48	2.39	0.100	0.498
Spleen index	1.09	1.164	1.21	1.12	0.045	0.801
Bursa index	1.60	1.86	1.83	1.74	0.069	0.339
Blood Cell Counts						
WBC (10^3/µL)	26.7 [b]	28.3 [b]	31.5 [b]	39.3 [a]	3.82	0.042
RBC (10^6/µL)	2.24	1.86	1.93	1.71	0.29	0.126

[1] APEC_OMVs = avian pathogenic *Escherichia coli* O2-derived outer membrane vesicles. [2] ADFI = average daily feed intake; ADWG = average daily weight gain; FCR = feed conversion rate; WBC = white blood cells; RBC = red blood cells. [3] SE = Standard error of the mean. Growth performance were calculated from 7 to 21 days of age; immune organ index and blood cell counts were measured at 21 days (one week after the secondary vaccination). [a,b] Different superscript letters in the same row indicate significant difference ($p < 0.05$).

3.4. Vaccination with APEC_OMVs Was Protective against Homologous Infection in Broiler Chicks

The procedures for the vaccination and bacterial challenge are shown in Figure 3. As shown in Figure 4A, only 16.7% of chicks in the PBS-immunized group survived 10 days after the bacterial infection. The survival rates of 45.8% and 83.3% were observed for groups immunized with 10 and 50 µg of APEC_OMVs, respectively, which were significantly higher than those in the PBS-immunized group. However, an increase of the vaccination dose to 200 µg did not result in significant improvement of protective efficacy. Together with the results of experiment 2, the dose of 50 µg was selected as the final dosage for the following analyses. To further confirm the protective efficacy conferred by APEC_OMVs, bacterial loads in blood samples and proinflammatory cytokine production in serum samples were determined after bacterial challenge. As illustrated in Figure 4B, the APEC_OMV-immunized group showed significantly lower bacterial counts in the blood after 24 h post-infection compared with the control group, indicating that effective clearance of bacteria was induced by APEC_OMVs. Additionally, the levels of proinflammatory cytokines IL-1β and IL-6 in the APEC_OMV-immunized serum were significantly lower than those in the PBS-immunized serum (Figure 4C). These results revealed that vaccination with APEC_OMVs could reduce bacterial loads and proinflammatory cytokine production, and thus provided protection against homologous challenge.

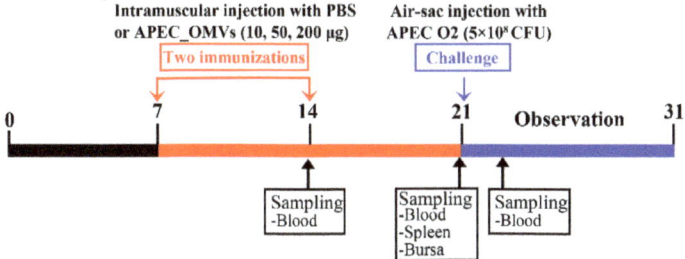

Figure 3. Timeline of APEC_OMV vaccination and bacterial challenge in broiler chick experiments. Four groups of broiler chicks (n = 30; 6 replicates per group with 5 birds per replicate) were intramuscularly immunized with PBS (as a control) and various doses of APEC_OMVs at 7 and 14 days of age, respectively, and challenged by the air sac route at 21 days of age. Blood and spleen samples were collected from PBS- and APEC_OMV-immunized chicks at indicated times.

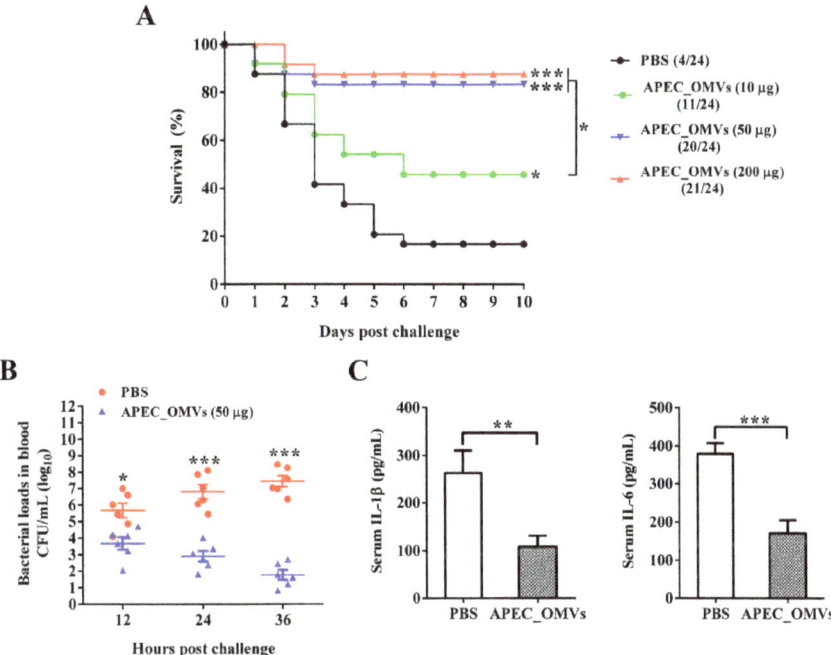

Figure 4. Protective efficacy conferred by APEC_OMV vaccination against homologous challenge in broiler chicks. (**A**) Survival rates of PBS- and APEC_OMV-immunized birds after bacterial challenge (n = 24). The number of surviving chicks in each group was recorded daily for 10 consecutive days after bacterial challenge. (**B**) Bacterial loads in peripheral blood collected from PBS- and APEC_OMV (50 μg)-immunized chicks at indicated times after bacterial challenge (n = 6). (**C**) The production of proinflammatory cytokines (IL-1β and IL-6) in the serum collected from PBS- and APEC_OMV (50 μg)-immunized chicks at 22 days of age (24 h after bacterial challenge) (n = 6). Data are presented as mean ± SE. * $p < 0.05$; ** $p < 0.01$; *** $p < 0.001$, versus the respective control.

3.5. APEC_OMVs Activated Innate Immune Responses In Vitro

Macrophages are not only important players in the clearance of pathogens but also function as antigen-presenting cells (APCs) to recognize and process foreign antigens, linking the innate and adaptive immune responses. We first examined whether chicken HD11 macrophages recognize and respond to APEC_OMVs in vitro. After co-incubation with HD11 cells for 4 h, these DiI-labeled vesicles (red signals) were observed in the cytoplasms of these cells, suggesting that APEC_OMVs were internalized by HD11 cells (Figure 5A). Furthermore, stimulation with APEC_OMVs dramatically enhanced the expression of MHC IIβ and cytokines TNF-α and IL-6 in a dose-dependent manner (Figure 5B). These results indicated that APEC_OMVs could provoke innate immune responses in APCs, which can activate T cell responses.

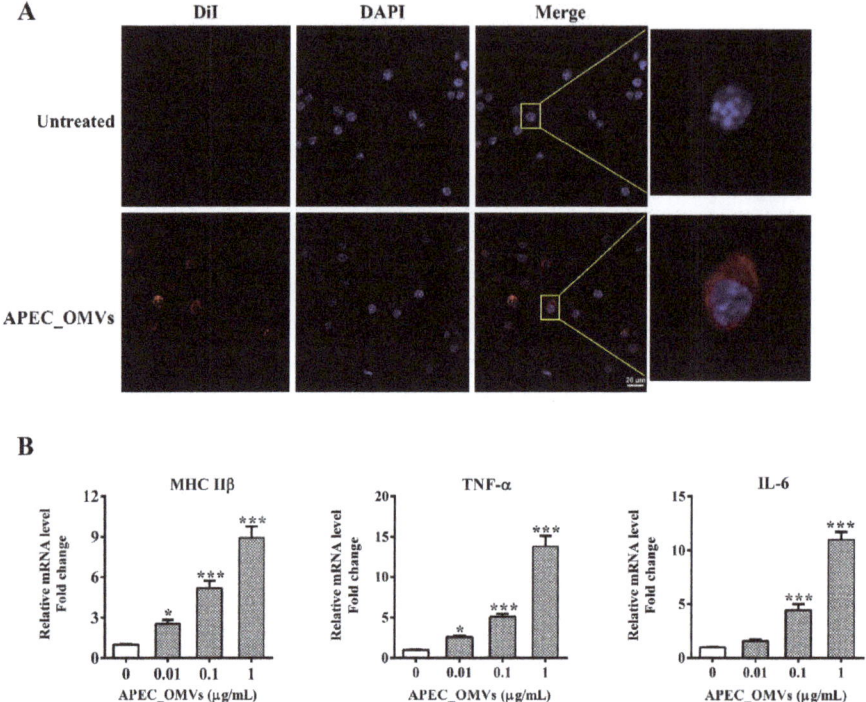

Figure 5. Innate immune responses induced by APEC_OMVs in chicken macrophages in vitro. (**A**) Visualization of internalization of APEC_OMVs by chicken HD11 macrophages using a confocal microscope. Row 1 was a non-stimulated treatment. Row 2 was stimulated with 5 μg/mL of DiI-labeled APEC_OMVs (red signal) for 6 h at 37 °C followed by cell nucleus staining with 10 μg/mL of DAPI (blue signal). (**B**) qRT-PCR analysis for the expression of MHC IIβ, TNF-α and IL-6 in HD11 cells stimulated with various concentrations of APEC_OMVs for 16 h. Results are representatives of three independent experiments and expressed as mean ± SE. * $p < 0.05$; ** $p < 0.01$; *** $p < 0.001$, versus the control.

3.6. Vaccination with APEC_OMVs Improved Serum Non-Specific Immune Factor Activities

We next evaluated the vaccination effect of APEC_OMVs on the serum non-specific immune factor activities. As shown in Figure 6, vaccination with 50 μg of APEC_OMVs significantly improved the lysozyme, complement 3, respiratory burst and SOD activities after both primary and secondary vaccinations. Moreover, the activity of these non-specific immune factors was significantly higher after the secondary booster vaccination than after the primary vaccination.

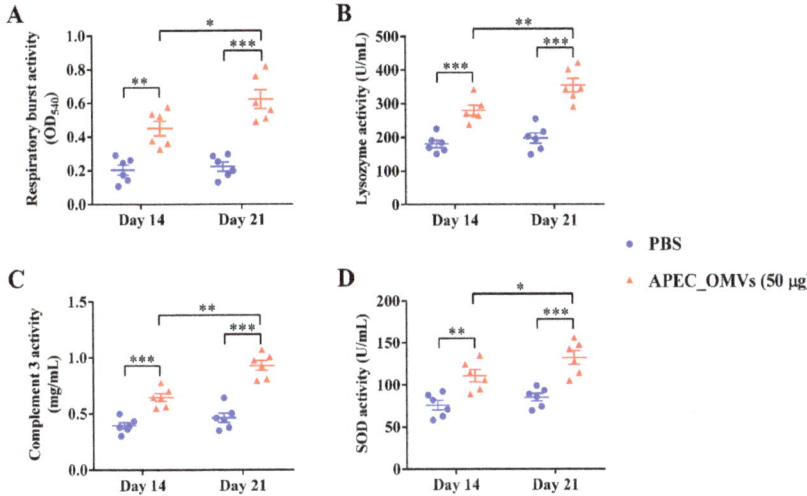

Figure 6. Effects of APEC_OMV vaccination on non-specific immune factor activities in the serum. Serum samples were collected from PBS- and APEC_OMV (50 μg)-immunized chicks at 14 and 21 days of age (one week after the primary and secondary immunization, respectively) before the secondary APEC_OMV immunization or bacterial challenge to determine the activities of the following immune factors: (**A**) lysozyme; (**B**) complement 3; (**C**) respiratory burst; (**D**) SOD. Data are presented as mean ± SE (n = 6). * $p < 0.05$; ** $p < 0.01$; *** $p < 0.001$.

3.7. APEC_OMV-Induced Protection Was Associated with Elevated Antibody Responses

To identify adaptive immune responses involved in APEC_OMV-induced protection, we first detected the specific antibody responses one week after the primary and secondary vaccinations. The levels of APEC_OMV-reactive IgY and APEC-reactive IgY were significantly elevated when chicks were immunized with APEC_OMVs (Figure 7A,B). The secondary booster vaccination significantly enhanced the antibody responses compared to the primary vaccination. Furthermore, APEC_OMV-immunized serum samples showed higher bactericidal activities after both primary and secondary vaccinations compared with PBS-immunized serum samples (Figure 7C).

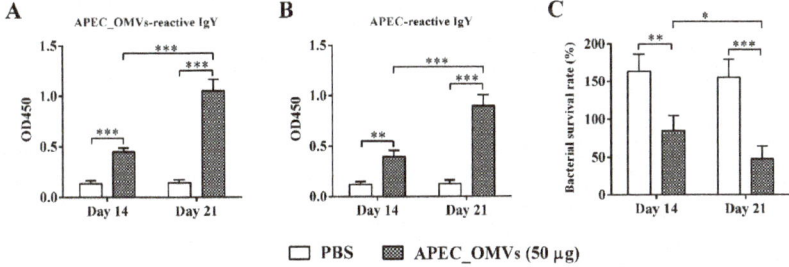

Figure 7. Specific IgY levels and bactericidal activities of serum samples from APEC_OMV-immunized chicks. Serum samples were collected from PBS- and APEC_OMV (50 μg)-immunized chicks at 14 and 21 days of age (one week after primary and secondary vaccination, respectively) before the secondary APEC_OMV vaccination or bacterial challenge. The production of APEC_OMV-reactive IgY (**A**) and APEC-reactive IgY (**B**) was estimated by ELISA assays. (**C**) Bacteria killing assay by the APEC_OMV-immunized serum. The APEC O2 strain was incubated with PBS- and APEC_OMV (50 μg)-immunized serum samples at 37 °C for 1 h and then the bacterial survival rate was measured. Data are presented as mean ± SE (n = 6). * $p < 0.05$; ** $p < 0.01$; *** $p < 0.001$.

3.8. Vaccination with APEC_OMVs Induced Lymphocyte Proliferation and a Predominant Th1 Response

We finally identified cellular responses associated with protection conferred by APEC_OMVs. As shown in Figure 8A, APEC_OMV vaccination significantly enhanced the proliferation of both spleen lymphocytes and peripheral blood lymphocytes in response to mitogen. To determine which T-cell responses were involved in APEC_OMV-induced protection, spleen lymphocytes were isolated from the immunized chicks one week after the secondary vaccination and re-stimulated with APEC_OMVs. The results showed that re-stimulation with APEC_OMVs significantly upregulated the expression of IFN-γ (a representative Th1 cytokine) and IL-17A (a representative Th17 cytokine); the expression of IL-4 (a representative Th2 cytokine) remained unchanged between PBS- and APEC_OMV-immunized groups. Meanwhile, the degree of IFN-γ upregulation (over 12-fold change compared with the control) was much higher than that of IL-17A upregulation (only 3.8-fold change compared with the control), suggesting that IFN-γ-mediated Th1 response may play a predominant role.

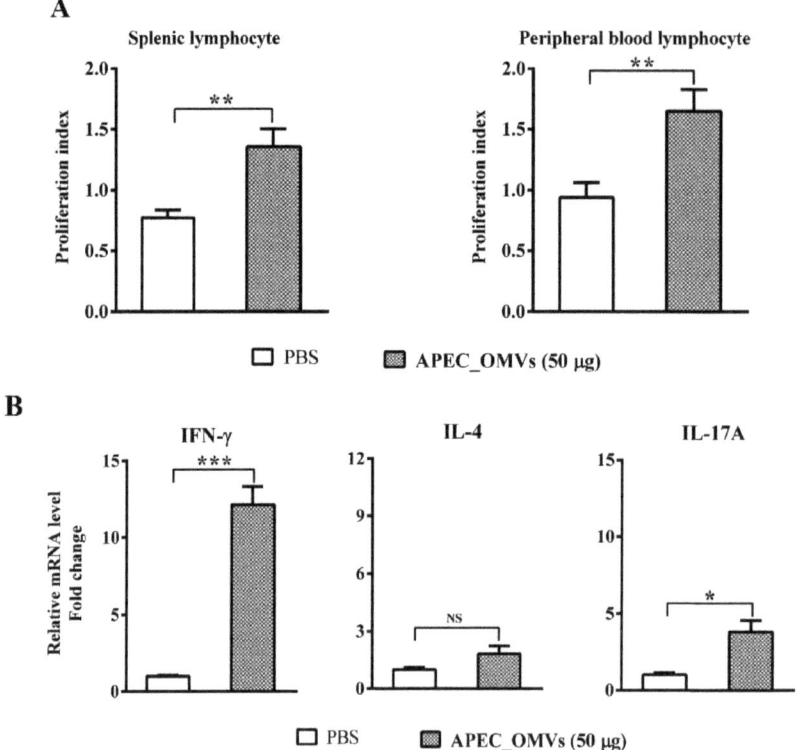

Figure 8. Lymphocyte proliferation and cytokine responses induced by APEC_OMVs. At 21 days of age (one week after secondary vaccination) before the bacterial challenge, splenic lymphocytes and peripheral blood lymphocytes were isolated from PBS- and APEC_OMV (50 μg)-immunized chicks. (**A**) Proliferation indexes of MTT assays for the splenic lymphocytes and peripheral blood lymphocytes re-stimulated with mitogen (ConA). (**B**) Analysis of mRNA expression of Th1 cytokine (IFN-γ), Th2 cytokine (IL-4) and Th 17 cytokine (IL-17) in the splenic lymphocytes re-stimulated with APEC_OMVs (5 μg/mL) for 24 h. Data are presented as mean ± SE. * $p < 0.05$; ** $p < 0.01$; *** $p < 0.001$; NS, not significant.

4. Discussion

Vaccination has proved to be the most practical and effective strategy to control bacterial infections. Bacterial OMVs are becoming increasingly attractive as effective immune-stimulating materials for the development of novel vaccines and adjuvants [20]. Avian colibacillosis, caused by APEC strains, is one of the most severe diseases leading to large economic losses in the global poultry industry [45]. In the present study, we confirmed that vaccination with 50 μg of APEC_OMVs showed no adverse effects and effectively protected chicks against homologous APEC infection by reducing bacterial loads and proinflammatory cytokine production. These protective effects were mediated through activations of both innate and adaptive immune responses elicited by APEC_OMVs, which mainly included serum non-specific immune factors, a specific antibody-mediated humoral immune response and an IFN-γ-mediated cellular immune response.

OMV-based vaccines hold several advantages over the current inactivated and attenuated live APEC vaccines. First, a large number of studies and reviews have revealed that OMVs are membranous vesicles with nanoscale sizes in the range of 20–250 nm, which enables them highly biocompatible and capable of delivering interior molecules in concentrated and protected forms [13,46,47]. Consistent with these previous results, electron microscopic and NTA analyses in our work showed that APEC_OMVs were intact spherical bilayer nanoparticles with a mean size of 89 nm in diameter. These structural characteristics allow OMVs to be more effectively delivered throughout intracellular compartments and efficiently taken-up by APCs. Second, OMVs carry various immune-stimulating molecules from the outer membrane, such as LPS and outer membrane proteins and lipids [13]. Many of these components are immunogenic and act as natural adjuvants, which have the potential to be both multi-antigen carriers and vaccine adjuvants [33,34,48]. These immunological characteristics of these OMV-based vaccines provide great advantages in vaccine efficacy compared to the current single-antigen vaccines. Third, in addition to being easily prepared from natural bacteria, OMVs can be conveniently loaded with specific antigens using bioengineered bacteria [49,50]. Finally, they showed better safety within a certain dose range than attenuated live vaccines due to their nonliving and acellular features, largely reducing the risk of bacterial transmission. However, it should be noted that injection with high doses of OMVs might be toxic because they contain various virulence-associated factors. In this study, we determined that a dose of 50 μg for APEC_OMVs not only showed no side effects but also induced effective protection. Therefore, extra considerations should be made in the window between efficacy and toxicity for OMV immunization on animals and humans in the future.

Innate immunity is recognized to be the first line of host defense against pathogen-associated invasion. Previous in vitro studies have demonstrated that OMVs could activate the innate immune responses of dendritic cells and macrophages and induce the production of cytokines that regulate the adaptive immune responses [25,33]. As an essential cellular component in the innate immune system, macrophages are not only directly involved in the elimination of pathogens, but also can be used as APCs to recognize and process antigens [51]. Consistent with these findings, in this study, we observed that APEC_OMVs were effectively taken-up by the chicken HD11 macrophage cell line in vitro and enhanced the expression of MHC IIβ, TNF-α and IL-6. MHC IIβ, mainly expressed in APCs, can assist these cells in presenting exogenous antigen to CD4 T cells, which can activate specific B- and T-cell immune responses [52]. IL-6 is known to induce adaptive immune responses in mammalian Th17 and play an important role in fighting bacterial invasion [33]. It is important to note, however, that these results were derived from a macrophage cell line, and future studies will be needed to investigate whether similar results are expected from primary cells. Additionally, non-specific immune factors in serum are essential for the elimination of pathogens. Lysozyme plays an essential role in the host's innate immune system against bacterial challenge by cleaving cell wall peptidoglycan [53]. The complement molecule is an important innate immune component that can initiate innate responses and modulate adaptive immune responses [54]. Respiratory burst is an oxygen-dependent mechanism by which neutrophils kill invading pathogens [55]. SOD can effectively alleviate inflammatory responses by reducing oxidative stress during bacterial infection [56]. The activities of these non-specific immune factors were significantly enhanced during APEC_OMV vaccination, which may be due to the enhanced pathogen clearance accompanied by the involvement of the increased leukocytes [57].

The adaptive immune response plays a very important role in host defense against bacterial infections. Specific antibody and T-cell immune responses induced by bacterial OMVs have been demonstrated in both in vitro and in vivo mouse studies [25,33,58]. However, it is unclear which immune response plays a major role. Some studies have shown that antibody-mediated humoral immunity is the most important factor [26], while other studies have suggested that cellular immunity mediated by cytokines, especially IFN-γ and IL-17, is essential for the protection [25]. In the current study, the ELISA results showed that vaccination with APEC_OMVs could elevate the production of anti-APEC_OMVs and anti-APEC antibodies in the APEC_OMV-immunized serum. These enhanced responses of specific antibody induced by APEC_OMVs were also confirmed by bactericidal activity assays. These findings are consistent with the recent study showing that OMVs derived from APEC O78 induced similar protective efficacy in an antibody-dependent manner [35]. However, cytokine-mediated cell responses to APEC_OMV vaccination have not previously been determined. Previous studies performed in mice have indicated that the IFN-γ-mediated Th1 response plays an important role in the protection against bacterial infections by enhancing the bactericidal activity of phagocytes [33,59]. Moreover, the protective effect of vaccines against bacterial challenge requires Th17-mediated immunity by promoting neutrophil recruitment to the site of infection [60]. Meanwhile, our study indicated that APEC_OMVs promoted splenic and peripheral blood lymphocyte proliferation during vaccination. We further identified that APEC_OMVs activated the expression of IFN-γ and IL-17A but not IL-4 in splenic lymphocytes. These results are in accordance with the previous study performed in mice with pathogenic *E. coli*-derived OMVs [33]. It is worth noting that the upregulation of IFN-γ induced by APEC_OMVs was visibly higher than that of IL-17, implying that the IFN-γ-mediated Th1 response may play a dominant role. However, at present, we could not rule out whether other cell types, such as NK cells and γ-δ T cells, are involved in the protection because these cells can also produce IFN-γ and IL-17. The exact cell responses to APEC_OMVs require further exploration. Taken together, although further study is needed, our present work reveals that vaccination with APEC_OMVs induces protective immunity against homologous bacterial infection mainly through the induction of specific antibody and IFN-γ-mediated immune responses.

APEC_OMV-induced protection was well-evidenced in this study, but it is challenging to identify which specific molecules are most essential because APEC_OMVs contain a variety of immunogenic components. Many reviews have illustrated that protein is the most important component of bacterial OMVs and mediates multiple functions [13,61]. Large-scale proteomic studies of various Gram-positive bacteria-derived OMVs have indicated that outer membrane proteins account for the majority of vesicular proteins [14,62]. Many outer membrane proteins have been proved to contribute to bacterial pathogenesis and are used as protective antigens to induce effective protection against bacterial infections [63,64]. Several outer membrane proteins with high abundance, mainly OmpA, OmpX and OmpW, are commonly found in OMVs secreted by APEC strains and other *E. coli* and can elicit strong protective immunity [35,65,66]. These conserved outer membrane proteins give APEC_OMVs the ability to confer a certain degree of cross-protection. The cross-protective effects of several pathogens-derived OMVs have been demonstrated in mice [30,32]. Further investigations are required to confirm whether APEC_OMVs protect against heterologous infections. Additionally, OMVs carry various non-protein antigens, such as LPS, which also participate in the APEC_OMV-induced protective immunity [61]. It is the combination of these diverse antigens that give OMVs their extensive immunogenicity.

Although our present study may be useful to developing a new APEC vaccine, there remain several shortcomings which shall lead us to future work. First, APEC_OMV vaccination using the intramuscular route is less likely to be feasible for practical use in large flocks. Further studies can focus on the development of oral OMV-based nanovaccines for poultry, which may be more competitive and attractive for commercial use in broilers. Second, vaccinating twice for broiler chickens can be costly compared to the currently available vaccine. Third, we did not evaluate the stability and uniformity of APEC_OMVs preparation. Fourth, we did not investigate whether APEC_OMVs could provide broad protection against heterologous challenges. It is believed that single-serogroup APEC_OMVs may not provide enough protective efficacy against chicken colibacillosis caused by multiple APEC serogroups. Therefore, it is still necessary to develop multi-serogroup APEC_OMVs or bioengineered APEC_OMVs with highly expressed heterologous antigens as broadly-protective vaccine candidates against multiple APEC serogroups in the future. Finally, some important investigations of APEC_OMVs as a vaccine candidate were not carried out. For example, antibody responses were not determined after the APEC challenge, the survival of chickens and bacterial load until slaughter age (day 42) were not monitored and the APEC lesions in the internal organs were also not investigated. Further studies, including investigations of the protective efficiency and long-term protection of APEC_OMVs, more detailed protection mechanisms associated with bacterial clearance in multiple organs, pathological changes of internal organs and cytokine responses, etc., will be considered in our future research programs. In conclusion, we revealed that vaccination with APEC_OMVs protected broiler chicks against homologous infection by enhancing bacterial clearance and reducing proinflammatory cytokine production. We further demonstrated that APEC_OMVs could activate innate immune responses in HD11 macrophages in vitro and enhanced activities of serum non-specific immune factors. We also identified that APEC_OMV vaccination could induce both specific antibody responses and a predominant IFN-γ-mediated cellular immune response. Our findings provide broader knowledge to better understand the immunological basis of APEC_OMV-mediated protection and offer a novel strategy for the development of cross-protective nanovaccines to control various APEC serogroups in the future.

Supplementary Materials: The following are available online at http://www.mdpi.com/2079-4991/10/11/2293/s1, Table S1: Primers used for quantitative real-time PCR in this study.

Author Contributions: Conceptualization, R.H., Y.G. and M.Y.; methodology, R.H., J.L. and H.L.(Hua Lin); formal analysis, R.H., H.L.(Haojing Liu), M.W. and M.L.; investigation, R.H., J.L., H.L. (Haojing Liu) and M.L.; writing—original draft preparation, R.H.; writing—review and editing, Y.G. and M.Y.; supervision, Y.G. and M.Y. All authors have read and agreed to the published version of the manuscript.

Funding: This work was supported by the National Natural Sciences Foundation of China (grant numbers 31,672,437 and 31,372,343). The funding organization was not involved in the design of the study, analysis or interpretation of data, or writing of the manuscript.

Acknowledgments: We would like to thank the Life Science Core Services facility at Northwest A&F University for microscopic imaging electron microscope analyses.

Conflicts of Interest: The authors declare no conflict of interest.

References

1. Antao, E.M.; Glodde, S.; Li, G.; Sharifi, R.; Homeier, T.; Laturnus, C.; Diehl, I.; Bethe, A.; Philipp, H.C.; Preisinger, R.; et al. The chicken as a natural model for extraintestinal infections caused by avian pathogenic *Escherichia coli* (APEC). *Microb. Pathog.* **2008**, *45*, 361–369. [PubMed]
2. Sadeyen, J.-R.; Kaiser, P.; Stevens, M.P.; Dziva, F. Analysis of immune responses induced by avian pathogenic *Escherichia coli* infection in turkeys and their association with resistance to homologous re-challenge. *Vet. Res.* **2014**, *45*, 19. [PubMed]
3. Ievy, S.; Islam, M.S.; Sobur, M.A.; Talukder, M.; Rahman, M.B.; Khan, M.F.R.; Rahman, M.T. Molecular detection of avian pathogenic *Escherichia coli* (APEC) for the first time in layer farms in Bangladesh and their antibiotic resistance patterns. *Microorganisms* **2020**, *8*, 1021.
4. Sadeyen, J.-R.; Wu, Z.; Davies, H.; van Diemen, P.M.; Milicic, A.; La Ragione, R.M.; Kaiser, P.; Stevens, M.P.; Dziva, F. Immune responses associated with homologous protection conferred by commercial vaccines for control of avian pathogenic *Escherichia coli* in turkeys. *Vet. Res.* **2015**, *46*, 5. [PubMed]
5. Wang, S.; Peng, Q.; Jia, H.M.; Zeng, X.F.; Zhu, J.L.; Hou, C.L.; Liu, X.T.; Yang, F.J.; Qiao, S.Y. Prevention of *Escherichia coli* infection in broiler chickens with *Lactobacillus plantarum* B1. *Poult. Sci.* **2017**, *96*, 2576–2586.

6. Redweik, G.A.J.; Stromberg, Z.R.; Van Goor, A.; Mellata, M. Protection against avian pathogenic *Escherichia coli* and *Salmonella Kentucky* exhibited in chickens given both probiotics and live *Salmonella* vaccine. *Poult. Sci.* **2020**, *99*, 752–762.
7. Bélanger, L.; Garenaux, A.; Harel, J.; Boulianne, M.; Nadeau, E.; Dozois, C.M. *Escherichia coli* from animal reservoirs as a potential source of human extraintestinal pathogenic *E. coli*. *FEMS Immunol. Med. Microbiol.* **2011**, *62*, 1–10.
8. Ghunaim, H.; Abdelhamid, M.A.; Kariyawasam, S. Advances in vaccination against avian pathogenic *Escherichia coli* respiratory disease: Potentials and limitations. *Vet. Microbiol.* **2014**, *172*, 13–22.
9. Hoelzer, K.; Bielke, L.; Blake, D.P.; Cox, E.; Cutting, S.M.; Devriendt, B.; Erlacher-Vindel, E.; Goossens, E.; Karaca, K.; Lemiere, S.; et al. Vaccines as alternatives to antibiotics for food producing animals. Part 2: New approaches and potential solutions. *Vet. Res.* **2018**, *49*, 70.
10. Han, Y.; Liu, Q.; Willias, S.; Liang, K.; Li, P.; Cheng, A.C.; Kong, Q.K. A bivalent vaccine derived from attenuated *Salmonella* expressing O-antigen polysaccharide provides protection against avian pathogenic *Escherichia coli* O1 and O2 infection. *Vaccine* **2018**, *36*, 1038–1046.
11. Ebrahimi-Nik, H.; Bassami, M.R.; Mohri, M.; Rad, M.; Khan, M.I. Bacterial ghost of avian pathogenic *E. coli* (APEC) serotype O78: K80 as a homologous vaccine against avian colibacillosis. *PLoS ONE* **2018**, *13*, 0194888.
12. Brown, L.; Wolf, J.M.; Prados-Rosales, R.; Casadevall, A. Through the wall: Extracellular vesicles in Gram-positive bacteria, mycobacteria and fungi. *Nat. Rev. Microbiol.* **2015**, *13*, 620–630. [PubMed]
13. Schwechheimer, C.; Kuehn, M.J. Outer-membrane vesicles from Gram-negative bacteria: Biogenesis and functions. *Nat. Rev. Microbiol.* **2015**, *13*, 605–619. [PubMed]
14. Lee, J.; Kim, O.Y.; Gho, Y.S. Proteomic profiling of Gram-negative bacterial outer membrane vesicles: Current perspectives. *Proteom. Clin. Appl.* **2016**, *10*, 897–909.
15. Wai, S.N.; Lindmark, B.; Soderblom, T.; Takade, A.; Westermark, M.; Oscarsson, J.; Jass, J.; Richter-Dahlfors, A.; Mizunoe, Y.; Uhlin, B.E. Vesicle-mediated export and assembly of pore-forming oligomers of the enterobacterial ClyA cytotoxin. *Cell* **2003**, *115*, 25–35. [PubMed]
16. Lusta, K.A. Bacterial outer membrane nanovesicles: Structure, biogenesis, functions, and application in biotechnology and medicine. *Appl. Biochem. Microbiol.* **2015**, *51*, 485–493.
17. Avalos-Gómez, C.; Reyes-López, M.; Ramírez-Rico, G.; Díaz-Aparicio, E.; Zenteno, E.; González-Ruiz, C.; de la Garza, M. Effect of apo-lactoferrin on leukotoxin and outer membrane vesicles of *Mannheimia haemolytica* A2. *Vet. Res.* **2020**, *51*, 36.
18. Kim, J.H.; Lee, J.; Park, J.; Gho, Y.S. Gram-negative and Gram-positive bacterial extracellular vesicles. *Semin. Cell Dev. Biol.* **2015**, *40*, 97–104.
19. Kaparakis-Liaskos, M.; Ferrero, R.L. Immune modulation by bacterial outer membrane vesicles. *Nat. Rev. Immunol.* **2015**, *15*, 375–387.
20. Collins, B.S. Gram-negative outer membrane vesicles in vaccine development. *Discov. Med.* **2011**, *12*, 7–15.
21. Huang, W.W.; Wang, S.J.; Yao, Y.F.; Xia, Y.; Yang, X.; Li, K.; Sun, P.Y.; Liu, C.B.; Sun, W.J.; Bai, H.M.; et al. Employing *Escherichia coli*-derived outer membrane vesicles as an antigen delivery platform elicits protective immunity against *Acinetobacter baumannii* infection. *Sci. Rep.* **2016**, *6*, 37242. [PubMed]
22. Jain, S.; Pillai, J. Bacterial membrane vesicles as novel nanosystems for drug delivery. *Int. J. Nanomed.* **2017**, *12*, 6329–6341.
23. Liu, Y.; Smid, E.J.; Abee, T.; Notebaart, R.A. Delivery of genome editing tools by bacterial extracellular vesicles. *Microb. Biotechnol.* **2019**, *12*, 71–73. [PubMed]
24. Vogel, U.; Claus, H. Vaccine development against *Neisseria meningitidis*. *Microb. Biotechnol.* **2011**, *4*, 20–31. [PubMed]
25. Lee, W.H.; Choi, H.I.; Hong, S.W.; Kim, K.S.; Gho, Y.S.; Jeon, S.G. Vaccination with *Klebsiella pneumoniae*-derived extracellular vesicles protects against bacteria-induced lethality via both humoral and cellular immunity. *Exp. Mol. Med.* **2015**, *47*, e183. [PubMed]
26. Wang, Z.; Lazinski, D.W.; Camilli, A. Immunity provided by an outer membrane vesicle cholera vaccine is due to O-antigen-specific antibodies inhibiting bacterial motility. *Infect. Immun.* **2017**, *85*, e00626-16.
27. Bottero, D.; Gaillard, M.E.; Zurita, E.; Moreno, G.; Martinez, D.S.; Bartel, E.; Bravo, S.; Carriquiriborde, F.; Errea, A.; Castuma, C.; et al. Characterization of the immune response induced by pertussis OMVs-based vaccine. *Vaccine* **2016**, *34*, 3303–3309.

28. Micoli, F.; Rondini, S.; Alfini, R.; Lanzilao, L.; Necchi, F.; Negrea, A.; Rossi, O.; Brandt, C.; Clare, S.; Mastroeni, P.; et al. Comparative immunogenicity and efficacy of equivalent outer membrane vesicle and glycoconjugate vaccines against nontyphoidal *Salmonella*. *Proc. Natl. Acad. Sci. USA* **2018**, *115*, 10428–10433.
29. Irene, C.; Fantappiè, L.; Caproni, E.; Zerbini, F.; Anesi, A.; Tomasi, M.; Zanella, I.; Stupia, S.; Prete, S.; Valensin, S.; et al. Bacterial outer membrane vesicles engineered with lipidated antigens as a platform for *Staphylococcus aureus* vaccine. *Proc. Natl. Acad. Sci. USA* **2019**, *116*, 21780–21788.
30. Baker, S.M.; Davitt, C.J.; Motyka, N.; Kikendall, N.L.; Russell-Lodrigue, K.; Roy, C.J.; Morici, L.A. A *Burkholderia pseudomallei* outer membrane vesicle vaccine provides cross protection against inhalational glanders in mice and non-human primates. *Vaccines* **2017**, *5*, 49.
31. Bae, E.-H.; Seo, S.H.; Kim, C.-U.; Jang, M.S.; Song, M.-S.; Lee, T.-Y.; Jeong, Y.-J.; Lee, M.-S.; Park, J.-H.; Lee, P. Bacterial outer membrane vesicles provide broad-spectrum protection against Influenza virus infection via recruitment and activation of macrophages. *J. Innate Immun.* **2019**, *11*, 316–329. [PubMed]
32. Raeven, R.H.M.; Rockx-Brouwer, D.; Kanojia, G.; Van Der Maas, L.; Bindels, T.H.E.; Have, R.T.; Van Riet, E.; Metz, B.; Kersten, G.F.A. Intranasal immunization with outer membrane vesicle pertussis vaccine confers broad protection through mucosal IgA and Th17 responses. *Sci. Rep.* **2020**, *10*, 7396. [PubMed]
33. Kim, O.Y.; Hong, B.S.; Park, K.-S.; Yoon, Y.J.; Choi, S.J.; Lee, W.H.; Roh, T.-Y.; Lotvall, J.; Kim, Y.-K.; Gho, Y.S. Immunization with *Escherichia coli* outer membrane vesicles protects bacteria-induced lethality via Th1 and Th17 cell responses. *J. Immunol.* **2013**, *190*, 4092–4102. [PubMed]
34. Park, K.-S.; Choi, K.-H.; Kim, Y.-S.; Hong, B.S.; Kim, O.Y.; Kim, J.H.; Yoon, C.M.; Koh, G.-Y.; Kim, Y.-K.; Gho, Y.S. Outer membrane vesicles derived from *Escherichia coli* induce systemic inflammatory response syndrome. *PLoS ONE* **2010**, *5*, e11334.
35. Wang, H.; Liang, K.; Kong, Q.; Liu, Q. Immunization with outer membrane vesicles of avian pathogenic *Escherichia coli* O78 induces protective immunity in chickens. *Vet. Microbiol.* **2019**, *236*, 108367.
36. Hu, R.; Lin, H.; Li, J.; Zhao, Y.; Wang, M.; Sun, X.; Min, Y.; Gao, Y.; Yang, M. Probiotic *Escherichia coli* Nissle 1917-derived outer membrane vesicles enhance immunomodulation and antimicrobial activity in RAW264.7 macrophages. *BMC Microbiol.* **2020**, *20*, 268.
37. Hu, R.; Li, J.; Zhao, Y.; Lin, H.; Liang, L.; Wang, M.; Liu, H.; Min, Y.; Gao, Y.; Yang, M. Exploiting bacterial outer membrane vesicles as a cross-protective vaccine candidate against avian pathogenic *Escherichia coli* (APEC). *Microb. Cell Factories* **2020**, *19*, 119.
38. Prados-Rosales, R.; Brown, L.; Casadevall, A.; Montalvo-Quirós, S.; Luque-Garcia, J.L. Isolation and identification of membrane vesicle-associated proteins in Gram-positive bacteria and mycobacteria. *MethodsX* **2014**, *1*, 124–129.
39. Natt, M.P.; Herrick, C.A. A new blood diluent for counting the erythrocytes and leucocytes of the chicken. *Poult. Sci.* **1952**, *31*, 735–738.
40. Beug, H.; von Kirchbach, A.; Döderlein, G.; Conscience, J.-F.; Graf, T. Chicken hematopoietic cells transformed by seven strains of defective avian leukemia viruses display three distinct phenotypes of differentiation. *Cell* **1979**, *18*, 375–390.
41. Nicola, A.M.; Frases, S.; Casadevall, A. Lipophilic dye staining of *Cryptococcus neoformans* extracellular vesicles and capsule. *Eukaryot. Cell* **2009**, *8*, 1373–1380. [PubMed]
42. Dan, X.-M.; Zhang, T.-W.; Li, Y.-W.; Li, A.-X. Immune responses and immune-related gene expression profile in orange-spotted grouper after immunization with *Cryptocaryon irritans* vaccine. *Fish Shellfish Immunol.* **2013**, *34*, 885–891. [PubMed]
43. Verma, A.; Prasad, K.N.; Singh, A.K.; Nyati, K.K.; Gupta, R.K.; Paliwal, V.K. Evaluation of the MTT lymphocyte proliferation assay for the diagnosis of neurocysticercosis. *J. Microbiol. Methods* **2010**, *81*, 175–178.
44. Livak, K.J.; Schmittgen, T.D. Analysis of relative gene expression data using real-time quantitative PCR and the $2^{-\Delta\Delta Ct}$ method. *Methods* **2001**, *25*, 402–408.
45. Alber, A.; Morris, K.M.; Bryson, K.J.; Sutton, K.M.; Monson, M.S.; Chintoan-Uta, C.; Borowska, D.; Lamont, S.J.; Schouler, C.; Kaiser, P.; et al. Avian pathogenic *Escherichia coli* (APEC) strain-dependent immunomodulation of respiratory granulocytes and mononuclear phagocytes in CSF1R-reporter transgenic chickens. *Front. Immunol.* **2020**, *10*, 3055. [PubMed]
46. Kulp, A.; Kuehn, M.J. Biological functions and biogenesis of secreted bacterial outer membrane vesicles. *Annu. Rev. Microbiol.* **2010**, *64*, 163–184.

47. Vanaja, S.K.; Russo, A.J.; Behl, B.; Banerjee, I.; Yankova, M.; Deshmukh, S.D.; Rathinam, V.A.K. Bacterial outer membrane vesicles mediate cytosolic localization of LPS and caspase-11 activation. *Cell* **2016**, *165*, 1106–1119.
48. Fransen, F.; Boog, C.J.; van Putten, J.P.; van der Ley, P. Agonists of toll-like receptors 3, 4, 7, and 9 are candidates for use as adjuvants in an outer membrane vaccine against *Neisseria meningitidis* serogroup B. *Infect. Immun.* **2007**, *75*, 5939–5946.
49. Chen, D.J.; Osterrieder, N.; Metzger, S.M.; Buckles, E.; Doody, A.M.; DeLisa, M.P.; Putnam, D. Delivery of foreign antigens by engineered outer membrane vesicle vaccines. *Proc. Natl. Acad. Sci. USA* **2010**, *107*, 3099–3104.
50. Kim, O.Y.; Choi, S.J.; Jang, S.C.; Park, K.S.; Kim, S.R.; Choi, J.P.; Lim, J.H.; Lee, S.W.; Park, J.; Di Vizio, D.; et al. Bacterial protoplast-derived nanovesicles as vaccine delivery system against bacterial infection. *Nano Lett.* **2015**, *15*, 266–274.
51. Varin, A.; Gordon, S. Alternative activation of macrophages: Immune function and cellular biology. *Immunobiology* **2009**, *214*, 630–641. [PubMed]
52. Juul-Madsen, H.R.; Nielsen, O.L.; Krogh-Maibom, T.; Rontved, C.M.; Dalgaard, T.S.; Bumstead, N.; Jorgensen, P.H. Major histocompatibility complex-linked immune response of young chickens vaccinated with an attenuated live infectious bursal disease virus vaccine followed by an infection. *Poult. Sci.* **2002**, *81*, 649–656. [PubMed]
53. Ragland, S.A.; Criss, A.K. From bacterial killing to immune modulation: Recent insights into the functions of lysozyme. *PLoS Pathog.* **2017**, *13*, e1006512.
54. Franciosini, M.P.; Bietta, A.; Moscati, L.; Battistacci, L.; Pela, M.; Tacconi, G.; Davidson, I.; Proietti, P.C. Influence of different rearing systems on natural immune parameters in broiler turkeys. *Poult. Sci.* **2011**, *90*, 1462–1466. [PubMed]
55. Genovese, K.J.; He, H.; Swaggerty, C.L.; Kogut, M.H. The avian heterophil. *Dev. Comp. Immunol.* **2013**, *41*, 334–340. [PubMed]
56. Ishfaq, M.; Chen, C.; Bao, J.; Zhang, W.; Wu, Z.; Wang, J.; Liu, Y.; Tian, E.; Hamid, S.; Li, R.; et al. Baicalin ameliorates oxidative stress and apoptosis by restoring mitochondrial dynamics in the spleen of chickens via the opposite modulation of NF-κB and Nrf2/HO-1 signaling pathway during *Mycoplasma gallisepticum* infection. *Poult. Sci.* **2019**, *98*, 6296–6310.
57. Zhu, B.; Liu, G.L.; Gong, Y.X.; Ling, F.; Wang, G.X. Protective immunity of grass carp immunized with DNA vaccine encoding the vp7 gene of grass carp reovirus using carbon nanotubes as a carrier molecule. *Fish Shellfish Immunol.* **2015**, *42*, 325–334.
58. Liu, Q.; Liu, Q.; Yi, J.; Liang, K.; Liu, T.; Roland, K.L.; Jiang, Y.L.; Kong, Q.K. Outer membrane vesicles derived from *Salmonella Typhimurium* mutants with truncated LPS induce cross-protective immune responses against infection of *Salmonella enterica* serovars in the mouse model. *Int. J. Med. Microbiol.* **2016**, *306*, 697–706.
59. Roberts, L.M.; Davies, J.S.; Sempowski, G.D.; Frelinger, J.A. IFN-γ, but not IL-17A, is required for survival during secondary pulmonary *Francisella tularensis* live vaccine stain infection. *Vaccine* **2014**, *32*, 3595–3603.
60. Ross, P.J.; Sutton, C.E.; Higgins, S.; Allen, A.C.; Walsh, K.; Misiak, A.; Lavelle, E.C.; McLoughlin, R.M.; Mills, K.H. Relative contribution of Th1 and Th17 cells in adaptive immunity to *Bordetella pertussis*: Towards the rational design of an improved acellular pertussis vaccine. *PLoS Pathog.* **2013**, *9*, 1003264.
61. Jan, A.T. Outer membrane vesicles (OMVs) of gram-negative bacteria: A perspective update. *Front. Microbiol.* **2017**, *8*, 1053. [PubMed]
62. Scorza, F.B.; Doro, F.; Rodriguez-Ortega, M.J.; Stella, M.; Liberatori, S.; Taddei, A.R.; Serino, L.; Moriel, D.G.; Nesta, B.; Fontana, M.R.; et al. Proteomics characterization of outer membrane vesicles from the extraintestinal pathogenic *Escherichia coli* ΔtolR IHE3034 mutant. *Mol. Cell Proteom.* **2008**, *7*, 473–485.
63. Shahin, R.; Brennan, M.; Li, Z.; Meade, B.; Manclark, C. Characterization of the protective capacity and immunogenicity of the 69-kD outer membrane protein of *Bordetella* pertussis. *J. Exp. Med.* **1990**, *171*, 63–73. [PubMed]
64. Pillai, S.; Howell, A.; Alexander, K.; Bentley, B.E.; Jiang, H.Q.; Ambrose, K.; Zhu, D.Z.; Zlotnick, G. Outer membrane protein (OMP) based vaccine for *Neisseria meningitidis* serogroup B. *Vaccine* **2005**, *23*, 2206–2209.

65. Lee, E.-Y.; Bang, J.Y.; Park, G.W.; Choi, D.-S.; Kang, J.S.; Kim, H.-J.; Park, K.-S.; Lee, J.-O.; Kim, Y.-K.; Kwon, K.-H.; et al. Global proteomic profiling of native outer membrane vesicles derived from *Escherichia coli*. *Proteomics* **2007**, *7*, 3143–3153. [PubMed]
66. Pore, D.; Mahata, N.; Pal, A.; Chakrabarti, M.K. Outer membrane protein A (OmpA) of *Shigella flexneri* 2a, induces protective immune response in a mouse model. *PLoS ONE* **2011**, *6*, e22663.

Publisher's Note: MDPI stays neutral with regard to jurisdictional claims in published maps and institutional affiliations.

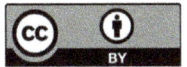 © 2020 by the authors. Licensee MDPI, Basel, Switzerland. This article is an open access article distributed under the terms and conditions of the Creative Commons Attribution (CC BY) license (http://creativecommons.org/licenses/by/4.0/).

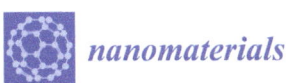

Article

Primary and Memory Response of Human Monocytes to Vaccines: Role of Nanoparticulate Antigens in Inducing Innate Memory

Mayra M. Ferrari Barbosa [1], Alex Issamu Kanno [1], Leonardo Paiva Farias [2], Mariusz Madej [3,†], Gergö Sipos [3], Silverio Sbrana [4], Luigina Romani [5], Diana Boraschi [3,6,*], Luciana C. C. Leite [1,*] and Paola Italiani [3,6,*]

1. Laboratório de Desenvolvimento de Vacinas, Instituto Butantan, São Paulo, SP 05503-900, Brazil; mayra_mara@msn.com (M.M.F.B.); alex.kanno@butantan.gov.br (A.I.K.)
2. Laboratório de Inflamação e Biomarcadores, Instituto Gonçalo Moniz, Fundação Oswaldo Cruz, Salvador, BA 40296-710, Brazil; leonardo.farias@fiocruz.br
3. Istituto di Biochimica e Biologia Cellulare, Consiglio Nazionale delle Ricerche, 80131 Napoli, Italy; mariusz.madej@ocello.nl (M.M.); gergoosipos@hotmail.com (G.S.)
4. Istituto di Fisiologia Clinica, Consiglio Nazionale delle Ricerche, 54100 Massa, Italy; silverio.sbrana@ifc.cnr.it
5. Dipartimento di Medicina e Chirurgia, University of Perugia, 06132 Perugia, Italy; luigina.romani@unipg.it
6. Stazione Zoologica Anton Dohrn, 80121 Napoli, Italy
* Correspondence: diana.boraschi@ibbc.cnr.it (D.B.); luciana.leite@butantan.gov.br (L.C.C.L.); paola.italiani@ibbc.cnr.it (P.I.)
† Current address: OcellO B.V., 2333 CH Leiden, The Netherlands.

Abstract: Innate immune cells such as monocytes and macrophages are activated in response to microbial and other challenges and mount an inflammatory defensive response. Exposed cells develop the so-called innate memory, which allows them to react differently to a subsequent challenge, aiming at better protection. In this study, using human primary monocytes in vitro, we have assessed the memory-inducing capacity of two antigenic molecules of *Schistosoma mansoni* in soluble form compared to the same molecules coupled to outer membrane vesicles of *Neisseria lactamica*. The results show that particulate challenges are much more efficient than soluble molecules in inducing innate memory, which is measured as the production of inflammatory and anti-inflammatory cytokines (TNFα, IL-6, IL-10). Controls run with LPS from *Klebsiella pneumoniae* compared to the whole bacteria show that while LPS alone has strong memory-inducing capacity, the entire bacteria are more efficient. These data suggest that microbial antigens that are unable to induce innate immune activation can nevertheless participate in innate activation and memory when in a particulate form, which is a notion that supports the use of nanoparticulate antigens in vaccination strategies for achieving adjuvant-like effects of innate activation as well as priming for improved reactivity to future challenges.

Keywords: innate immunity; innate memory; *Schistosoma mansoni*; monocytes; macrophages; vaccination

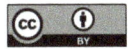

1. Introduction

In vaccine development, antigen-specific immune responses, and the development of long-term protective immunological memory are currently sought by exploiting technological platforms to construct vaccines that allow for appropriate antigen presentation. No vaccines are currently available for the parasite *Schistosoma mansoni*, which is the causative agent of schistosomiasis that is one of the most devastating parasitic diseases in terms of public health and socio-economic impact [1]. Among the most promising *S. mansoni* antigens that are currently considered for vaccine development are the two surface proteins SmCD59.2 and SmTSP-2. SmCD59.2 is a GPI-anchor tegument surface-exposed immunogenic protein [2] orthologue of human CD59 [3], whose function remains to be established [2–4]. At variance with human CD59, SmCD59.2 does not show any activity on complement [3]. Whether SmCD59.2 could interact with innate receptors, as it has been shown for the human orthologue [5], is currently unknown. SmTSP-2 is an immunogenic tetraspanin protein [2] essential in schistosomula development [4], with structural properties in cell membrane orgnization and in the parasite's tegument [6]. Based on its similarity with human tetraspanins, it is hypothesized that SmTSP-2 could interact with integrins and MHC-II on human cell membranes [4]. Both molecules have been suggested as potential vaccine candidates, although the results to date indicate the need to increase their immunogenicity [7–9]. To this end, these proteins were expressed in recombinant form in fusion with the biotin-binding protein rhizavidin and coupled to biotin-labeled Outer Membrane Vesicles (OMV) of *Neisseria lactamica*, thereby generating antigen-decorated OMV that were more effective in inducing antigen-specific humoral and cellular immunity in mice compared to the soluble protein alone [10,11]. In fact, mice immunized with the antigen-decorated OMV could generate an antigen-specific IgG antibody response much more potent than that induced by the soluble antigen or by the mixture of soluble antigen with bare OMV, the antibody production being paralleled by antigen-specific activation of $CD4^+$ and $CD8^+$ T lymphocytes in the spleen [10,11].

In assessing the efficacy of vaccine candidates, it is also important to evaluate the effects on innate immunity, i.e., the host response that, although not directly responsible for antigen-specific recognition, reaction, and specific protective memory, has a central role in amplifying antigen-specific responses and in establishing effective long-term immunity. In this perspective, the role of vaccine adjuvants is that of activating innate immunity to improve vaccine efficacy. Similar to adaptive immunity, innate immunity can display memory, i.e., a variation in the secondary response to a challenge, which depends on the host being previously exposed to/primed with the same or other agents [12–16]. At variance with adaptive memory, which is antigen-specific, innate memory is largely non-specific in mammals, with exposure to a given stimulus (e.g., bacterial LPS) causing a secondary memory response that is the same to a variety of different agents [12–16]. Innate memory responses aim at shaping the innate/inflammatory response to secondary challenges in a way that is more protective and less damaging than the first reaction, as in the case of LPS tolerance that limits the extent of the local inflammatory reaction, which would cause significant damage to the affected tissue, while maintaining the production of chemokines and alarmins that initiate the defensive immune reaction [12,17–22]. Most interestingly, vaccination with several whole live attenuated vaccines (*B. pertussis*, BCG, poliovirus, smallpox, measles, measles–mumps–rubella) was shown to induce long-term resistance not only to the specific immunizing microorganism but also to different pathogens [23–26], suggesting that vaccine-induced non-specific innate memory can amplify vaccine-induced protection by extending it to non-related infections. It is notable that particulate agents are very efficient in inducing innate memory, to underline the fact that cells of the innate immune system, in particular mononuclear phagocytes such as monocytes and macrophages, can recognize size/shape in addition to molecular patterns [27].

In this study, we have used an in vitro system based on human primary monocytes to assess the capacity of *S. mansoni* antigens, either soluble or displayed on the OMV surface, to induce innate primary and memory responses, in order to examine the possible contribution of innate immunity in the overall efficacy of the anti-*S. mansoni* candidate vaccines. Our data show that the soluble Sm antigens do not induce significant innate activation of either monocytes or monocyte-derived macrophages in terms of production of the inflammatory cytokines TNFα and IL-6, and of the anti-inflammatory cytokine IL-10, while both bare and antigen-displaying OMV are effective although to different extents. Priming with soluble rSmTSP-2 or rSmCD59.2 did not induce memory to either the same or an unrelated challenge (LPS). Priming with bare or antigen-decorated OMV induced a significant tolerance in terms of TNFα production and a significant IL-10 production in response to LPS but no substantial changes in response to the homologous stimuli. As a control for assessing the role of size in inducing innate memory, the primary and memory TNFα response of human monocytes and macrophages to LPS from *Klebsiella pneumoniae* was compared to that to whole *K. pneumoniae* bacteria. Although LPS is a potent stimulus of innate responses, also in this case the memory response induced by whole bacteria was more pronounced than that induced by purified LPS.

2. Materials and Methods

2.1. Synthesis and Characterization of rRzv:SmCD59.2 and rRzv:SmTSP-2 OMV Complexes

The recombinant fusion proteins between rhizavidin from *Rhizobium etli* and *S. mansoni* CD59.2 and TSP-2 (rRzvSmCD59.2 and rRzvSmTSP-2) were produced in *E. coli*, purified, and characterized as previously described in detail [10,11]. The elimination of possible contaminating LPS was performed with the Triton X-114 wash method [28], yielding recombinant proteins with an LPS contamination <8.0 EU/mg, as evaluated by the LAL gel-clot assay (Lonza Group Ltd., Basel, Switzerland). OMV were obtained from *Neisseria lactamica* 799/98, purified and detoxified by treatment with sodium deoxycholate, and shown to reduce the LPS content by 95% [29]. LPS in membranes is considered 100x less toxic than free LPS [30]; thus, the LPS activity rather than amount was always measured to meet the quality control criteria for OMV vaccines that set the limit of LPS activity to <400 EU/µg. However, the 2-keto-3-deoxy-D-mannooctanoic acid (KDO) measurement (see below) performed on some OMV samples confirmed the presence of an amount of LPS that matched the measured activity, i.e., 1 EU = 0.1 nanogram. Biotinylated OMV were obtained as previously described [10]. Briefly, 25 mg OMV were incubated with 10 mg biotin in sodium phosphate buffer, 150 mM NaCl, 3% sucrose, and 0.1 M *N*-(3-dimetylaminopropyl)-*N*'-ethylcarbodiimide hydrochloride, and re-purified by gel filtration chromatography [10]. Recombinant proteins were coupled to biotinylated OMV by exploiting biotin–rhizavidin affinity binding, as previously described for the Multiple Antigen Presenting Strategy (MAPS) [31]. Avidin binding to biotin is the strongest non-covalent interaction known in nature, and it has been extensively developed and approved for many therapeutic applications, including cancer treatments [32,33]. Biotinylated OMV were incubated with rRzvSmCD59.2 or rRzvSmTSP-2 for 18 h at 4 °C at a 5:1 mass ratio and then purified by size exclusion chromatography on Sephacryl S-200 in endotoxin-free conditions [10]. The antigen to OMV protein mass ratio after conjugation was 1:10–1:20 [11].

The OMV-protein complexes, displaying SmCD59.2 (OMV:D) or displaying SmTSP-2 (OMV:T) and the unconjugated purified biotinylated OMV (OMV), were characterized by transmission electron microscopy (TEM) using a JEM-1230 microscope (JEOL Ltd., Tokyo, Japan), and for electrophoretic mobility, and for hydrodynamic size/polydispersion by dynamic light scattering (DLS) with a Zetasizer Nano ZS90 instrument (Malvern Panalytical Ltd., Malvern, UK) with a fixed scattering angle of 173° at 25 °C in triplicate [9]. Endotoxin/LPS contamination was assessed with the gel clot LAL assay (Lonza Group Ltd., Basel, Switzerland) and with the 2-keto-3-deoxy-D-mannooctanoic acid (KDO) assay.

2.2. Human Monocyte Isolation and Differentiation of Monocyte-Derived Macrophages

Blood was obtained from healthy donors upon informed consent and in agreement with the Declaration of Helsinki. The protocol was approved by the Regional Ethics Committee for Clinical Experimentation of the Tuscany Region (Ethics Committee Register n. 14,914 of 16 May 2019). Monocytes were isolated by CD14 positive selection with magnetic microbeads (Miltenyi Biotec, Bergisch Gladbach, Germany) from peripheral blood mononuclear cells (PBMC), obtained by Ficoll–Paque gradient density separation (GE Healthcare, Bio-Sciences AB, Uppsala, Sweden), as previously described in detail [34]. Monocyte preparations used in the experiments were >95% viable and >95% pure (assessed by trypan blue exclusion and cytosmears). Isolated monocytes included the subpopulations of classical, intermediate, and non-classical monocytes at the same percentages as present in PBMC, as indicated by the manufacturer and confirmed in-house by cytofluorimetric analysis of CD14- and CD16-expressing cells (Supplementary Figure S1). The staining procedure and flow cytometric analysis are reported in detail in the Supplementary Materials.

Monocytes were cultured in culture medium (RPMI 1640 + Glutamax-I; GIBCO by Life Technologies, Paisley, UK) supplemented with 50 µg/mL gentamicin sulfate (GIBCO) and 5% heat-inactivated human AB serum (Sigma-Aldrich, Inc., St. Louis, MO, USA). Cells (5–7.5×10^5) were seeded in a final volume of 1.0 mL in wells of 24-well flat bottom plates (well internal diameter 15.6 mm; Corning® Costar®; Corning Inc. Life Sciences, Oneonta, NY, USA) at 37 °C in moist air with 5% CO_2. Monocyte stimulation was performed after overnight resting.

Freshly isolated monocytes were differentiated into tissue-like macrophages by culturing them in culture medium containing 50 ng/mL macrophage colony-stimulating factor (M-CSF; R&D Systems, Minneapolis, MN, USA) for 6 days (with one medium change on the third day). Differentiation and M2-like polarization, typical of tissue resident macrophages, was assessed morphologically and by the decreased expression of CD14 and increased expression of CD206. No significant mortality or increase in cell number was observed at the end of the differentiation period.

2.3. Human Cell Activation and Induction of Innate Memory

For assessing the primary response to stimulation, monocytes or macrophages were exposed for 24 h to LPS (positive control; from *E. coli* O55:B5 or *K. pneumoniae*; Sigma-Aldrich, Inc., St. Louis, MO, USA) or to increasing concentrations of rSmCD59.2, rSmTSP-2, unconjugated OMV, OMV:D, OMV:T, heat-killed *K. pneumoniae* (clinical isolates of both wild-type and carbapenemase-producing bacteria), or left untreated (medium/negative control).

For memory experiments, after the first exposure to stimuli for 24 h and supernatant collection, cells were washed and cultured with fresh culture medium for 6 additional days (one medium change after 3 days), to allow for the extinction of the activation induced by the previous stimulation. After this resting phase, the supernatant was collected, and cells were challenged for 24 h with fresh medium alone or containing a ten-fold higher concentration of stimuli. All supernatants (after the first stimulation, after the resting phase and after the challenge phase) were frozen at -20 °C for subsequent cytokine analysis. By visual inspection, cell viability and cell number did not substantially change in response to the different treatments.

2.4. Cytokine Analysis

The levels of the human inflammatory cytokines TNFα and IL-6 and of the anti-inflammatory factor IL-10 were assessed by ELISA (R&D Systems), using a Cytation 3 imaging multi-mode reader (BioTek, Winooski, VT, USA).

2.5. Statistical Analysis

Data were analyzed using the GraphPad Prism6.01 software (GraphPad Inc., La Jolla, CA, USA). For cytokine production, results are presented as ng produced cytokine/10^6 plated monocytes. Results are reported as mean ± SD of values from 2 to 4 replicates from the same donor or from 2 to 4 different donors. Statistical significance of differences is indicated by *p* values, which were calculated using one-way non-parametric ANOVA with *post hoc* Tukey's multiple comparison test and one-tailed unpaired *t* test.

3. Results

3.1. Particle Characterization

Unconjugated OMV and OMV–antigen complexes were characterized for their size, polydispersity, presence of recombinant antigens, and LPS content.

The results in Figure 1 show that the three particles have similar characteristics, with an average size between 150 and 250 nm (corresponding to a hydrodynamic size of 200–400 nm) and a negative ζ-potential. All OMV preparations show polydispersity, which is likely due to both particle size heterogeneity and to aggregates [11], as confirmed by TEM. The presence of the recombinant antigens on the surface of OMV:D and OMV:T was confirmed to be about 1:10–1:20 vs. OMV proteins. A more complete characterization of the

OMV, from isolating to the OMV–antigen conjugates, has been published elsewhere [10]. After detoxification, all OMV still displayed a residual LPS activity, which was at least 30 EU/μg in unconjugated OMV, 8 EU/μg in OMV:D, and 80 EU/μg in OMV:T. Since 1 EU roughly corresponds to 100 pg LPS, we can infer the presence of 3 ng LPS per μg particles in unconjugated OMV, 0.8 ng/μg in OMV:D, and 8 ng/μg in OMV:T (the latter value was confirmed by KDO assessment). It should be noted that the OMV complexes comply with the quality control criteria for OMV vaccines that require a residual LPS activity of <400 EU/μg.

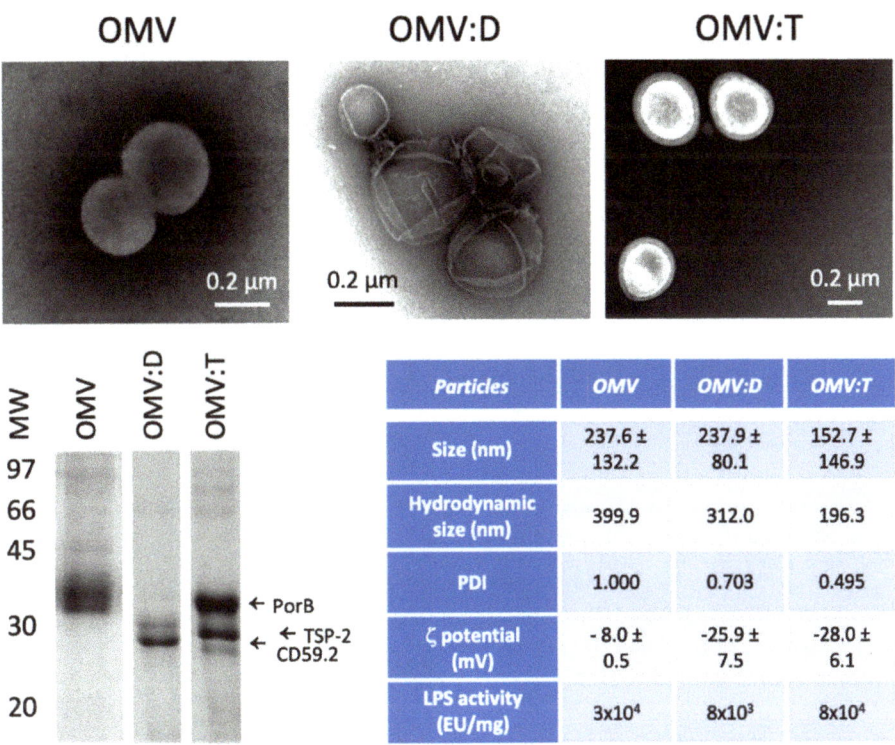

Figure 1. Characterization of Outer Membrane Vesicles (OMV) and OMV–antigen complexes. TEM images of unconjugated biotinylated OMV of *N. lactamica* (OMV, upper left), OMV conjugated with rRzvSmCD59.2 (OMV:D, upper center) and OMV conjugated with rRzvSmTSP-2 (OMV:T, upper right). Lower left panel: electrophoretic mobility of OMV and OMV–antigen complexes. Left arrows indicate the position of the main *N. lactamica* protein PorB, of SmTSP-2 in OMV:T and of SmCD59.2 in OMV:D (the two antigens having a calculated MW of 27.2 kDa for rRzvSmTSP-2 and 26.9 kDa for rRzvSmCD59.2). Lower right table: Summary of the OMV characteristics of size (measured in TEM, mean ± SD of 16–131 particles), hydrodynamic size, polydispersity, ζ-potential (mean of 3 determinations ± SD) (all measured by dynamic light scattering (DLS)) and LPS activity (measured with the LAL assay). PDI, polydispersity index.

3.2. Innate Response of Innate Immune Cells to S. mansoni Antigens

The capacity of recombinant *S. mansoni* antigens to stimulate the production of inflammatory (TNFα, IL-6) and anti-inflammatory (IL-10) cytokines was assessed on fresh human blood monocytes and on monocyte-derived macrophage (Figure 2). Both soluble antigens and antigens coupled to OMV were examined in parallel to unconjugated OMV and to the prototypical inflammatory stimulus LPS.

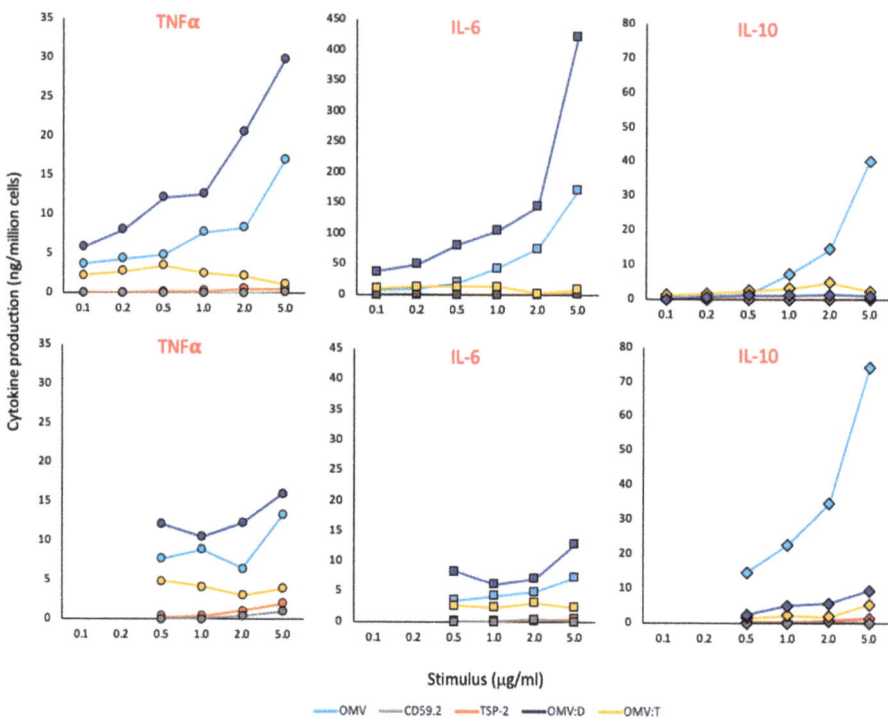

Figure 2. Primary response of human monocytes and macrophages to *S. mansoni* antigens. The production of TNFα (left panels, round symbols), IL-6 (center panels, square symbols) and IL-10 (right panels, diamond symbols) was assessed in human fresh blood monocytes (upper panels) and monocyte-derived macrophages (lower panels) stimulated for 24 h with increasing concentrations of unconjugated OMV (light blue), rSmCD59.2 (gray), rSmTSP-2 (red), OMV:D (dark blue), or OMV:T (yellow). The negative and positive controls (culture medium alone and LPS 10 ng/mL) are the following: TNFα in monocytes 0.03 and 2.23 ng/10^6 cells; TNFα in macrophages 0.00 and 3.06; IL-6 in monocytes 0.04 and 5.00; IL-6 in macrophages 0.00 and 1.84; IL-10 in monocytes 0.00 and 0.16; IL-10 in macrophages 0.02 and 0.30. Data are from one donor of 2–4 tested (data from other donors are reported in the Supplementary Table S1). The SD of technical replicates was always <10% and is not reported. Statistical significance is reported in the Supplementary Table S2.

As shown in Figure 2, soluble antigens have little/no activity (gray and red symbols). Conversely, unconjugated OMV (light blue symbols) have a strong capacity of inducing inflammatory cytokines in monocytes and, to a lesser extent, in macrophages, while they are very potent inducers of IL-10 in monocytes and even more in macrophages. OMV:D (dark blue symbols) are more potent than unconjugated OMV in inducing inflammatory cytokines while essentially unable to induce IL-10. On the other hand, OMV:T (yellow symbols) have little/no activity, which is similar to the soluble recombinant protein. A possible interfering role for biotin, present on all OMV preparations for antigen ligation, is likely to be minimal/null, since the three OMV types showed variable qualitative and quantitative differences in the induction of different cytokines while containing the same amount of biotin.

The concentrations indicated in Figure 2 are those of the recombinant proteins, either alone or coupled to OMV; e.g., 1 µg OMV:T is the amount of OMV:T that contains 1 µg of SmTSP-2 (the amount of OMV being about 10× higher, i.e., 10 µg). Likewise, for 1 µg of unconjugated OMV, it is intended that the amount of OMV contained in complexes displaying 1 µg of Sm antigens (again 10 µg). Data in Figure 2 are from one donor, which are representative of two to four tested (the results from all donors are reported in the Supplementary Table S1).

3.3. Innate Memory of Human Monocyte/Macrophages to S. mansoni Antigens

Monocytes were exposed for 24 h to a low concentration of Sm antigens, OMV, and OMV–antigen complexes (0.1 µg antigen/mL) or LPS as control (1 ng/mL) and cultured for an additional 6 days in fresh medium (one medium change after 3 days) to allow for return to a quiescent state. This was assessed by measuring the release of cytokines in the last 3-day supernatant, which was always undetectable (data not shown). At this time, monocytes had spontaneously differentiated in culture into macrophages. Cells were re-exposed to stimuli for 24 h, the challenge being a 10x higher concentration of LPS (10 ng/mL, as control) or the Sm antigens, OMV, and OMV–antigen complexes (1 µg antigen/mL). The inflammatory cytokine TNFα and the anti-inflammatory cytokine IL-10 were measured. The results in Figure 3 show the memory-induced variation in the cell response to different challenges, which are indicated with different colors. The data in Figure 3 refer to cells from a single donor out of three tested. Given the donor-to-donor quantitative variability of responses, the data could not be averaged (the results from each donor are reported in the Supplementary Table S2). In Figure 3, the response of unprimed cells is reported in the line indicated as "medium" in the horizontal axis "PRIMING", and it shows that cells produce significant amounts of TNFα in response to LPS (orange), OMV (gray), and OMV–antigen complexes (green and dark blue), while the response to soluble rSmCD59.2 (yellow) and rSmTSP-2 (light blue) is limited. For IL-10 production, it is notable that unprimed cells do not respond well to LPS, while the response to OMV is very high. OMV–antigen complexes also induce IL-10 production, although to a lesser extent than bare OMV. This pattern of response reflects quite precisely the response of macrophages to a primary stimulation depicted in Figure 2.

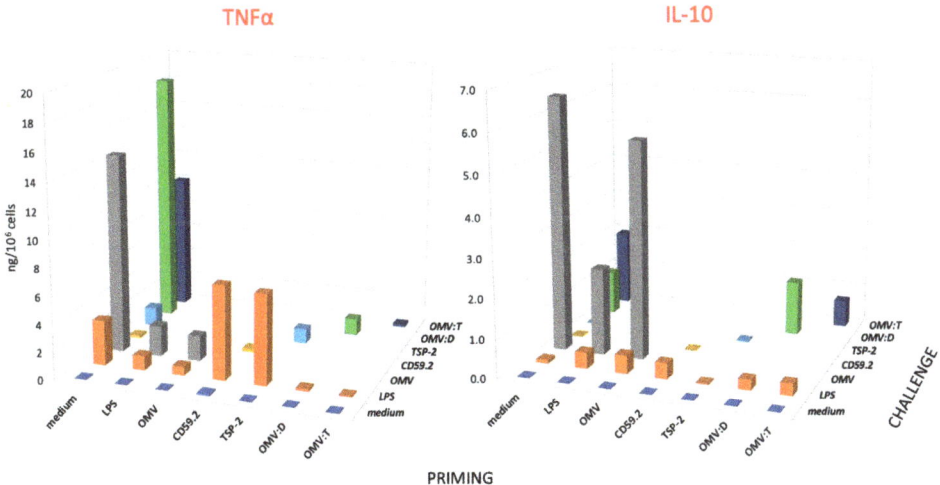

Figure 3. Secondary response of human monocytes to challenge with *S. mansoni* antigens. Production of TNFα (left panel) and IL-10 (right panel) of human monocytes that had been previously exposed (PRIMING in the horizontal axis) to culture medium alone (medium), LPS (1 ng/mL), unconjugated OMV (OMV), rSmCD59.2 (CD59.2), rSmTSP-2 (TSP-2), OMV:D, or OMV:T (all at 0.1 µg antigen/mL). After 6 days of resting, cells were challenged (see depth axis CHALLENGE) with a 10x higher concentration of stimuli; medium (purple), LPS (orange), OMV (gray), rSmCD59.2 (yellow), rSmTSP-2 (light blue), OMV:D (green) and OMV:T (dark blue). LPS was used as control challenge for cells primed with every kind of stimuli. Data are the values of the 24-h cytokine production by cells from one donor representative of three examined (see Supplementary Table S3 for the values of individual donors). SD of technical replicates were always <10% and are not shown. Statistical significance is reported in the Supplementary Table S4.

When examining the memory response in terms of inflammatory TNFα production (Figure 3, left), we can observe that, as expected, priming with LPS induces a clear tolerance (decrease of response) to an LPS challenge, which is a phenomenon that can be observed also in cells primed with unconjugated OMV and OMV–antigen complexes, whereas priming with soluble Sm antigens slightly increased the secondary response to LPS (see orange columns, LPS challenge). Challenge with unconjugated OMV (gray columns) or with OMV–antigen complexes (green and dark blue columns) showed the same trend, i.e., a decreased TNFα production in cells primed with particulate agents as compared to unprimed cells. Conversely, the soluble Sm antigens triggered in primed cells the same low TNFα production as in unprimed control cells (yellow and blue columns). Thus, our data show that the particulate agents induce a tolerance-type memory in human monocytes/macrophages, which reduces the production of the inflammatory factor TNFα upon a secondary challenge (both identical and unrelated), while the soluble antigens do not have a significant effect. However, it should be noted that OMV also display a significant amount of LPS, roughly corresponding to the LPS control, which may imply that the tolerance effect of priming with OMV could be actually due to LPS.

Quite different is the picture of memory-induced modulation of the anti-inflammatory cytokine IL-10 (Figure 3, right). As already mentioned, challenge with LPS could induce a very limited production of IL-10 in unprimed cells, which was slightly increased in primed cells (except after rSmTSP-2 priming). In the case of priming with particulate agents (OMV, OMV:D, OMV:T), at variance with the results with TNFα, priming did not induce a clear tolerance-type response to challenge with either LPS or the identical agents, with only a partial decrease observed in the case of OMV:T homologous challenge. Thus, the memory response of particle-primed cells results in a significant decrease of the production of the inflammatory factor and no/little decrease of the anti-inflammatory factor, leading to a secondary response that is less inflammatory than that of unprimed cells. In the case of OMV:D, the response of unprimed cells to the complex (18.4 ng TNFα/10^6 cells and 1.1 ng IL-10) was strongly rebalanced in OMV:D-primed cells (1.2 ng TNFα and 1.4 ng IL-10). In addition, in the case of OMV:T, the response of unprimed cells (10.0 ng TNFα and 1.9 ng IL-10, less inflammatory than the response to OMV:D) was significantly shifted toward anti-inflammation in primed cells (0.2 ng TNFα and 0.7 ng IL-10).

3.4. Innate and Memory Responses of Human Monocytes and Macrophages to Klebsiella pneumoniae LPS vs. Whole Bacteria

To assess the possible role of size on the capacity of microbial agents to stimulate innate responses and memory, we have tested the production of TNFα by human monocytes and monocyte-derived macrophages in response to LPS from Klebsiella pneumoniae in comparison to the whole inactivated bacteria, which display LPS on their surface. LPS concentrations were selected to correspond to those present on bacteria, considering that 1 EU (corresponding to about 100 pg LPS) is the amount of LPS displayed by 10^5 bacteria. The results in Figure 4 (upper panels) show that the primary response of monocytes to LPS was 7–10× higher than that of macrophages, while the response of macrophages to K. pneumoniae was only half of that of monocytes at the highest concentration.

When examining the secondary memory response, both for LPS and for the whole bacteria, a tolerance-type memory response was evident, with the production of TNFα was much lower in primed vs. unprimed cells (Figure 4, lower panels). The secondary response of monocytes (lower left panel) represents the memory response of effector monocytes that entered an infected tissue and developed memory afterwards, whereas the secondary response of macrophages (lower right panel) represents the memory response of tissue-resident macrophages. The results show that the secondary response of monocytes, which respond to whole bacteria more potently than to isolated LPS, displays a potent tolerance when cells had been primed with whole bacteria, which is a tolerance that is already maximal at the lowest bacterial priming dose (ratio bacteria to monocytes 0.1 to 1). Conversely, tolerance to LPS depends on the LPS priming dose, being minimal at the lowest dose (0.1 ng LPS/10^6 monocytes, corresponding to a bacteria to monocyte ratio of 0.1 to 1) and well evident only at a priming ratio of 10 to 1. A similar trend, although less pronounced, can be observed in the secondary response of tissue-like macrophages, in which the tolerance to challenge is significantly more pronounced in macrophages primed with increasing doses of bacteria in comparison to isolated LPS.

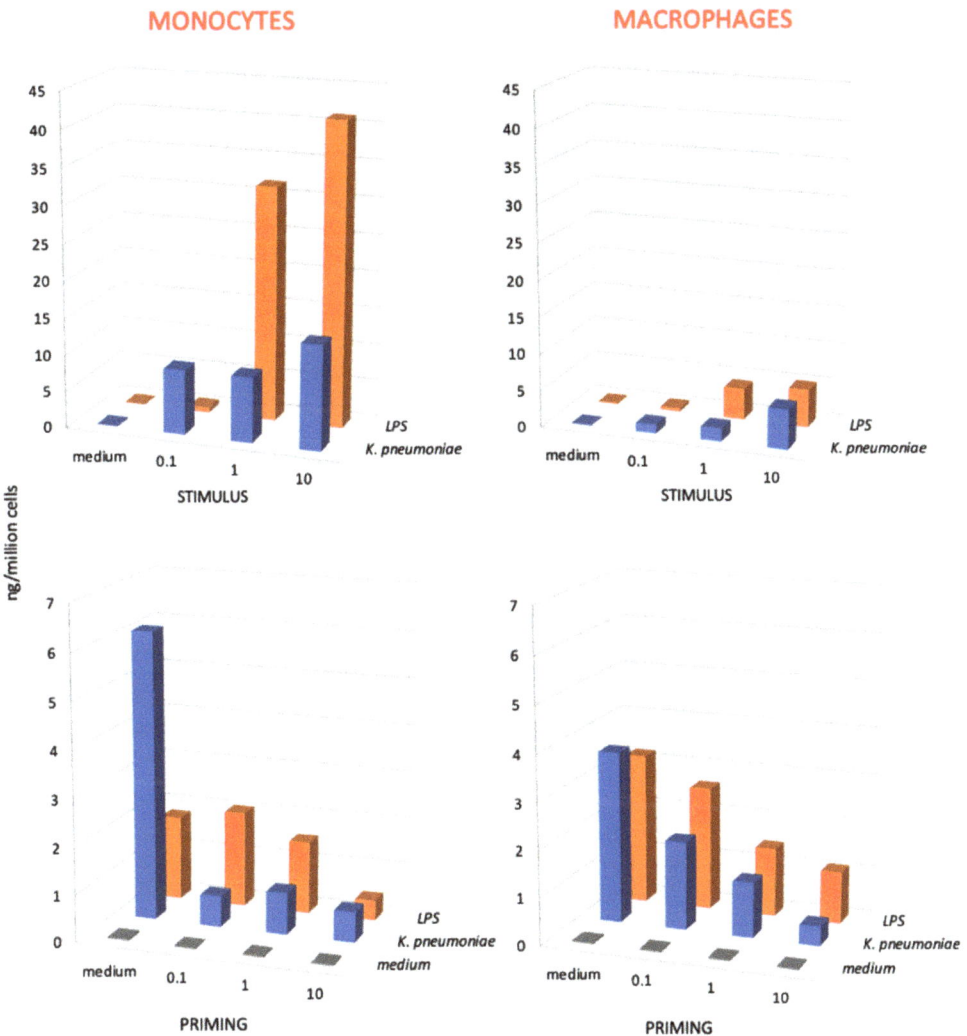

Figure 4. Primary and secondary innate response of monocytes and macrophages to *Klebsiella pneumoniae* bacteria vs. *K. pneumoniae* LPS. The primary response (upper panels) of monocytes (left panels) and monocyte-derived macrophages (right panels) was measured in terms of TNFα production upon stimulation with increasing concentrations of killed *K. pneumoniae* bacteria (0.1, 1, and 10 bacteria per each monocyte/macrophage; blue columns) and to LPS from *K. pneumoniae* (0.1, 1, and 10 ng/10^6 monocytes/macrophages; orange columns). The secondary response (lower panels) of unprimed control cells (medium, in the horizontal axis; gray columns) and cells primed with increasing concentrations of *K. pneumoniae* bacteria (blue columns) or *K. pneumoniae* LPS (LPS; orange columns) was again measured in terms of TNFα production after a challenge of 24 h with the highest challenge concentration (10 bacteria per monocyte/macrophage; 10 ng LPS/10^6 monocytes/macrophages). Only homologous priming/challenge combinations are shown (in the depth axis). Results are the average of two to four replicates from two different donors. SD were <20% and are not shown. Statistical analysis is reported in the Supplementary Table S5.

It should be said that in these experiments, we have used both wild-type *K. pneumoniae* and carbapenemase-producing *K. pneumoniae* isolates with identical results (the data in Figure 4 are the average values obtained in experiments with different isolates), which suggests that innate immunity and innate memory responses are not affected by the development of antibiotic resistance.

4. Discussion

The hypothesis that vaccination with a number of bacterial and viral vaccines, in particular those based on live attenuated microorganisms, may increase resistance to a number of unrelated diseases, in addition to the specific disease against which the vaccine is designed, is currently attracting significant attention for the possible positive impact on public health [24]. The biological basis for the non-specific effect of vaccination is most likely residing in the immunological phenomenon known as innate immune memory (or trained immunity), which is well known in plants and invertebrates and also present in vertebrates. Innate memory (also defined as "trained immunity") implies a more efficient innate immune response to a challenge by organisms/cells previously exposed to the same or another agent [13–16,35–37]. In vaccine formulations, the specific immune response to antigens and the development of protective long-term adaptive immunological memory is facilitated by the use of adjuvants, which are agents that non-specifically induce a local inflammatory/innate immune reaction that creates the right conditions for the development of a potent and effective immunization against the vaccine antigens [38]. Indeed, epidemiological evidence supports the hypothesis that recurrent exposure to infectious stimuli is at the basis of a long-term protective immune memory that can be independent of T and B cells, thereby pointing at innate immune cells [39]. Thus, current research on vaccines aims at assessing the capacity of vaccine formulations (in particular their adjuvant components) not only to induce the immediate innate/inflammatory reaction required for optimal specific immunization but also to devise adjuvant strategies able to induce a non-specific innate memory that would increase the host resistance to a wider range of infections/diseases [22–26,40–43]. The concept of vaccination based on innate memory ("trained immunity" vaccines) is being further developed by the notion that organ/tissue-resident innate cells (in particular macrophages) can strongly contribute to innate memory-biased defensive responses to subsequent organ-specific infections [44–48].

In this study, we have investigated the possible role of innate memory, specifically focusing on mononuclear phagocytes (monocytes and macrophages), in the human reactivity to candidate vaccine formulations for *S. mansoni*. In fact, two promising parasite proteins (SmCD59.2 and SmTSP-2) are being developed in particulate formulations that provide excellent immunogenicity in experimental animals, with high production of antigen-specific antibodies and antigen-specific activation of CD4$^+$ and CD8$^+$ T lymphocytes [10,11]. The vaccine constructs imply the use of OMV from *N. lactamica*, which has been detoxified to decrease their endotoxin content below the acceptable limits for human use, and, using the MAPS technology, biotinylated and conjugated to recombinant fusion proteins encompassing the parasite protein in fusion with rhizavidin [10,11]. The particulate form, which is often used in vaccination strategies as effective antigen carrier, is known to be particularly effective in the interaction with macrophages, which react to particles by proliferating and by readily ingesting the particulate agents, thereby favoring their presentation to T lymphocytes for initiating adaptive immune responses (as macrophages are, together with dendritic cells, efficient antigen-presenting cells) [27,49,50]. Therefore, it is expected that particles, in addition to carrying the vaccine antigens, can have a direct capacity to initiate innate immune responses, at the basis of their adjuvant effect and, consequently, to induce the generation of an innate memory that can contribute to the vaccine efficacy.

The aim of this study was to examine the capacity of the two vaccine formulations for *S. mansoni* not only to activate innate immunity, i.e., to display an intrinsic adjuvant effect, but in particular if and how they can induce an innate immune memory able to contribute to long-term vaccine efficacy and non-specific resistance. To this end, we have examined the two *S. mansoni* antigens coupled with OMV (OMV:D and OMV:T) compared to unconjugated OMV and to the unconjugated SmCD59.2 and SmTSP-2 recombinant proteins. We should be aware of the fact that detoxified OMV still display endotoxin levels that, although below the threshold for regulatory approval, are detectable and active in our in vitro assays on human monocytes. Specifically, based on its activity the endotoxin levels may be of about 30 ng/mL for OMV, 8 ng/mL for OMV:D, and 80 ng/mL for OMV:T at the highest concentration used for challenge in memory experiments, i.e., 10 μg OMV (corresponding to 0.5–1.0 μg antigen)/mL, while 10x lower in the priming phase. Such endotoxin levels may be at least in part responsible for the capacity of OMV to induce an innate/inflammatory response and to establish a subsequent innate memory. The contribution of LPS in the innate/inflammatory activation of human monocytes and macrophages by OMV was assessed in comparison with similar amounts of purified LPS (from *E. coli*, since LPS from *N. lactamica* was not available; 1 ng/mL as priming and 10 ng/mL as challenge).

The results show different behaviors of OMV in inducing innate immune activation that cannot be exclusively attributed to LPS (see Figure 2). Indeed, OMV:T induced a primary response comparable to that induced by isolated LPS, but it was much lower than that triggered by unconjugated OMV and OMV:D. This is true for all inflammation-related factors examined, i.e., the inflammatory cytokines TNFα and IL-6 and the anti-inflammatory cytokine IL-10. Interestingly, OMV:D are more efficient than unconjugated OMV in inducing the two inflammatory factors, both in monocytes and macrophages, whereas the unconjugated particles are significantly more effective in inducing the anti-inflammatory factor IL-10, while LPS and all the other antigens show much lower effects. Thus, the innate reaction to OMV:T is low, in terms of induction of both inflammatory and anti-inflammatory factors, and at similar levels as the response induced by isolated LPS, while the soluble antigens do not induce any significant innate reaction. Interestingly, the unconjugated OMV induced a significant production of inflammatory factors but were also very effective in inducing the anti-inflammatory IL-10, suggesting that their innate immune activation potential and adjuvant effect may be limited. On the other hand, OMV:D are very efficient in inducing the inflammatory factors but not the anti-inflammatory cytokine, suggesting an efficient adjuvant effect. The inflammatory activation induced by the particles turns out to be transient, as expected for a safe adjuvant. Indeed, cell activation is completely extinguished after six additional days in culture, and cells have returned to a baseline quiescent state (again assessed in terms of cytokine production). Thus, we have shown that OMV induce a primary innate/inflammatory activation in both human monocytes and macrophages in culture that goes far beyond their content of LPS, in particular in quantitative terms, with only OMV:T showing effects quantitatively comparable to those of isolated LPS.

To stress the difference between the effect of LPS and that of LPS-bearing particles, we have also compared the innate activation induced in human monocytes and macrophages by different concentrations of LPS from *K. pneumoniae* in comparison to the entire *K. pneumoniae* bacteria displaying corresponding amounts of LPS on their surface (Figure 4, upper panels). In this case as well, bacteria have effects that are not superimposable to those of their LPS, as shown by the dose-independent activation of monocytes by whole bacteria compared to the strongly dose-dependent activation induced by isolated LPS. This causes a lack of response to a low dose of LPS, while the same dose of bacteria induces a significant response, and a very high response to intermediate and high LPS doses, while the response to the corresponding doses of bacteria is essentially identical to that triggered by the low dose and much lower than the response to LPS.

As already mentioned, the hypothesis that a priming of innate immunity could result in the establishment of a longer-term "innate memory" that contributes to an improved secondary reaction to a challenge (an infection, a second vaccine dose) has been recently explored by several groups and proposed as a very promising development in the vaccine field, in particular because of the non-specific effects of innate immunity that may afford protection against a wide spectrum of infections [22–26,40–45,47]. We have examined the possible role of innate memory upon challenge with the candidate *S. mansoni* vaccines by exploiting an in vitro system based on human primary monocytes that are exposed to the vaccine antigens twice in a priming–extinction–challenge sequence. Essentially, cells exposed in culture to the vaccine antigens for 24 h were subsequently allowed to rest for 6 additional days, so that their primary activation was extinguished and cells were again in a resting state. Then, cells were challenged with the same antigen (or LPS as control), and the response of antigen-primed cells was compared to that of cells that were not previously exposed (unprimed controls). In our study, we have examined the memory response in terms of production of two representative innate cytokines with opposing effects, the inflammatory TNFα and the anti-inflammatory IL-10, in order to have a realistic picture of the secondary innate reaction that includes the balance between inflammation and anti-inflammation. It should be noted that in this study, we have used a single low dose of each compound as priming stimulus, and a higher dose as challenge. This schedule derives from previous studies that have determined it to be the optimal way for assessing priming-induced innate memory, the concept being that memory induced by a lower-level primary stimulation (as in the case of vaccines) can induce a memory effect protective in the case of a strong challenge (e.g., an infection). To assess whether induction of innate memory is an hormesis phenomenon, i.e., whether low vs. high doses of a priming stimulus could afford opposite effects, we had examined the effect of different doses of priming stimuli on the ability to induce innate memory in vitro in human monocytes/macrophages, and we found that the memory effect was the same (tolerance) and dose-dependent, with increasing effect obtained with increasing priming doses, which was a finding that was true for a soluble stimulus, LPS, as well as for a particulate one, zymosan [50].

Examining the memory response in terms of TNFα production, we observed that priming with OMV (either unconjugated or coupled to antigens) results in a tolerance-like response to both a homologous challenge and to LPS. This means that the secondary response of primed cells is significantly lower than that of unprimed controls. This is the same kind of secondary response observed in LPS-primed cells, which reproduces the well-known phenomenon of LPS tolerance, aiming at preserving the host tissues from damage due to excessive inflammation upon repeated challenges [21,22]. Conversely, priming with the soluble antigens does not induce a different response to homologous challenge when compared to unprimed cells, whereas a potentiation of the response to LPS could be observed. The memory response in terms of production of the anti-inflammatory factor IL-10 shows a very different picture. Challenge with OMV (bare or antigen-decorated) can induce a potent production of IL-10 in control unprimed cells, which is an event that is not mimicked by LPS, showing that the OMV effect is most likely due to their particulate form rather than to their LPS content. Challenge with OMV also triggered a significant production of IL-10 in OMV-primed cells (homologous challenge), which was practically identical to that induced in unprimed cells (except for a partial decrease in OMV:D primed/challenged cells). Thus, while the particle-induced memory results in a tolerance effect for the inflammatory cytokine, the production of the anti-inflammatory cytokine is essentially not affected, suggesting an overall balance toward anti-inflammation in the secondary response. In fact, the TNFα/IL-10 ratios in unprimed vs. primed cells challenged with OMV:D are 16.7 vs. 0.9, and the TNFα/IL-10 ratios in unprimed vs. primed cells in response to OMV:T are 5.3 vs. 0.3, these figures being similar to those obtained with bare OMV (TNFα/IL-10 ratios in unprimed vs. primed cells in response to OMV are 2.2 vs. 0.3). Indeed, even in the case of LPS (a very good adjuvant apart from its toxicity), the TNFα/IL-10 ratio goes toward reduced inflammation in primed cells, being 33.0 (highly inflammatory) in unprimed cells challenged with LPS, and being significantly reduced to 2.5 in LPS-primed cells challenged with LPS. The priming effect of LPS is apparently changed by its presentation to monocytes/macrophages by whole bacteria, as shown in the experiments with *K. pneumoniae*. Monocyte priming with whole bacteria, even at the lowest dose, achieved a very profound tolerance effect (in terms TNFα production), whereas the tolerance induced by LPS was dose-dependent irrespective of the intensity of the primary response, suggesting that the LPS-bearing whole bacteria induce a more profound memory than the isolated agent.

The present study did not yet address the mechanisms underlying the observed memory effects (studies currently ongoing), which is an issue of particular interest since the observed effects were different (increased vs. decreased production) depending on the cytokine under evaluation, implying concomitant changes at different levels, likely including epigenetic and metabolic regulation [51–55].

5. Conclusions

These findings indicate that the OMV-based antigens can exploit the adjuvant effects of both the particulate form of OMV and the presence of non-toxic amounts of LPS, for shaping innate immunity and generating innate memory toward the amplification of immune responses with a safe, non-inflammatory long-term innate reactivity. Understanding the mechanisms at the basis of beneficial innate memory would allow us to modulate them in a controlled fashion in order to obtain the desired memory effects in future vaccination strategies as well as in therapeutic immunomodulation. Notably, the innate memory effects appear to be strongly dependent on the donor, which is most likely a consequence of their "immunobiography", i.e., the cumulative effects of their individual history of exposure to repeated and different challenges during the lifetime [56]. This indicates the need for an individual immune memory profile as the basis for a personalized selection of the most appropriate (most effective and safer) preventive and therapeutic strategies.

Supplementary Materials: The following are available online at https://www.mdpi.com/article/10.3390/nano11040931/s1: Supplementary Materials and Methods (Staining Procedure, Flow Cytometric Analysis); Figure S1, Monocyte subsets before and after positive isolation with CD14 magnetic beads; Table S1, Primary cytokine production by human monocytes in response to *S. mansoni* antigens; Table S2, Statistical analysis of primary cytokine production by human monocytes in response to *S. mansoni* antigens; Table S3, Memory response of human monocytes from different donors primed with *S. mansoni* antigens; Table S4, Statistical analysis of memory responses of human monocytes primed with *S. mansoni* antigens; Table S5, Statistical analysis of primary and memory responses to *K. pneumoniae* bacteria and their LPS.

Author Contributions: M.M.F.B. produced the antigens and performed the experiments; A.I.K., L.P.F., M.M., G.S., and S.S. performed the experiments; L.R. provided microbiological reagents and expertise; D.B., L.C.C.L. and P.I. devised the study, analyzed the results, and wrote the manuscript. All authors have read and agreed to the published version of the manuscript.

Funding: This study was funded by the European Commission FP7 project HUMUNITY (GA 316383), the Horizon 2020 projects PANDORA (GA 671881), and ENDONANO (GA 812661), the Italian MIUR Flagship InterOmics project MEMORAT, the PRIN project 20173ZECCM, the CNR Italy-Brazil Joint Laboratory initiative, the FAPESP grant 2017/24632-6 (to L.C.C.L.) and Fundação Butantan. M.M.F.B. received a CAPES fellowship.

Institutional Review Board Statement: The study was conducted according to the guidelines of the Declaration of Helsinki, and the protocol was approved by the Regional Ethics Committee for Clinical Experimentation of the Tuscany Region (Ethics Committee Register n. 14,914 of 16 May 2019). C57BL/6 mice were kept under appropriate conditions during the study according to the Animal Care and Ethics Committee of the institution, under protocol 3314160715.

Informed Consent Statement: Informed consent was obtained from all subjects involved in the study.

Data Availability Statement: The data presented in this study are available in this article and its Supplementary Materials.

Acknowledgments: The authors wish to thank Paola Migliorini (University of Pisa, Italy) for her help in the coordination and ethical monitoring of the study, and Richard Malley (Boston Children's Hospital, Harvard, MA, USA) for help with the MAPS technology, including kindly providing the plasmid for expression of proteins in fusion with rhizavidin.

Conflicts of Interest: The authors declare no conflict of interest.

References

1. Tebeje, B.M.; Harvie, M.; You, H.; Loukas, A.; McManus, D.P. Schistosomiasis vaccines: Where do we stand? *Parasites Vectors* **2016**, *9*, 528. [CrossRef]
2. Tran, M.H.; Pearson, M.S.; Bethony, J.M.; Smyth, D.J.; Jones, M.K.; Duke, M.; Don, T.A.; McManus, D.P.; Correa-Oliveira, R.; Loukas, A. Tetraspanins on the surface of *Schistosoma mansoni* are protective antigens against schistosomiasis. *Nat. Med.* **2006**, *12*, 835–840. [CrossRef] [PubMed]
3. Farias, L.P.; Krautz-Peterson, G.; Tararam, C.A.; Araujo-Montoya, B.O.; Fraga, T.R.; Rofatto, H.K.; Silva, F.P., Jr.; Isaac, L.; Da'dara, A.A.; Wilson, R.A.; et al. On the three-finger protein domain fold and CD59-like proteins in *Schistosoma mansoni*. *PLoS Negl. Trop. Dis.* **2013**, *7*, e2482. [CrossRef]
4. Tran, M.H.; Freitas, T.C.; Cooper, L.; Gaze, S.; Gatton, M.L.; Jones, M.K.; Lovas, E.; Pearce, E.J.; Loukas, A. Suppression of mRNAs Encoding Tegument Tetraspanins from *Schistosoma mansoni* Results in Impaired Tegument Turnover. *PLoS Pathog.* **2010**, *6*, e1000840. [CrossRef]
5. Marcenaro, E.; Augugliaro, R.; Falco, M.; Castriconi, R.; Parolini, S.; Sivori, S.; Romeo, E.; Millo, R.; Moretta, L.; Bottino, C.; et al. CD59 is physically and functionally associated with natural cytotoxicity receptors and activates human NK cell-mediated cytotoxicity. *Eur. J. Immunol.* **2003**, *33*, 3367–3376. [CrossRef] [PubMed]
6. Jia, X.; Schulte, L.; Loukas, A.; Pickering, D.; Pearson, M.; Mobli, M.; Jones, A.; Rosengren, K.J.; Daly, N.L.; Gobert, G.N.; et al. Solution Structure, Membrane Interactions, and Protein Binding Partners of the Tetraspanin Sm-TSP-2, a Vaccine Antigen from the Human Blood Fluke *Schistosoma mansoni*. *J. Biol. Chem.* **2014**, *289*, 7151–7163. [CrossRef] [PubMed]
7. Egesa, M.; Hoffmann, K.F.; Hokke, C.H.; Yazdanbakhsh, M.; Cose, S. Rethinking schistosomiasis vaccine development: Synthetic vesicles. *Trends Parasitol.* **2017**, *33*, 918–921. [CrossRef]
8. Fonseca, C.T.; Oliveira, S.C.; Alves, C.C. Eliminating Schistosomes through Vaccination: What are the Best Immune Weapons? *Front. Immunol.* **2015**, *6*, 95. [CrossRef]
9. Wilson, R.A.; Li, X.H.; Castro-Borges, W. Schistosome vaccines: Problems, pitfalls and prospects. *Emerg. Top. Life Sci.* **2017**, *1*, 641–650. [CrossRef] [PubMed]
10. Barbosa, M.M.F.; Kanno, A.I.; Barazzone, G.; Rodrigues, D.; Pancakova, V.; Trentini, M.; Faquim-Mauro, E.L.; Freitas, A.; Khouri, M.I.; Lobo da Silva, J.; et al. Robust humoral and cellular responses induced by *Schistosoma mansoni* TSP-2 antigen coupled to outer membrane vesicles. *Int. J. Nanomed.* **2021**. under review.
11. Barbosa, M.M.F.; Kanno, A.I.; Pancakova, V.; Gonçalves, V.M.; Malley, R.; Faria, L.P.; Leite, L.C.C. Expression and purification of *Schistosoma mansoni* antigens in fusion with rhizavidin for vaccine development. *Mol. Biotechnol.* **2021**. under review.
12. Beeson, P.B. Development of Tolerance to Typhoid Bacterial Pyrogen and its Abolition by Reticulo-Endothelial Blockade. *Exp. Biol. Med.* **1946**, *61*, 248–250. [CrossRef]
13. Howard, J.G.; Biozzi, G.; Halpern, B.N.; Stiffel, C.; Mouton, D. The effect of *Mycobacterium tuberculosis* (BCG) infection on the resistance of mice to bacterial endotoxin and *Salmonella enteritidis* infection. *Br. J. Exp. Pathol.* **1959**, *40*, 281–290.
14. Bistoni, F.; Vecchiarelli, A.; Cenci, E.; Puccetti, P.; Marconi, P.; Cassone, A. Evidence for macrophage-mediated protection against lethal *Candida albicans* infection. *Infect. Immun.* **1986**, *51*, 668–674. [CrossRef] [PubMed]
15. Netea, M.G.; Quintin, J.; Van Der Meer, J.W.M. Trained Immunity: A Memory for Innate Host Defense. *Cell Host Microbe* **2011**, *9*, 355–361. [CrossRef] [PubMed]
16. Netea, M.G.; Schlitzer, A.; Placek, K.; Joosten, L.A.B.; Schultze, J.L. Innate and Adaptive Immune Memory: An Evolutionary Continuum in the Host's Response to Pathogens. *Cell Host Microbe* **2019**, *25*, 13–26. [CrossRef]
17. Fan, H.; Cook, J.A. Molecular mechanisms of endotoxin tolerance. *J. Endotoxin Res.* **2004**, *10*, 71–84. [CrossRef]
18. Cavaillon, J.-M.; Adib-Conquy, M. Bench-to-bedside review: Endotoxin tolerance as a model of leukocyte reprogramming in sepsis. *Crit. Care* **2006**, *10*, 233. [CrossRef] [PubMed]
19. Seeley, J.J.; Ghosh, S. Molecular mechanisms of innate memory and tolerance to LPS. *J. Leukoc. Biol.* **2017**, *101*, 107–119. [CrossRef]
20. Foster, S.L.; Hargreaves, D.C.; Medzhitov, R. Gene-specific control of inflammation by TLR-induced chromatin modifications. *Nature* **2007**, *447*, 972–978. [CrossRef] [PubMed]
21. Ifrim, D.C.; Quintin, J.; Joosten, L.A.B.; Jacobs, C.; Jansen, T.; Jacobs, L.; Gow, N.A.R.; Williams, D.L.; Van Der Meer, J.W.M.; Netea, M.G. Trained Immunity or Tolerance: Opposing Functional Programs Induced in Human Monocytes after Engagement of Various Pattern Recognition Receptors. *Clin. Vaccine Immunol.* **2014**, *21*, 534–545. [CrossRef]
22. Töpfer, E.; Boraschi, D.; Italiani, P. Innate Immune Memory: The Latest Frontier of Adjuvanticity. *J. Immunol. Res.* **2015**, *2015*, 478408. [CrossRef] [PubMed]
23. Blok, B.A.; Arts, R.J.W.; Van Crevel, R.; Benn, C.S.; Netea, M.G. Trained innate immunity as underlying mechanism for the long-term, nonspecific effects of vaccines. *J. Leukoc. Biol.* **2015**, *98*, 347–356. [CrossRef]
24. Jensen, K.J.; Benn, C.S.; van Crevel, R. Unravelling the nature of non-specific effects of vaccines—A challenge for innate immunologists. *Semin. Immunol.* **2016**, *28*, 377–383. [CrossRef]
25. Cauchi, S.; Locht, C. Non-specific effects of live attenuated pertussis vaccine against heterologous infections and inflammatory diseases. *Front. Immunol.* **2018**, *9*, 2872. [CrossRef] [PubMed]

26. Aaby, P.; Benn, C.S. Developing the concept of beneficial non-specific effect of live vaccines with epidemiological studies. *Clin. Microbiol. Infect.* **2019**, *25*, 1459–1467. [CrossRef] [PubMed]
27. Jain, N.; Möller, J.; Vogel, V. Mechanobiology of Macrophages: How Physical Factors Coregulate Macrophage Plasticity and Phagocytosis. *Annu. Rev. Biomed. Eng.* **2019**, *21*, 267–297. [CrossRef]
28. Liu, S.; Tobias, R.; McClure, S.; Styba, G.; Shi, Q.; Jackowski, G. Removal of Endotoxin from Recombinant Protein Preparations. *Clin. Biochem.* **1997**, *30*, 455–463. [CrossRef]
29. Frasch, C.E.; van Alphen, L.; Holst, J.; Poolman, J.T.; Rosenqvist, E. Outer membrane protein vesicle vaccines for meningococcal disease. In *Methods in Molecular Medicine, Meningococcal Vaccines*; Pollard, A.J., Maiden, M.C.J., Eds.; Humana Press: Totowa, NJ, USA, 2001; pp. 83–106.
30. Tsai, C.-M.; Frasch, C.; Rivera, E.; Hochstein, H. Measurements of lipopolysaccharide (endotoxin) in meningococcal protein and polysaccharide preparations for vaccine usage. *J. Biol. Stand.* **1989**, *17*, 249–258. [CrossRef]
31. Zhang, F.; Lu, Y.-J.; Malley, R. Multiple antigen-presenting system (MAPS) to induce comprehensive B- and T-cell immunity. *Proc. Natl. Acad. Sci. USA* **2013**, *110*, 13564–13569. [CrossRef]
32. Lesch, H.P.; Kaikkonen, M.U.; Pikkarainen, J.T.; Ylä-Herttuala, S. Avidin-biotin technology in targeted therapy. *Expert Opin. Drug Deliv.* **2010**, *7*, 551–564. [CrossRef]
33. Paganelli, G.; Bartolomei, M.; Grana, C.; Ferrari, M.; Rocca, P.; Chinol, M. Radioimmunotherapy of brain tumor. *Neurol. Res.* **2006**, *28*, 518–522. [CrossRef] [PubMed]
34. Italiani, P.; Mazza, E.M.C.; Lucchesi, D.; Cifola, I.; Gemelli, C.; Grande, A.; Battaglia, C.; Bicciato, S.; Boraschi, D. Transcriptomic profiling of the development of the inflammatory response in human monocytes *in vitro*. *PLoS ONE* **2014**, *9*, e87680. [CrossRef]
35. Reimer-Michalski, E.-M.; Conrath, U. Innate immune memory in plants. *Semin. Immunol.* **2016**, *28*, 319–327. [CrossRef] [PubMed]
36. Milutinović, B.; Kurtz, J. Immune memory in invertebrates. *Semin. Immunol.* **2016**, *28*, 328–342. [CrossRef]
37. Boraschi, D.; Italiani, P. Innate Immune Memory: Time for Adopting a Correct Terminology. *Front. Immunol.* **2018**, *9*, 799. [CrossRef]
38. Awate, S.; Babiuk, L.A.; Mutwiri, G. Mechanisms of Action of Adjuvants. *Front. Immunol.* **2013**, *4*, 114. [CrossRef]
39. Zinkernagel, R.M. What if protective immunity is antigen-driven and not due to so-called "memory" B and T cells? *Immunol. Rev.* **2018**, *283*, 238–246. [CrossRef] [PubMed]
40. Goodridge, H.S.; Ahmed, S.S.; Curtis, N.; Kollmann, T.R.; Levy, O.; Netea, M.G.; Pollard, A.J.; Van Crevel, R.; Wilson, C.B. Harnessing the beneficial heterologous effects of vaccination. *Nat. Rev. Immunol.* **2016**, *16*, 392–400. [CrossRef]
41. Mourits, V.P.; Wijkmans, J.C.; Joosten, L.A.; Netea, M.G. Trained immunity as a novel therapeutic strategy. *Curr. Opin. Pharmacol.* **2018**, *41*, 52–58. [CrossRef]
42. De Bree, L.C.J.; Koeken, V.A.C.M.; Joosten, L.A.B.; Aaby, P.; Benn, C.S.; van Crevel, R.; Netea, M.G. Non-specific effects of vaccines: Current evidence and potential implications. *Semin. Immunol.* **2018**, *39*, 35–43. [CrossRef] [PubMed]
43. Sánchez-Ramón, S.; Conejero, L.; Netea, M.G.; Sancho, D.; Palomares, Ó.; Subiza, J.L. Trained Immunity-Based Vaccines: A New Paradigm for the Development of Broad-Spectrum Anti-infectious Formulations. *Front. Immunol.* **2018**, *9*, 2936. [CrossRef]
44. Rasid, O.; Cavaillon, J.-M. Compartment diversity in innate memory reprogramming. *Microbes Infect.* **2018**, *20*, 156–165. [CrossRef]
45. Xing, Z.; Afkhami, S.; Bavananthasivam, J.; Fritz, D.K.; D'Agostino, M.R.; Vaseghi-Shanjani, M.; Yao, Y.; Jeyanathan, M. Innate immune memory of tissue-resident macrophages and trained innate immunity: Re-vamping vaccine concept and strategies. *J. Leukoc. Biol.* **2020**, *108*, 825–834. [CrossRef]
46. Weavers, H.; Evans, I.R.; Martin, P.; Wood, W. Corpse Engulfment Generates a Molecular Memory that Primes the Macrophage Inflammatory Response. *Cell* **2016**, *165*, 1658–1671. [CrossRef] [PubMed]
47. Chan, L.C.; Rossetti, M.; Miller, L.S.; Filler, S.G.; Johnson, C.W.; Lee, H.K.; Wang, H.; Gjertson, D.; Fowler, V.G., Jr.; Reed, E.F.; et al. MRSA Systems Immunobiology Group Protective immunity in *Staphylococcus aureus* infection reflects localized immune signatures and macrophage-conferred memory. *Proc. Natl. Acad. Sci. USA* **2018**, *115*, E11111–E11119. [CrossRef]
48. Wendeln, A.-C.; Degenhardt, K.; Kaurani, L.; Gertig, M.; Ulas, T.; Jain, G.; Wagner, J.; Häsler, L.M.; Wild, K.; Skodras, A.; et al. Innate immune memory in the brain shapes neurological disease hallmarks. *Nat. Cell Biol.* **2018**, *556*, 332–338. [CrossRef]
49. Hamilton, J.A.; Byrne, R.; Whitty, G. Particulate adjuvants can induce macrophage survival, DNA synthesis, and a synergistic proliferative response to GM-CSF and CSF-1. *J. Leukoc. Biol.* **2000**, *67*, 226–232. [CrossRef] [PubMed]
50. Madej, M.P.; Töpfer, E.; Boraschi, D.; Italiani, P. Different Regulation of Interleukin-1 Production and Activity in Monocytes and Macrophages: Innate Memory as an Endogenous Mechanism of IL-1 Inhibition. *Front. Pharmacol.* **2017**, *8*, 335. [CrossRef] [PubMed]
51. Van der Heijden, C.D.C.C.; Noz, M.P.; Joosten, L.A.B.; Netea, M.G.; Riksen, N.P.; Keating, S.T. Epigenetics and trained immunity. *Antioxid. Redox Signal.* **2018**, *29*, 1023–1040. [CrossRef]
52. Domínguez-Andrés, J.; Fanucchi, S.; Joosten, L.A.B.; Mhlanga, M.M.; Netea, M.G. Advances in understanding molecular regulation of innate immune memory. *Curr. Opin. Cell Biol.* **2020**, *63*, 68–75. [CrossRef]
53. Arts, R.J.W.; Carvalho, A.; La Rocca, C.; Palma, C.; Rodrigues, F.; Silvestre, R.; Kleinnijenhuis, J.; Lachmandas, E.; Gonçalves, L.G.; Belinha, A.; et al. Immunometabolic Pathways in BCG-Induced Trained Immunity. *Cell Rep.* **2016**, *17*, 2562–2571. [CrossRef] [PubMed]

54. Arts, R.J.W.; Novakovic, B.; Ter Horst, R.; Carvalho, A.; Bekkering, S.; Lachmandas, E.; Rodrigues, F.; Silvestre, R.; Cheng, S.C.; Wang, S.Y.; et al. Glutaminolysis and fumarate accumulation integrate immunometabolic and epigenetic programs in trained immunity. *Cell Metabol.* **2016**, *24*, 807–819. [CrossRef] [PubMed]
55. Italiani, P.; Della Camera, G.; Boraschi, D. Induction of innate immune memory by engineered nanoparticles in monocytes/macrophages: From hypothesis to reality. *Front. Immunol.* **2020**, *11*, 566309. [CrossRef] [PubMed]
56. Franceschi, C.; Salvioli, S.; Garagnani, P.; De Eguileor, M.; Monti, D.; Capri, M. Immunobiography and the Heterogeneity of Immune Responses in the Elderly: A Focus on Inflammaging and Trained Immunity. *Front. Immunol.* **2017**, *8*, 982. [CrossRef] [PubMed]

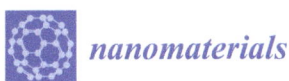

Review

Cross-Species Comparisons of Nanoparticle Interactions with Innate Immune Systems: A Methodological Review

Benjamin J. Swartzwelter [1], Craig Mayall [2], Andi Alijagic [3], Francesco Barbero [4], Eleonora Ferrari [5], Szabolcs Hernadi [6], Sara Michelini [7], Natividad Isabel Navarro Pacheco [8], Alessandra Prinelli [9], Elmer Swart [10] and Manon Auguste [11,*]

1. Institute of Biochemistry and Cell Biology, National Research Council, 80131 Napoli, Italy; swartzwe@colorado.edu
2. Department of Biology, Biotechnical Faculty, University of Liubljana, 1000 Ljubljana, Slovenia; craig_mayall@hotmail.co.uk
3. Institute for Biomedical Research and Innovation, National Research Council, 90146 Palermo, Italy; andialijagic@gmail.com
4. Institut Català de Nanociència i Nanotecnologia (ICN2), Bellaterra, 08193 Barcelona, Spain; fra.barbero@gmail.com
5. Center for Plant Molecular Biology–ZMBP Eberhard-Karls University Tübingen, 72076 Tübingen, Germany; eleonora.ferrari2018@gmail.com
6. School of Biosciences, Cardiff University, Cardiff CF10 3AX, UK; hernadi222@gmail.com
7. Department of Biosciences, Paris-Lodron University Salzburg, 5020 Salzburg, Austria; sara.michelini@sbg.ac.at
8. Institute of Microbiology of the Czech Academy of Sciences, 142 20 Prague, Czech Republic; natividad.pacheco@biomed.cas.cz
9. AvantiCell Science, Ltd., Ayr KA6 5HW, UK; alessandra.prinelli@gmail.com
10. UK Centre for Ecology and Hydrology, Wallingford OX10 8BB, UK; elmswa@ceh.ac.uk
11. Department of Earth Environment and Life Sciences, University of Genova, 16126 Genova, Italy
* Correspondence: manon.auguste@edu.unige.it

Citation: Swartzwelter, B.J.; Mayall, C.; Alijagic, A.; Barbero, F.; Ferrari, E.; Hernadi, S.; Michelini, S.; Navarro Pacheco, N.I.; Prinelli, A.; Swart, E.; et al. Cross-Species Comparisons of Nanoparticle Interactions with Innate Immune Systems: A Methodological Review. *Nanomaterials* **2021**, *11*, 1528. https://doi.org/10.3390/nano11061528

Academic Editors: Diana Boraschi and David M Brown

Received: 18 February 2021
Accepted: 7 June 2021
Published: 9 June 2021

Publisher's Note: MDPI stays neutral with regard to jurisdictional claims in published maps and institutional affiliations.

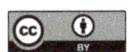

Copyright: © 2021 by the authors. Licensee MDPI, Basel, Switzerland. This article is an open access article distributed under the terms and conditions of the Creative Commons Attribution (CC BY) license (https://creativecommons.org/licenses/by/4.0/).

Abstract: Many components of the innate immune system are evolutionarily conserved and shared across many living organisms, from plants and invertebrates to humans. Therefore, these shared features can allow the comparative study of potentially dangerous substances, such as engineered nanoparticles (NPs). However, differences of methodology and procedure between diverse species and models make comparison of innate immune responses to NPs between organisms difficult in many cases. To this aim, this review provides an overview of suitable methods and assays that can be used to measure NP immune interactions across species in a multidisciplinary approach. The first part of this review describes the main innate immune defense characteristics of the selected models that can be associated to NPs exposure. In the second part, the different modes of exposure to NPs across models (considering isolated cells or whole organisms) and the main endpoints measured are discussed. In this synergistic perspective, we provide an overview of the current state of important cross-disciplinary immunological models to study NP-immune interactions and identify future research needs. As such, this paper could be used as a methodological reference point for future nano-immunosafety studies.

Keywords: environmental models; human cells; innate immunity; markers; NPs testing

1. General Introduction: The Need for Studying Nanoparticle–Immune System Interactions

Over the last twenty years, there has been a significant growth in the research, development, and production of engineered NPs [1]. When materials are downsized to the nanoscale, novel physical and chemical properties emerge, conferring them with new and unique behaviors. Depending on their nature (e.g., composition, size, shape, surface state), these materials have remarkable optical, magnetic, electrical, catalytic, structural, and chemical properties, which can be exploited in many different sectors such as automotive, agricultural, pharmaceutical, and biomedical fields [2–5]. It is estimated that the global nanomaterial production in 2014 was between 0.3 and 1.6 million tons, with SiO_2, TiO_2 and ZnO nanomaterials being the most abundantly produced [6].

The wide utilization and increasing production of NPs has inevitably lead to an increase in humans and environmental exposure to these materials although exposure routes are not necessarily identical for different organisms. The expected increased exposure in human and environmental organisms has given rise to concerns regarding potential safety risks. The main exposure routes to NPs in both humans and environmental species are highlighted and summarized in Figure 1.

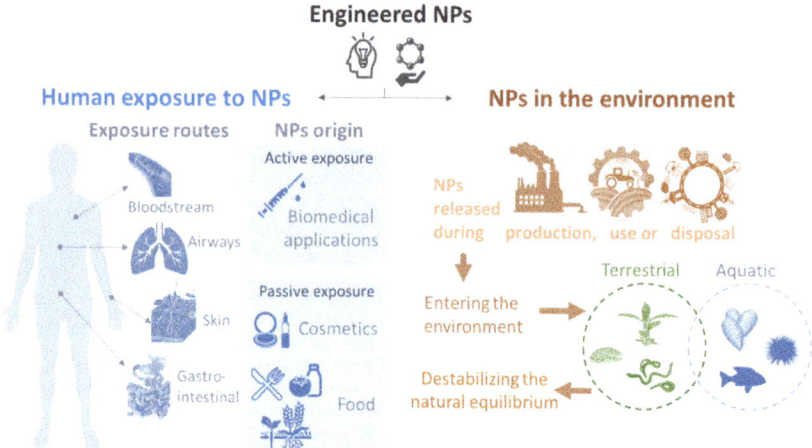

Figure 1. The different exposure pathways of engineered NPs that can interact with human or environmental species.

In humans, the first main exposure pathway is via intentional introduction of NPs, for instance during medical administration. The ability of some NPs to interact with molecular and cellular processes and to be target specific makes their use in drug delivery an attractive application. They have long been known to play an effective role in vaccination, acting not only as antigen carriers, but also as adjuvants that activate innate immunity and thereby increase the efficacy of antigen presentation [7]. They can also be valuable tools in medical imaging and diagnosis, and innovative new therapies [8]. Alongside the potential benefits of nanoparticle-based therapies, there is also a risk associated with parenteral introduction of novel substances, and thus there is a need to ensure that NPs will not negatively impact the normal functioning of the immune system [9–13]. Other interactions can arise from passive exposure such as through cosmetic products or food. Although NPs will likely first interact with epithelial and mucosal barriers, in some cases they are able to cross these barriers or potentially cause adverse effects, for example by interacting with the natural gut microbiome [14].

Although most NPs are not directly applied in the environment, many NPs used in consumer products or industry are expected to be released into the environment during production, use or during the disposal of products containing NPs [15]. Over the past decade, an increasing number of products containing NPs have been introduced into agricultural practices with the aim of increasing crop yield and reducing production costs [16]. In addition, the use of wastewater treatment plant biosolids as crop fertilizers can facilitate release of NPs into the terrestrial environment leading to exposure in soil organisms [17]. NPs can also reach aquatic environments, including seashores, through landfill leachates, or direct disposal of wastes (e.g., consumer products containing plastics) [18]. Once in the water, NPs can remain in suspension in the water column, interacting with planktonic organisms, or due to interactions with organic matter and/or their higher density, NPs can aggregate and deposit on the seafloor. This has been reflected by several models predicting NP concentrations within different regions which showed higher concentrations of NPs in sediments than surface water [19]. Therefore, benthic and sediment dwelling organisms are expected to be exposed to NPs, due to their feeding habit (e.g., filter, deposit feeders) [20]. In addition, some marine invertebrates possess an open (or semiopen) circulatory system, which is in direct contact with the external environment, eventually contributing to increased exposure.

Considering the many possible exposure and entry routes of NPs, defining common parameters for assessing organism-NP interactions is fundamental for allowing comparisons at different taxonomic levels. Innate immunity is a shared feature for every multicellular organism and the effector mechanisms of the innate immune system are the first line of defense that detect and protect the body from nonself objects such as NPs [21–23]. As is the case for natural pathogens, NPs have the potential to induce an immune response. In cases where NPs can elicit an immune response, there is a need to study the type and degree of this response, and the NP-immune interaction mechanisms rather than remaining limited to only measurements of acute toxicity. Comparative immunology, by its multidisciplinary approach may unravel fundamental mechanisms activated by NPs and help further global understanding regarding the effects of NPs.

Experiments in a laboratory are first necessary to allow the understanding of basic mechanisms under controlled conditions. However, carefully chosen models and assessment parameters are important with regard to future translocation to more realistic environmental exposure. To this end, models within this review have been selected which can be good indicators and representatives of their regional and global distribution and which are easy to maintain under laboratory conditions. Environmental models can be therefore compared across taxa and even to human cells, through both in vitro and/or in vivo approaches according to the model possibilities (Figure 2). Plant models are a compelling place to begin for assessment of NP-immune interactions. In particular *Arabidopsis thaliana*, a small flowering plant belonging to the Brassicaceae family, which is widely used in crop science studies and was also the first plant genome to be fully sequenced [24–26]. Among terrestrial invertebrates, earthworms belonging to the family Lumbricidae *(Eisenia fetida)* are abundant in the soil and play an essential role in soil formation, by facilitating nutrient cycling, fragmenting biomass and aeration of soil through bioturbation [27,28]. Similarly, terrestrial isopods, such as *Porcelio scaber*, are crustaceans which evolved to live on land, inhabiting the top-soil level. They are decomposers and play an important role in returning nutrients to the soil [29–31]. Their feeding habits makes it likely they will come into contact with environmental pollutants, including NPs, and thus represent interesting model species to study these interactions. The Mediterranean mussel *Mytilus galloprovincialis* and the sea urchin *Paracentrotus lividus* are both sessile marine invertebrates. Mussels are able to filter large quantities of water which they use for breathing and feeding, while sea urchins graze on the seafloor layer. These qualities, as well as the ease with which they can be harvested along seashores, make these good models in which to study invertebrate interactions with NPs [20,32–34].

This work is supported by the EU PANDORA project [35], which devoted effort to study the effects and mechanisms of action of NPs on the innate immunity of different models from across the tree of life. The general outcomes of the project were previously reported, summarizing the main findings but also to set future perspective and research direction in this field [21,36]. The remainder of this review will focus on the translatable aspects of experimental methodology, parameters and endpoints used, the suitably of the selected models when considering investigating NP effects, and the possibilities regarding research at the whole organism level (in vivo) or with isolated cells (in vitro).

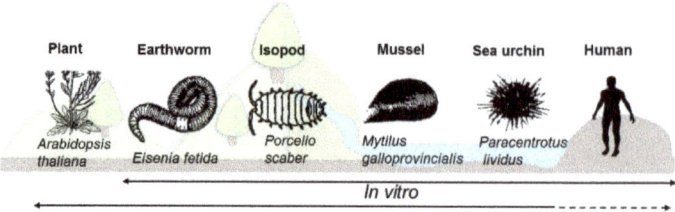

Figure 2. The different models discussed in the current review, and their main experimental usage in the laboratory: in vivo (whole organism experiments) and in vitro (isolated cells or cell lines).

Here we aim to: (i) give a short overview of the characteristics of various relevant innate immune models from across tree of life; and (ii) provide a comparative analysis of the methods used to study the interaction of NPs with these innate immune models.

2. Short Description of the Innate Immune System for the Models of Interest
2.1. Generalities and Conserved Innate Immune Traits across the Selected Models

The ability to mount an immune response against external threats is a characteristic of every living organism. While increasing levels of immune complexity are found in higher organisms, at every stage of evolution there is present a basic initial host defense that has been characterized as innate immunity. Innate immunity is a fast, standardized, nonspecific response which includes multiple levels of defense mechanisms, beginning with physicochemical barriers (e.g., shell, mucosal or epithelial barrier) [37,38]. Further mechanisms of defense rely on dual components of the immune system, the immune cells (e.g., monocytes, macrophages for vertebrates, or hemocytes, coelomocytes for invertebrates) and the production of humoral factors. Innate immune cells found in the circulating fluids of invertebrates can have different names and the cellular portion of their innate immunity relies on these unique cells. These cells can be subdivided into different cell populations, such as granular or hyaline cells, and they have distinct roles and can trigger a specific response upon encountering threatening nonself material. Only plants lack these specialized immune cells, but in plants all the cells are believed to be able to mount a defensive response to foreign attack [39]. Complex machinery, including cells and humoral factors is involved in recognition of nonself material, and especially in detecting domains called pathogen/microbe associated molecular patterns (PAMPs/MAMPs) that are typically displayed on the surface of bacterial, fungal, and parasitic organisms and virus-infected cells. Host recognition of nonself will involve a large range of cell membrane bound and scattered pattern recognition receptors (PRRs). Although the distinctive PRRs can vary between models, the main concept is consistent, and different PRRs share a similar role upon recognition of nonself particles. PRRs in humans, much like their invertebrate homologues, are responsible for initiating innate immune cell responses including the initiation of phagocytosis or endocytosis, cellular motility, and beginning the processes leading to inflammatory reactions [40]. Upon successful recognition, the pathogen detecting cell will initiate a process of destruction or sequestration to eliminate eventual danger, and later repair the stress or damage caused by this unexpected material. Most invertebrate immune cells, similarly to human macrophages or monocytes, are involved in phagocytosis, which remains one of the most efficient mechanisms to clear nonself material. The induction of some global defense mechanisms can be easily observed across different models, such as the production of reactive oxygen species (ROS) and nitrogen radicals (RNS), synthesis and secretion of antibacterial and antifungal proteins, cytokine-like proteins, and hydrolytic enzymes. Antimicrobial peptides (AMPs—small cationic, amphipathic molecules) are very well studied and highly involved in invertebrate immunity. They can tag objects or induce direct destruction by destabilizing biological membranes, which make them effective against large range of unicellular organisms like bacteria, yeast, fungi, and also some protozoans and enveloped viruses [41]. Circulating fluid also contains a large panel of enzymes (released by immune cells) with hemolytic, proteolytic and cytotoxic roles (one of the most common being lysozyme).

The encapsulation of foreign objects and activation of enzymatic cascades that regulate melanization and coagulation of hemolymph are also common defense mechanisms encountered in invertebrates. Indeed, phenoloxidase is considered among the most important components of the invertebrate immune system, especially in insects and crustaceans. The phenoloxidase cascade produces the antimicrobial molecule melanin, as well as inducing multiple potent bioactive agents such as peroxinectin and ROS, that aid in phagocytosis and cell adhesion. Melanization is essential in wound healing, encapsulation, and nodulation. Proper modulation of this enzyme is crucial to ensure survival of the organism. The majority of species activate the phenoloxidase cascade using the proPO enzyme [42–44].

Although general immune features are conserved across the previously described models and organisms, adaptations exist in each case that address the organism particular vulnerabilities and environmental stresses. These adaptations occur according to the organism's lifestyle, habits and need, which might cause certain parameters to be more important than others in some species to deal with threats some models are more likely to encounter. In line with this, the next section aims to report the main mechanisms and characteristics of innate immune responses for the selected models, and in particular those known to be activated upon exposure to NPs. A summary is presented in Table 1.

Table 1. Summary of the main defense mechanisms involved in innate immunity at different levels of the models discussed.

Name	Innate Immune Cell Types	Whole Organism Level Defense	Cellular Response	Humoral/Extracellular Factors	Recognition & Activation
Plant *Arabidopsis thaliana*	All cells	Cell wall Waxy epidermal cuticle	MAMP-triggered immunity Effector triggered Immunity Hypersensitive response	ROS production Hormones (ethylene, JA, SA) Antimicrobial secreted peptides	PRRs: RLKs RLPs NLRs
Earthworm *Eisenia fetida*	Amoebocytes (granular and hyaline) Eleocytes	Skin Mucus Expulsion by dorsal pore Autotomy	Phagocytosis Agglutination-encapsulation ProPO cascade → melanization	AMPs (lumbricin I) Bacteriolytic enzyme (lysozyme) Hemolytic, proteolytic and cytotoxic proteins (fetidin and lysenins) ROS production	PRRs: CCF (lectinlike domain) TLR LBP/BPI
Terrestrial isopod *Porcelio scaber*	Hemocyte Granular and hyaline	Cuticle	Phagocytosis Encapsulation ProPO cascade → melanization	AMPs ROS/NO production	PRRs: TLR
Marine mussel *Mytilus galloprovincialis*	Hemocyte Granular and hyaline	Shell barrier Mucus layer Pseudo-feces	Phagocytosis Encapsulation ProPO	AMPs (mytilin, myticin, mytimicin), Defensins Complement system (C1qDC) Bacteriolytic enzyme-Lysozyme ROS/NO production	PRRs: lectins PGRPS TLR C1qDC FRED

Table 1. Cont.

Name	Innate Immune Cell Types	Whole Organism Level Defense	Cellular Response	Humoral/Extracellular Factors	Recognition & Activation
Sea urchin *Paracentrotus lividus*	Macrophage-like phagocytes, amoebocytes (colorless, red); vibratile cells	Test Gut barrier Faeces	Phagocytosis Encapsulation	ROS production, AMPs (strongylocins, centrocins, paracentrin 1), lysozyme	PRRs: TLRs NLRs SRCR domain-containing proteins
Human	Monocytes Macrophages DCs Granulocytes [1]	Epithelial and mucosal tissue	Phagocytosis Inflammation Granulocyte recruitment Antigen presentation	Complement antibodies, AMPs NETs, ROS/NO	PRRs:TLRs, NLRs, Scavenger Receptors, RLRs, CLRs,

[1] Other innate cell types exist that are not discussed, including natural killer cells and innate lymphoid cells. Refer to the main text for the meaning of the abbreviations.

2.2. Model Specific Immune System Characteristics

2.2.1. Plants

Plants lack specialized mobile immune cells, and every cell is believed to be capable of initiating an immune defense against pathogens and invaders. Two layers of innate immune responses, i.e., pattern triggered immunity (PTI) and effector-triggered immunity (ETI), provide an efficient defense that keeps most pathogens and external attacks under control [39,45]. The activation of PTI relies on PRRs perceptions of MAMPs/PAMPs to trigger complex immune responses. PRRs are solely on the cell surface of plant cells and among them the most studied is the plant flagellin receptor-FLS2 [46–51]. The second line of defense, ETI, is mediated by nucleotide-binding domain leucine-rich repeat (NB-LRR) disease resistance proteins (NLR), which induce defense responses leading to a hypersensitive programmed cell death [52]. NLRs can detect effectors directly or by indirect surveillance of the effector action on other host target proteins [39]. Both lines of defense share parts of their defense signaling pathways [53,54]. After pathogen detection, multiple morphological and physiological responses are induced, such as ion fluxes over the plasma membrane, including Ca^{2+}- and H^+-influx; production of ROS and antimicrobial compounds (phytoalexins); activation of mitogen-activated protein kinases (MAPKs) and calcium-dependent protein kinases (CDPKs). In consequence, the transcriptome will be reprogramed by activation of a subset of transcription factors; callose deposition; stomatal closure; restriction of nutrient transfer from the cytosol to the apoplast and programmed cell death [55,56]. Phytohormones such as salicylic acid, abscisic acid, jasmonic acid, and ethylene have a critical role in the plant's responses to specific pathogens [57]. Defense hormones can be transported within and between plants to alert distant tissues and confer systemic immunity [55,58].

2.2.2. Earthworms

Earthworms are protostome animals that have large coelomic cavities throughout the length of the animal. The coelomic cavity is typically nonsterile, open to the outer environment through dorsal pores, allowing the entrance of fungi, bacteria, and protozoans. Coelomocytes can be classified into two major cell types: amoebocytes and eleocytes. Amoebocytes (hyaline and granular) are involved in various immune responses including phagocytosis, encapsulation, and the production of antimicrobial molecules [59,60]. Eleocytes display more nutritive and accessory functions [59,61]. Three types of PRRs have so far been identified: coelomic cytolytic factor (CCF) [62], toll-like receptors (TLR) [63], and lipopolysaccharide-binding protein/bacterial permeability-increasing protein (LBP/BPI) [64]. CCF has two recognition domains that can interact with bacterial or fungal MAMPs, which in turn triggers the proPO cascade [42,65]. A range of antimicrobial molecules including lysozyme and the hemolytic proteins fetidins and lysenins are involved in the elimination of the microorganisms [66–69].

2.2.3. Isopods

The hemocytes of *Porcellio scaber* originate in the hematopoietic glands located along the animals dorsal vessel, and can be split into granular and hyaline hemocytes [70,71]. Hyaline (absence of granules) hemocytes are mainly responsible for phagocytosis [71]. Semigranular cells also show some phagocytic ability but seem more involved in encapsulation and nodulation. Granular cells are predominantly involved with the phenoloxidase system [72], and along with semigranular cells are thought to produce AMPs and be involved in antioxidant defense [73,74]. In *P. scaber*, the PO cascade is initiated by hemocyanin [44]. In addition, for defense they are able to produce, RNS, ROS, and AMPs like other invertebrates [75,76]. Genomic mining of the terrestrial isopod, *Armadillidium vulgare*, revealed genes for specific AMPs including anti-lipopolysaccharide factor (ALF) 1 and 2, crustin 1, 2, and 3, and I type lysozyme, and pathogen recognition genes C-type lectins 1, 2, and 3 and peroxinectin-like A and B [77].

2.2.4. Mussels

The innate effector cells of *Mytilus*, hemocytes, are composed of granulocytes and hyalinocytes. Mature granulocytes are among the first lines of cell defense for the elimination of invaders via phagocytic processes [78]. In *Mytilus*, a large range of PRRs, anchored on the cell outer membrane and secreted are encountered, with lectins the most dominant group. Other classes of soluble PRRs are found, like C-terminal fibrinogen related domain-FReD-containing proteins, which have been shown to improve the rate of phagocytosis. TLRs and peptidoglycan recognition proteins-PGRPs, and others have been recently discovered but further study remains to be done to properly appraise their mechanisms of action (see [79] for more details). Moreover, *Mytilus* possesses the complement system pathway and relies on the involvement of C1qDC (C1q domain-containing) proteins [80]. Several signaling transduction pathways have been reported to be present in bivalves such as the mitogen-activated protein kinase (MAPK), nuclear factor-κB (NF-κB), the complement component, the toll pathways, and the JAK-STAT pathway (reviewed in [79]). Additionally, as with other species, hemocytes can trigger the production and release of several factors such as ROS, nitric oxide-NO, hydrolytic enzymes (e.g., lysozyme), and AMPs. Several AMPs have been identified in *Mytilus* such as mytilin, myticin, mytimicin (with an antifungal and/or antibacterial role) and defensins [81]. In extreme cases and for larger objects, hemocytes can encapsulate foreign matter via the coordination of several hemocytes and the release of cytotoxic products (enzymes or ROS) to degrade the material, followed by cellular reabsorption of the debris [82]. Finally, the proPO cascade, while present, remains relatively unstudied in bivalves [83].

2.2.5. Sea Urchins

Sea urchins contain circulating immune cells called coelomocytes which can be subdivided into four classes and are able to infiltrate into different tissues [84,85]. The macrophage-like phagocytes can encapsulate and internalize nonself particles, red amoebocytes release the bactericidal pigment echinochrome A, and white/colorless amoebocytes operate the cytotoxic/cytolytic response, while vibratile cells most probably degranulate and trigger immune cell aggregation [85]. Recently, their genome sequences have revealed the presence of a vast array of immune-related genes, including those coding for PRRs such as TLRs, NLRs or SRCR domain-containing proteins, and complement proteins (Complement C3 homologue) [86,87]. Moreover, lectins are also important in sea urchins and in addition to their role in opsonization, they show lytic functions, and are involved in wound repair [88]. Sea urchins contain several humoral factors including hemolysin and agglutinin which can be induced upon cell activation. ROS are also produced during immune responses. Echinoderms possess many different AMPs with various modes of action depending on the species, among them paracentrin 1 in *P. lividus*, showing an antimicrobial role [89]. Interestingly, the phagocytes can contain AMPs but they are not released into the extracellular medium, instead they play a role within the phagolysosome [88]. Finally, sea urchins belong to deuterostome lineage which makes them phylogenetically near to chordates, sharing several common traits with mammalians, especially with regard to cytokine production [90,91].

2.2.6. Human Cells

Human and other mammalian immune responses are organized within two branches: the innate immune response which is characteristic of all eukaryotes, and additionally a highly specific adaptive immune response, individualized for distinct pathogens. As NPs do not display highly specified and unique surface patterns, it is the innate branch of human immunity that is tasked with responses to NP exposure. Nonself particles and pathogenic threats that enter human circulation may activate humoral components such as AMPs and complement alongside innate immune cells. Cells participating in the human innate immune response include granulocytes, such as neutrophils (which primarily function to overwhelm pathogenic invaders through large numbers and phagocytic mechanisms), and myeloid-derived cells, including monocytes, macrophages, and dendritic cells (DCs). Monocytes represent about 2–8% of the leukocytes in circulation at any given time [92] and generally patrol the circulatory system for signs of foreign particles or internal damage. They can be recruited in tissue via resident cells releasing chemokines such as CCL2 [93]. As monocytes attempt to engulf foreign particles by phagocytosis, simultaneous chemokines and cytokines are secreted that signal for a broader inflammatory and immune response. They can be further involved in the resolution of an inflammatory reaction, assisting in tissue repair [94]. Macrophages, are tissue resident and represent up to 15% of the cells in a given tissue [95]. Functionally two broad classes of macrophage exist, M1 which display a more inflammatory phenotype involved in early immune response (killing and defending); and later M2, which display more phagocytic and tissue repair oriented traits [96–98]. Finally, DCs are known as antigen-presenting cells, acting as the bridge between human innate and adaptive immunity. They play a role in the generation of pathogen-specific T-cells and B-cell antibodies. Of the PRRs in humans, toll-like receptors (TLRs) play the most prominent role in the detection of extracellular pathogens [99], where they recognize substances such as bacterially associated carbohydrate patterns or RNA sequences associated with viruses [100]. Other PRRs that can be found on the membrane of human innate immune cells include scavenger receptors, which detect various polymers and lipoproteins [101], and C-type lectin receptors including dectin-1, which recognizes B-glucan components of various fungi [102]. In addition, they are some intracellular PRRs found in cytosol, such as NOD-like receptors (NLRs) and rig-I-like receptors (RLRs), which recognize a large range of PAMPs [103–105]. The most notable difference with invertebrates, is the diversity and number of types of cells involved in the immune response.

3. Parameters Assessed: From NPs to Innate Immune Responses

3.1. NPs: What to Consider When You Use a Biological System?

The physico-chemical characteristics of a NP and its behavior in different exposure media are fundamental considerations when attempting to understand the interactions of NPs within a biological model. It is important to take into account that the relatively large surface area to volume, the low coordination of atoms at the surface, and their colloidal nature cause NPs to display physical and chemical characteristics that differ from their bulk counterparts. It is also fundamental to understand the characteristics of the final object that living organisms will encounter and to correlate the pristine and final NP features with the potential effects on living organisms. The main NP characteristics to be considered are reported in Figure 3.

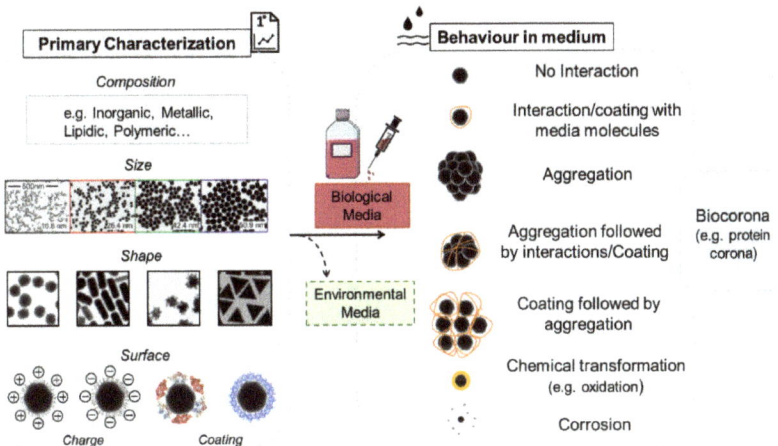

Figure 3. The different characteristics of NPs and parameters to investigate when they are in suspension media for laboratory experiments.

3.1.1. Primary Characterization

The first determination of primary characteristics includes the description of the material composition, the nominal size, shape, and surface charge (zeta potential). Moreover, characterization of NP coating and other surface modifications are crucial to consider (Figure 3 left panel).

3.1.2. Behavior in Medium

In addition to the known properties of a chosen NP following synthesis, once exposed to biological conditions (e.g., medium or circulating fluid), NPs can display unpredicted new characteristics. NPs can have a propensity to move towards a more stable thermodynamic state via different means: aggregation (which can mean escaping from the nanoscale), formation of a coating composed of various molecules, chemical transformations, particle corrosion, and dissolution [1]. All these transformations can change the identity of the NP or produce new chemical entities (e.g., reactive metal ions), modifying their behavior and their potential associated risk and interactions (Figure 3 right panel). Therefore, the determination of NP characteristics in exposure medium needs to be assessed. This generally includes the aggregation state (Z-average), the change in surface charge (zeta potential), and the dispersion index (PdI). Moreover, the evolution over time of these parameters can also be of value for a full appraisal of the NPs dynamic in the exposure medium. All these analyses are usually performed using DLS (dynamic light scattering) analysis, or electron microscopy (TEM and SEM) depending on the material being investigated. Additionally, careful controls have to be performed in order to avoid artifacts due to the presence of chemicals, often used to stabilize the particles [106,107], or contaminants, such as bacterial lipopolysaccharide (LPS), that can cause false positives in an immune assay [108].

Another routinely measured parameter is the presence and composition of the molecular biocorona, where components of biological fluids can be adsorbed by the NP, forming a corona on its surface. Usually, they are believed to be mostly constituted by proteins (protein corona -PC) but other macromolecules including lipids present in the medium can also contribute to its formation. The presence of this supplementary layer on top of the NPs can in turn affect the NPs behavior and interactions with the surrounding media. However, this corona depends on both the biological fluid (plasma, or otherwise) composition and the properties of the NPs, including size, curvature, surface functionalization, and charge. The composition of the corona is theoretically divided into the soft corona (weakly bound) and the hard corona (tightly bound), but it is dynamic and the ligand on the top can be exchanged and replaced over time, according to the affinity of the macromolecule for the NPs [109,110]. The PC is the biological identity of the NP and represents what cells "see" and with which they will interact [111–118]. Consequently, recognition by immune cells can be different and specific from one type of NP to another, which means that they will interact with the protein on the surface rather than the NP itself. This results in the triggering of defense mechanisms different from those observed in medium free of proteins. This does not apply only to mammalian plasma, but it has been demonstrated in the biological fluids of different terrestrial and marine invertebrates, including earthworms, bivalve, and sea urchins, in which the composition and effects on immune parameters appeared different for each NP type [119–122]. For these reasons, the PC is an important parameter to consider under laboratory conditions and needs to be characterized with precision during the exposure event.

All the previously cited characteristics can also be applied to environmental media [123–126]. The NPs will be subjected to other factors like abiotic physico-chemical parameters (such as pH, ionic strength, temperature) which can influence their dispersion, aggregation, agglomeration [127,128], interaction with molecules present in their environment, and adsorption to macro-organic matter (e.g., eco-corona) [117]. Scientific literature is being produced on the physico-chemical transformation of NPs due to their exposure to aquatic and terrestrial scenarios, correlating the environments and particle properties with the observed changes. Consideration of this should be taken into account in future studies working with environmental scenario experiments [129–132].

3.2. Models, Cell Culture and Mode of Exposure

In experimental science, the use of in vitro assays is being promoted as sustainable alternative for a large range of product testing, including NPs, following the 3R principle (replacement, reduction, and refinement). The extraction of immune cells, separation, culture and feasibility to maintain such isolated primary cells varies across models. To illustrate, a summary of the different methods of cell harvesting and exposure for both invertebrates and human primary cells are reported in Figures 4 and 5.

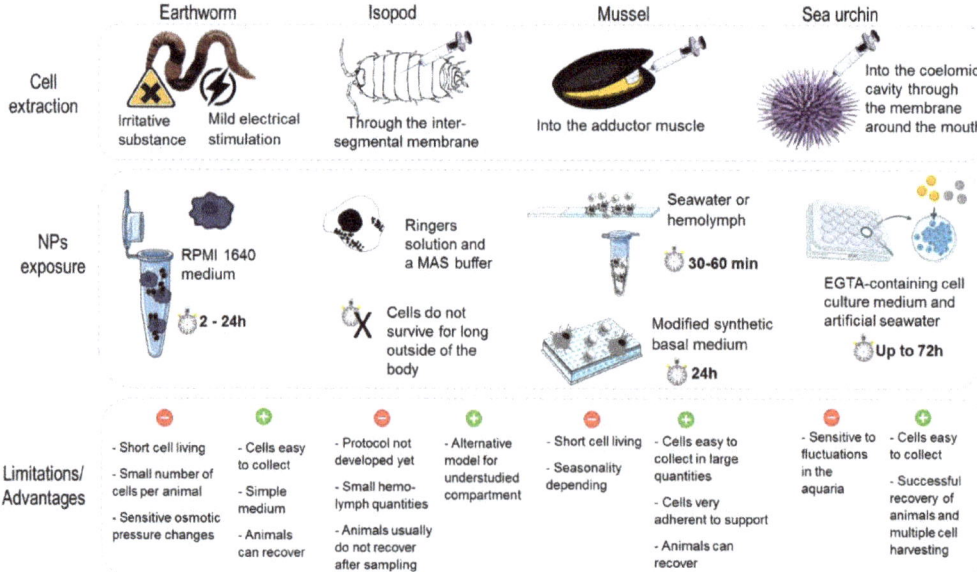

Figure 4. The different in vitro approaches and NPs exposure parameters encountered across the selected models.

3.2.1. Nonmammalian In Vitro Assays

In many invertebrates, coelomocytes/hemocytes act as the first line of defense against nonself objects. The induction of functional responses with these cells is often rapidly observed, helping to counteract the limitation of the relative short-term lifespan of cells in cultures (ranging from a few hours to a few days depending on the model). As a natural defense mechanism, earthworms can extrude their coelomic fluid, through dorsal pores. Therefore, coelomocytes can be extracted by mild electrical stimulation or by exposing the animals to an irritative substance [133,134]. Immediately upon collection, the coelomocytes need to be stabilized in a culture medium in order preserve cell viability. Recent studies show that RPMI 1640 medium is the optimal medium for earthworm coelomocytes culturing, as well as the assessment of NP toxicity towards coelomocytes [135,136]. Critical for the successful culturing of coelomocytes is the adjustment of osmolality of the medium so that it reflects that of the coelomic fluid [137–139]. Exposure time for in vitro assays depends on cell viability and may range from between 2 to 72 h, with 24 h being the optimum time for cell cultures in RPMI 1640, according to some investigations [136,137,140]. For terrestrial isopods, the culturing of hemocytes did not show hopeful results yet. Hemolymph can be collected by puncturing through the intersegmental membrane on the dorsal side of the isopod with a sterile needle and collecting the hemolymph with a micropipette. With the use of ringers solution and a MAS (mitochondrial assay solution) buffer, cells appeared to hardly survive for even a few hours outside the body. The selection of a suitable medium is still needed to be identified and adapted for keeping hemocytes alive without showing excessive levels of stress [141].

In marine invertebrates, in vitro experiments are much more abundant, in particular, experiments using hemocytes of the marine mussel *M. galloprovincialis* extracted via a non-invasive method. This method can provide a first line of investigation for testing several types of substances, including NPs [142–145]. *Mytilus* hemolymph is easy to collect via the adductor muscle and fluid quantities are sufficient (depending on the season, volume can be as high as several ml per animal) to perform various experiments [146]. Short-term exposures ($\leq$1 h) have shown rapid activation of hemocyte functional parameters but longer exposure times (up to 24 h) have shown the induction of further immune or stress parameters. For short experiments, hemocytes can be maintained in a natural hemolymph or seawater suspension, in tubes or as monolayers on glass slides. Longer culture times were more successful when modified synthetic basal medium (Basal Medium Eagle) was used in microwell plates. These in vitro experiments are possible due to the cells ability to quickly adhere to supports (<20 min) [147,148]. Ex-vivo tissue explant has also been used (e.g., gills) to study the first interactions and potential uptake of NPs [149].

The coelomocytes from sea urchin once extracted are placed in cell culture plates and kept in EGTA-containing cell culture medium and artificial seawater [84,85,150]. The coelomocytes can be kept for a long period of time (over two weeks), with regular medium replenishment and without the addition of the special growth factors or nutrients [90,151].

Finally, as plants do not possess specialized mobile immune cells, in vitro research is not typically suitable/realizable, and the main experiments in laboratories are made on the full plant or tissues excisions (see next section). Each piece of tissue should respond upon exposure as each single cell is able to launch an effective immune response [152].

3.2.2. Human Cell Models

The study of human cells offers a wide range of possibilities not currently developed for invertebrate models. Multiple cell types, coculture conditions, and cell maturation or differentiation programs exist to define more precisely the interactions with NPs. Several important models used in mammalian systems to test NP–immune system interactions are listed below.

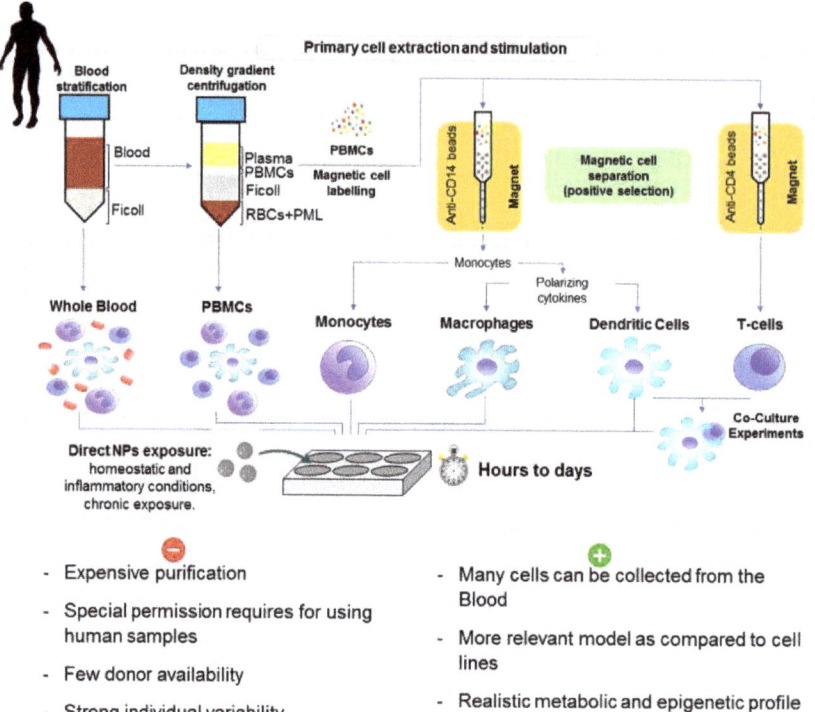

Figure 5. The different in vitro NP exposure possibilities available for human primary cells and the procedure of cell extraction and preparation (Reprinted with permission from Michelini et al. (2021) [153]. Copyright 2021, Copyright Royal Society of Chemistry).

In vitro modelling of human innate immunity is usually conducted using monocytes, macrophages, or dendritic cells, as these cells are responsible for directing the innate immune response from pathogen recognition to phagocytosis to inflammation, and even to eventual antigen presentation and induction of adaptive immunity. Cell lines for each of these cell types exist and are frequently used due to their easy experimental repeatability and scalability, with THP-1 (monocytes) and U937 (macrophages) being the most frequently reported [154]. However, cell lines are truly limited to the representative phenotype observed at the time of culture, and even this is susceptible to mutations that do not represent the true reactivity of healthy human cells. More robust models of innate immune responsiveness utilize primary cells, which are collected directly from donors and may be isolated using techniques that select for the desired cell type. Primary cells are representative of an individual's current in vivo condition, and lack the altered metabolic and epigenetic profile inherent to cell lines. Furthermore, as monocytes are found abundantly in circulation, and since they can be precursors for both macrophages and DCs, the differentiation of monocytes in culture into primary differentiated macrophages or DCs is an effective tool to create models of innate immune responses in vitro. However, models utilizing primary cells must contend with individual variability as the immune experience and capacity is different between donors [155].

The whole blood assay is one of the most simple and rapid tests for assessing the immune activating capacity of novel substances within a human system. Typically, blood is drawn from healthy donors and immediately exposed to the substance under investigation, with 250 µL of blood typically diluted in 750 µL of RPMI plus the tested material and incubated for 24–48 h [156]. Peripheral blood mononuclear cell (PBMCs) can also be isolated from the whole blood using Ficoll–Paque density gradient centrifugation [157]. Magnetic cell separation using some CD-4 beads can be used to isolate monocytes, and later growth factors can be added to differentiate macrophages such as macrophage colony stimulating factor (M-CSF) or DC GM-CSF and IL-4 [94,158].

The monocyte activation test (MAT) models (or using macrophage and DCs) can assess the exposure and response of monocytes to NPs, and many parameters may be assessed following activation [159–161]. Usually cells (in the range of ~500,000 cells/mL) in plate culture can be directly exposed to NPs added to the wells, and tests on monocyte/macrophage/DC activation are typically completed within 24 h. Oftentimes, PBMC culture is conducted in round bottom wells, which simulate a lymph node in which communication between myeloid cells and lymphocytes occurs.

Finally, NPs can also interact with other cells present in blood, such as DCs, which link with adaptive immunity. Similar principles of the MAT test can also be applied for testing NPs, but also cocultures with T-cells of self or foreign origin [153]. These types of test can mimic autoimmunity or the mixed lymphocytes reaction and are of interest for the use of NPs in vaccines and immunotherapy [162].

Experiments considering primary isolated cells offer other advantages by representing a simplified model, limiting interfering factors, which could help to spotlight NPs mechanisms of action before performing further experiments; e.g., coculture, tissue models, or even using whole-organism in vivo experiments. Moreover, these in vitro experimentations allow easier comparison between models, particularly, with human cells. In addition to the commonly known pros for in vitro assessment such as cheap cost, fewer animals used and relatively fast results, a list of the more important pros and cons for each model, with special input for in vitro assays, is presented in Figures 4 and 5, lower panel. Although they provide a simplified set up and can be used to try and understand some of the basic mechanisms, they do not represent the true exposure pathway. Additionally, large variations in the exposure time and the culture methods between different models persist. In invertebrates, the immune cells are usually easy to collect, except for isopods, and in large quantity. There are some species-specific difficulties in experimentation, such as molt cycles in isopods or seasonality with reproductive period in mussels that can impact immune measurements. Moreover, some cells are more sensitive and fragile to handle compared to others. Usually, the immune cells from invertebrates are viable for shorter times in culture, as basal parameters are quickly impacted. For humans, in addition to regulatory hurdles, donor availability is restricted for the obtaining of primary immune cells. Each donor is usually considered independently, which can reflect stronger variabilities in responses. However, from one whole blood sample many cells can be collected and offer a large range of possible assays after purification.

3.3. Whole Model Exposure Experiments

In vivo experiments allow for evaluation of the effects and mechanisms of action of NPs in organisms at different levels of biological organization (molecular, cellular, tissue level). They provide a realistic scenario of the exposure pathways as encountered under natural conditions. For controlled laboratory experiments, the mode of exposure to NPs needs to be adapted for each model; a summary is presented in Figure 6.

These tests are usually conducted in environmentally relevant mediums (soil or water), through feeding experiments or through breathing and filtering experiments for aquatic species. As the selected models are usually easy to maintain in laboratory conditions for long periods of time, requiring little space and maintenance (e.g., feeding), the exposure time (acute, semichronic and chronic exposure) can range from hours, to days and weeks.

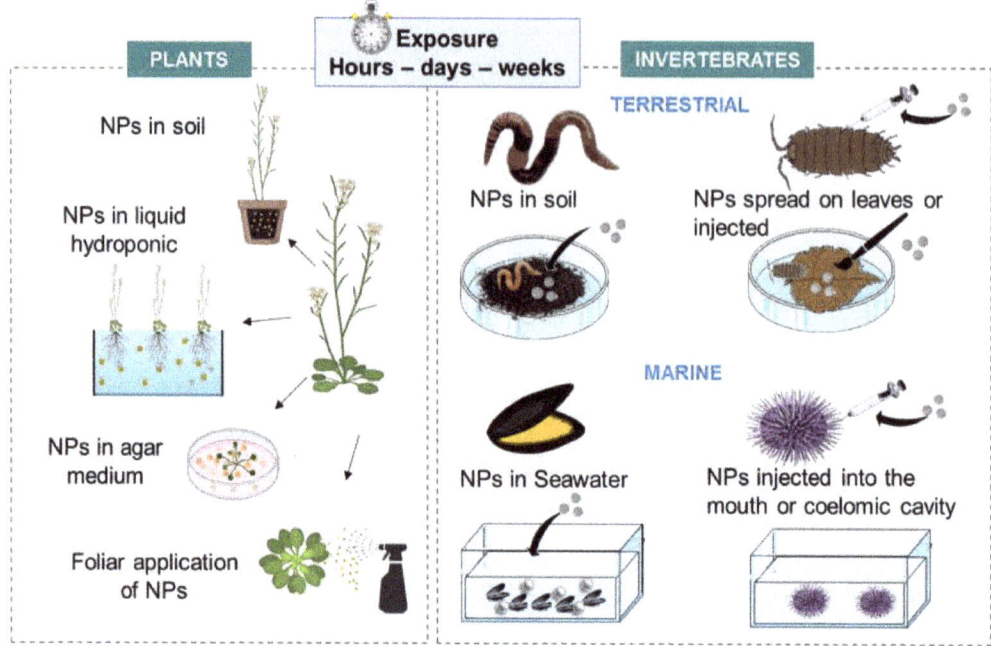

Figure 6. NP exposure approaches using the whole organism with the different exposure pathways across the selected models.

Plants can germinate and grow directly in the presence of the NP in the growth medium, i.e., soil, hydroponic nutrient solutions or agar-solidified agents, or they can be exposed at subsequent development stages. Despite the presence of cell walls, that can represent a barrier preventing NPs entering into the plant cell and cytoplasm, NPs might be absorbed through root or leaf and be potentially transported to the shoot or to other points through the phloem (vascular system) [163–166]. NPs can be also dispensed onto the plants surface by foliar spray application [167]. After entrance into the leaf tissue, NPs can diffuse into the intercellular space, the apoplast, or membranes and cause secondary effects. Moreover, temporality is important, and it is necessary to understand the course of plant growth and development, from seed germination to root elongation and shoot emergence, in relation to NP exposure [168]. The following investigations can assess the NP uptake by cells and further nanophytotoxicity, focusing on the toxicity symptoms of plants.

In vivo earthworm exposures are typically conducted in soils following well-described and standardized procedures (e.g., [27]) that can also be applied for NPs [140,169]. However, care must be taken when it comes to the mixing of NPs with soils, adjusting the parameters depending on the form (i.e., as solution dispersion or as powder) in which the NPs are supplied [170]. Furthermore, coexposures with infectious microbes are also important in order to establish whether an exposure to NPs has an effect on the ability of a host to maintain immunity [171]. A methodological approach to investigate the impact NPs have on the earthworm's ability to maintain immunity when coexposed with infectious bacteria has been recently established [140].

A major benefit of working with the terrestrial isopod, *P. scaber* is that they are able to be exposed to the NPs in a manner similar to how they would be exposed in nature. NP suspensions can be spread on leaves that *P. scaber* eat, and both the leaf and animal are then placed in a petri dish. During the experiment, feeding rate, defecation rate, and mortality can be monitored. This also allows for modelling of real-world impacts of NPs on the organism from behavioral changes, like feeding avoidance and mortality, to cellular immune responses. However, the gut of *P. scaber* is covered in a thick cuticle which is believed to stop the translocation of NPs from the gut into the hemocoel where the hemocytes are, so the immunological effects of the NPs might not be seen when ingested [172]. There is the possibility for an alternative exposure scenario, with injection experiments delivering substances directly into the animals hemocoel, allowing for the study of the direct interaction of a known concentration of NPs with the hemocytes. This ensures NP and immune cell interaction [141,173].

Mussels are suspension feeders and are able to filter large amounts of water (up to 3 L per hour) implying that, in a short period of time, they can easily uptake the NPs present in the seawater of experiment tanks. For this reason, the NPs can be directly added to the seawater and the ventilation system allows for constant movement of water within the tank. To study the first immune defense response, short term experiments (24 h to 96 h), have been shown to be sufficient to induce the activation of the immune system [142]. Moreover, the use of artificial seawater (ASW) implies the absence of organic matter or other substances that could interact with the NP suspension; together with a constant salt content and as such are reproducible for all periods of the year. The experiments are mainly conducted in the spring and summer periods where mussels are at their healthiest. During experiments, mussels are not fed and can readily survive several days without feeding [146]. This is necessary for NP experiments, as the presence of microalgae could interact with the NPs. In this context, the study relies only on the uptake of the NPs in seawater. To mimic a more realistic exposure, other studies have performed longer-period experiments to consider the interactions between food intake and the NPs, but this generally focused more on physiology and tissue changes and not strictly the immune response [148,174]. Biological uptake routes are dependent on NP properties and may occur as direct uptake in gill tissues and/or through transference from the cilia to the digestive system. Moreover, the agglomeration of particles in seawater has been shown to facilitate NP ingestion by suspension feeding bivalves, and their potential translocation from the gut to the circulatory system [175,176]. However, this internalization pathway seems to vary according to the NPs and some can be captured and excreted in pseudofaeces (mixture of mucus and undigested particles) before arriving to the stomach, resulting in lower tissue accumulation and higher depuration [177].

The existing in vivo studies utilizing sea urchins mainly focus on the immune status of the animal after exposure to NPs via the injection of the NP suspension into the mouth or directly into the coelomic cavity (through the soft peristomal membrane surrounding the mouth). Consequently, NPs injected orally partially cross the intestinal epithelium, invade the coelomic fluid and are then engulfed by phagocytes, while the remaining particles pass the digestive system and can be excreted [178]. On the other hand, NPs injected into the coelomic cavity can directly interact and be recognized by phagocytes [85,179].

In general, the in vivo passive exposure experiments consider more realistic exposure pathways (feeding, breathing) of NPs. However, for more simplistic set up and to be sure that NPs encounter immune cells, NP suspensions can be also injected into the animal. Results obtained from in vivo tests can provide a good proxy of interactions of immune cells in situ and thereby in vivo tests are crucial to resolve the issue of whether NPs pose an immune threat to living organisms. These models have been shown to be easy to maintain in the laboratory, and exposure experiments allow for the effects of NPs to be studied at different levels of the organism. For future experiments, mesocosms will help to mimic environmental scenarios before further studies in the environment.

3.4. Innate Immune Parameters of Interest

As highlighted in Figure 7, a variety of endpoints can be used to compare immune system–nanoparticle interactions between different models. This includes functional responses, which comprise the biochemical assessment of cellular and humoral responses, and molecular responses that aim to evaluate changes in the expression of immune-related genes. Because there are many methods available to quantify functional responses, here we provide a comparative overview of these methods to show which are most appropriate for the purpose of NP testing and cross-species comparisons (see Table 2).

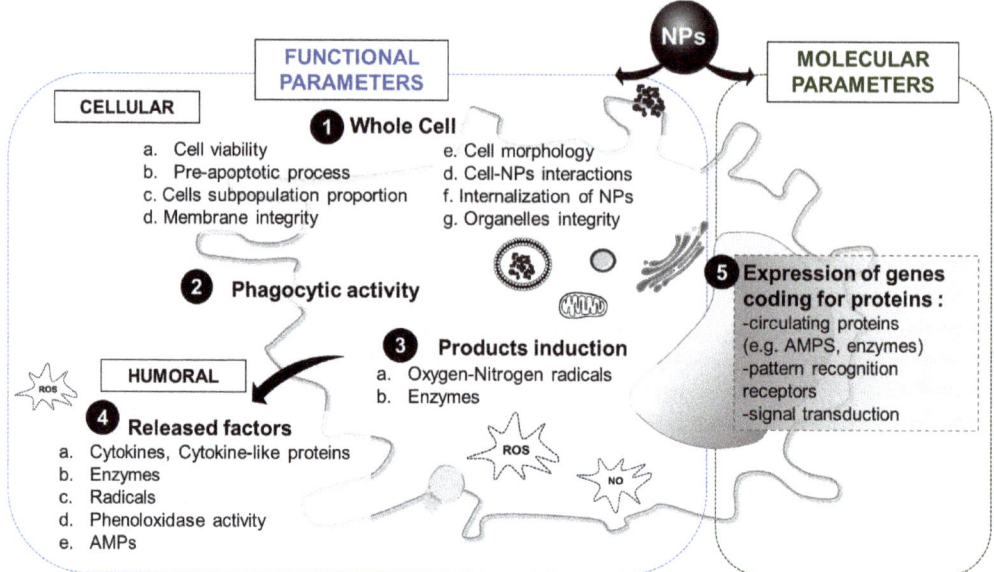

Figure 7. Summary of the different endpoints measured in immune cells after exposure to NPs.

Table 2. Overview of studies demonstrating the use of cellular and humoral parameters to characterize the immune responses of organisms.

	Plants	Earthworms	Isopods	Mussels	Sea Urchins	Human
		1. Whole cell				
Cell viability	✔	✔	✔	✔	✔	✔
LDH or ATP release	[180]	[181]				[153,182]
Fluorescent probes (FDA or PI)	[183,184]	[138,139]		[185,186]	[178]	[187]
Metabolic activity (MTT or CTB)	[188]	[181]		[189]		[153]
Blue tryptan	[190]	[191]	[173]	[192]	[193]	[194]
(Pre)-apoptosis (Annexin-V, DAPI, PI)	[195,196]	[138,139]	[141]	[197]	[121]	[198]
Cell subpopulation or polarization		[139,199]	[141,173]	[200,201]	[179]	[153,202]
NP internalization	✔	✔	✔	✔	✔	✔
TEM/SEM	[203,204]	[181,205]	[141]	[189,206–208]	[90,151,178]	[153,209]
Organelles	✔	✔	✘	✔	✔	✔
Neural red uptake/ release	[210,211]	[212]		[185,189]	[150,179]	[213]
Lysosome acidification	[214,215]			[200]	[179]	
Other organelles integrity (Trans-Golgi apparatus, Mitochondria)				[216]	[178,179]	

Table 2. Cont.

	Plants	Earthworms	Isopods	Mussels	Sea Urchins	Human
			2. Phagocytic activity			
Phagocytosis	✘	✔	✘	✔	✔	✔
Phagocytic activity (index, rate)		[139,181]		[174,216]	[150,217]	[218]
			3. Cytotoxic factors			
Oxygen and nitrogen radicals	✔	✔	✔	✔	✔	✔
ROS production	[219,220]	[139,205]		[146,208,221]	[151,222]	[223,224]
Lipid peroxidase activity	[220,225]	[138,139]		[226]		[227]
RNS (including NO) production	[228,229]	[230]	[173]	[185]		[231]
Hydrolytic enzymes	✔	✔	✘	✔	✔	✔
Lysozyme	[232]	[233]		[234]	[235,236]	[237]
Other species specific enzymes		lysenin [119]				
			4. Humoral factors			
Cytokines	✘	✘	✘	✘	✔	✔
IL, TNF, IF secretion					[151]	[94,238,239]
Melanization	✘	✔	✔	✔	✔	✘
Phenoloxidase activation		[230,240]	[44]	[83]	[241]	
			5. Gene expression			
Oxidative stress genes	✔	✔	✘	✔	✔	✘
Antioxidant defense and detoxification genes (e.g., CAT, SOD)	[242]	[140,195]		[176,200]	[243]	
Circulating protein genes	✘	✔	✘	✔	✘	✔
Signal transduction protein, enzymes, AMPs (general and species-specific)		Lysenin/Fetidin [141,170,192] CCF [181,244]		mytilin, myticin, EPp [176,200]		[231]
Receptor protein genes	✔	✔	✘	✔	✔	✔
TLR	[245]	[244]		[177]	[151,179]	[246]
LBP/BPI (LPS-binding protein/bacterial permeability-increasing protein)	[247]	[64]			[243]	

3.4.1. Whole Cell Response

Parameters looking at the whole immune cell concerns the immune cells viability, the membrane integrity, all the different types of interactions they can have with NPs, and their potential changes in morphology (Figure 7, first point). The first important cellular responses that can be used to investigate nanoparticle—immune system interactions is (immune) cell viability. Although cell death and apoptosis are part of a normal immune response, studies have shown that NPs are able to cause excessive mortality in immune cells with possible adverse effects on immunocompetence. There are several methods available that can measure cell viability (Table 2). A common method used in human cell lines is the measurement of the release of LDH or ATP through biochemical assays [153,182]. An alternative is the staining of living or dead cells using fluorescent probes (e.g., fluorescein diacetate–FDA or propidium iodide–PI) for observation using flow cytometry fluorescent microscopy. In some models, cell viability may also be studied by measuring metabolic activity through cell-permeable fluorescent reduction such as CTB or the colorimetric MTT. In some models the use of counter stain dye such as trypan blue or nigrosine [141,192] or the use of DNA-binding florescent dyes are alternative methods for assessing cell viability [150]. There are several methods available to measure the number of cells that are in the process of dying (apoptosis). Apoptosis and preapoptosis evaluation methods, which are available for several models, can be used as early markers for cell viability through the use of specific fluorescent dyes (e.g., annexin V binding, apostain, tetramethylrhodamine, ethylester perchlorate-TMRE or DAPI labelling) [139,197]. Cell viability is probably the best described immune parameter in most species (Table 2); therefore, this parameter is one of most relevant to assess in cross-species comparison. In addition to measuring the overall immune cell viability, quantifying changes in the ratios of different subpopulations of immune cells (e.g., total hemocyte counts-THC) can often give a more detailed view of the impact of NPs on immune cell viability [141,179,199,200]. In human cells, fluorescence-activated cell sorting (FACS) is a common method in which fluorescent antibody-tags can be used to determine a large range of parameters but also to discriminate sub-cell populations [153].

The subcellular effects of NP exposure can be identified via assessment of the integrity of organelles, membranes, and other cellular compartments. Lysosomal functional integrity is an evolutionarily conserved marker of stress (including NPs) and of an individuals' health status, and is commonly evaluated by measuring neural red retention or uptake [185,189,248]. Other approaches that can be used to assess the effects of NPs on organelles include methods measuring trans-golgi apparatus integrity and internal membrane polarization [178,179,200].

Another crucial step in the characterization of NP–immune system interactions is assessing whether immune cells are able to internalize NPs. The internalization of NPs has been observed for different types of NPs across the selected models and was recently reviewed in [36]. There are several techniques available to detect the internalization of NPs. These include transmission electron microscopy (TEM) which can image internalized particles and scanning electron microscopy (SEM) which helps to visualize membrane-bound particles and can give a direct image of the particles and cells following contact. They can also provide details on how the interaction occurs as well as the state of the NPs (e.g., agglomeration, aggregation, precipitation). These techniques when coupled to an EDX system (energy dispersive X-ray) can be used to perform chemical characterization of the NPs' surfaces. TEM and SEM are descriptive techniques that can provide valuable information but makes quantification difficult between models. Some research has reported the use of fluorescently labelled particles to help to measure particle uptake, although the use of such labelled particles requires additional controls to rule out any effects linked to the leakage of fluorescent dyes [249]. In general, NP internalization in human cells has been well reported but for invertebrate, similar methods often require adjustments to be made (as for example, the salt or osmotic concentrations during fixation) [90,141,153,205,206,209]. For plants, TEM can be used to verify the entry of NPs into the cells [203]. In addition, these kinds of techniques can reveal the change in cell morphologies and subcellular structures (e.g., vacuoles, phagosomes, endosomes) upon NP exposure and give hints regarding the general activation or damages that the cell has undergone [203,207].

3.4.2. Phagocytic Activity

While an immune response towards NPs could be part of normal immune functioning, overstimulation of the immune system resulting in damage or suppression leading to a compromised immune functioning may pose a threat to the organism. Such suppression of immune functioning caused by NPs could be studied via the assessment of the immune cells capacity to phagocytose and the consequent changes on index and rates (Figure 7, second point, Table 2). In earthworms, mussels, and sea urchins, phagocytosis can be evaluated by using fluorescence beads or yeast (using neutral red stained zymosan) [139,145,150,181,216,250].

3.4.3. Cytotoxic Factors

Upon contact with NPs, cells can be activated and produce cytotoxic factors inside the cells in order to help to remove internalized foreign particles (Figure 7, third point). Among them, the oxidative burst, which involves the production of several radicals from oxygen (ROS) and nitrogen (RNS) derivatives. To quantify ROS, several methods, including the use of fluorescent probes (e.g., DCF or calcein), UV-vis spectroscopy (e.g., cytochrome C reduction) or histochemical staining, can be used and many of which have been adjusted for use across the model organisms (Table 2). Moreover, lipid peroxidation can be measured as a proxy for the damages caused by oxidative stress to the membranes, even if it is more frequently analyzed in tissues than in individual cells [138,139]. As for the quantification of RNS and more commonly nitric oxide (NO), in isopods, mussels, and earthworms, NO levels in the hemolymph can be measured spectrophotometrically from hemolymph samples using Griess reagent [141,234,250].

Lysozyme is an evolutionary conserved enzyme that catalyzes the hydrolysis of peptidoglycan and plays a role in the innate immunity of many organisms including earthworms, mussels, sea urchins, and plants [67,234,251,252]. The quantification of the release of lysozyme into the extracellular medium is based on the lysis activity of *Micrococcus lysodeikticus* which can be determined spectrophotometrically. Fluorescent probes can be also used to monitor the evolution of the lysosomal compartment and acidification in the cell upon exposure to NPs [200].

3.4.4. Humoral Factors

Humoral immune responses play a crucial role in immunity by facilitating communication between immune cells and directing the extracellular destruction of foreign objects. Upon activation of the immune cells, some factors can be released into the extracellular medium (Figure 7, fourth point, Table 2). In mammals, cytokine production is a key driver of cellular immune responses [238]. Analyzing the extra- and intracellular concentration of cytokines secreted by (human) immune cells is a well-established method to test the effects and safety of NPs [253]. Many techniques have been developed to detect single or multiple cytokines and factors secreted by cells. These include classic methods such as western blot, ELISA, and bio-chemiluminescence assays, and many commercial possibilities for multiplex assays including legendplex or Ella multiplex technology [153,209,254]. Interestingly, in sea urchins, cytokine IL-6 can be detected in immune cells and secretome using western blot analysis after exposure to NPs [151].

Lysozyme and radicals can also be released by immune cells in the extracellular medium, to directly destruct foreign particles in close proximity to the cell. In addition, there are species specific released factors such as the hemolytic protein lysesin found in the coelomic fluid of earthworms.

Lastly, an important immunological parameter often analyzed in invertebrate models is the measurement of phenoloxidase (PO) activity. This enzyme, produced via the pro-PO cascade, is involved in the production of melanin [43,141]. Upon detecting a melanized pathogen or object, immune cells quickly encapsulate the material resulting in the elimination of the threat. PO activity can be assessed by monitoring the formation of a reddish-brown pigments in the hemolymph from an individual organism using spectrophotometry [44,173,240]. In bivalves, the presence of PO has been reported but its basal levels, the variation across species and especially its response to NP exposure remain poorly understood [83,255]. In the sea urchin *Strongylocentrotus nudus* coelomocytes, three proteins with PO-like activities have been identified using electrophoretic methods [241].

3.4.5. Molecular Response

Increasingly, humoral responses can be measured through genetic or omics approaches (e.g., quantitative PCR or full-transcriptome sequencing) (Table 2). A main advantage of using these approaches over biochemical ones is their high-throughput potential and increased specificity. Furthermore, genetic or omics approaches allow for the assessment of entire immunological pathways instead of focusing on specific biochemical endpoints. However, major limitations of these methods are that they require species specific primers and the availability of transcriptomes, which are currently lacking for many invertebrate species. Moreover, gene expression is highly regulated and time-dependent, so careful consideration must be given to the experimental model in terms of stimulation/exposure time, and cell collection technique.

Genes involved in different immune-related functions, such as oxidative stress response, humoral factors (e.g., AMPs), and receptor proteins, are available for some organisms and the main immune related genes known to be activated upon NP exposure are reported in Table 2.

A whole genome transcript is under development and will be available for *P. scaber*. Using this and genes previously annotated in other more commonly used crustacean species, primers specific for *P. scaber* immune-related genes can be designed (Hernadi, Mayall personal communication). Moreover, gene expression offers alternative possibilities to study several proteins involved in the immune response that biochemical tests that evaluate their activity or functionality are not feasible, such as the effects of NPs on AMP modulation. In plants, microarray-based studies are good tools to monitor the expression of candidate genes involved in the plant defense responses after interaction with NPs [204]. Additionally, an important future issue for environmental molecular biology is to establish whether an up- or downregulation of a certain gene correlates to a modification in the levels of related proteins [256]. The study of transcriptomic changes in cells, tissues, or full invertebrate organisms after exposure to NPs is now emerging but is still in its early phase. Transcriptome analysis can highlight pathways being activated but it should also be accompanied by the study of functional parameters for a fuller, deeper understanding [228,257,258]. In addition, changes in protein repertoires (proteomics approach) have shown interesting outcomes; however, studying of the combined immune response to NP exposure remains in its infancy [259–261].

4. Proposal for Future Cross-Species Evaluations and Conclusions

During the PANDORA project [35], several studies were conducted on the innate immune response of different models exposed to a large range of different NPs. Based on the outcomes of these studies, several conclusions can be made which may help to guide future (comparative) studies on nanoparticle–immune system interactions (Figure 8).

Because chemical conditions of mediums strongly affect the form and state of NPs and thereby the behavior of NPs, it is crucial to characterize the physico-chemical properties of NPs in the exposure medium as well as in their pristine form (e.g., after production). As the behavior and the interaction of NPs with immune systems are also time-dependent, experimental design will need to critically consider exposure duration as well. In vitro models can be considered as the prime focus for studying nanoparticle–immune system interactions. However, in vitro models are not available for all immune model species (e.g., isopods, plants), limiting comparative studies based on in vitro testing. In vivo experiments are crucial to study nanoparticle–immune system interactions under more realistic conditions. Studies using invertebrates, which are well-established and can be conducted on a routine basis, may serve as good alternatives to in vivo mammalian testing models such as mice or rats.

Here, exposure route and exposure concentration will need to be critically considered as these factors are likely to significantly affect immune cells and their interaction with the NPs.

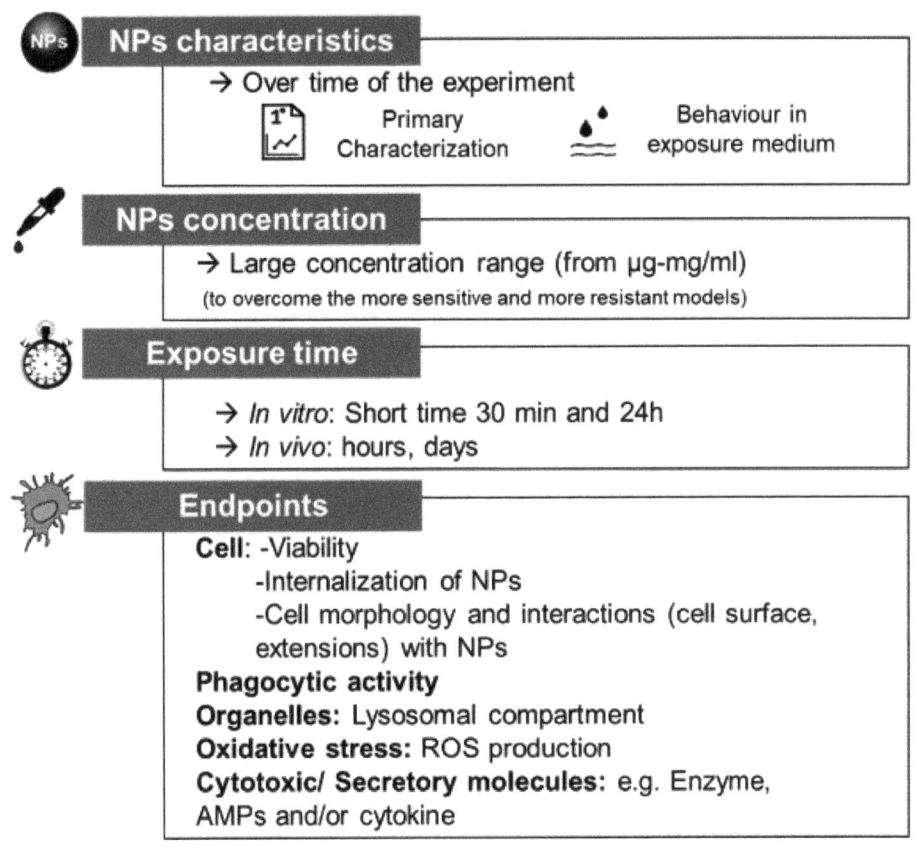

Figure 8. Proposal template for translatable NP experiments across the models of interest (plants, terrestrial and marine invertebrates, and human cells).

In this review, we provided an overview of the methods used to characterize nanoparticle immune responses in various organisms across the tree of life (Table 2). Among cellular parameters, it appears that methods to assess cell viability (including assessments of subpopulations) and NPs internalization by immune cells are well described in most organisms. Phagocytic activity is a crucial parameter to be evaluated for immune cells, however, some models lack the methods to study this parameter (e.g., isopods) or do not rely on this type of response (e.g., plants). Moreover, as methods for microscopy are universally available, measurements of the change in morphology and external interactions of NPs can be studied in most immune models.

Due to a lack of general knowledge on the composition and functioning of humoral immunity in most organisms other than mammal/human models, it remains difficult to identify the most relevant humoral parameter for cross-species evaluations. The exception being oxidative (and nitrosative) stress, for which methods are well described in most species.

Further work is needed to identify the interorganism comparability of otherwise species-specific markers, especially in invertebrates. In order to fully characterize NP-immune responses across species from the tree of life, there is a need for the identification of markers indicative for both pro- and anti-inflammatory responses, as are currently already available for human models (e.g., [253]). The development of such markers will require fundamental research on the innate immune systems of organisms other than human models. Thorough investigations in species from across the tree of life will help to understand how NPs interact with the innate immune system under different conditions and environments which may guide the future development of NPs that are immunologically safer-by-design.

Author Contributions: Conceptualization, B.J.S., C.M. and M.A.; writing—original draft preparation, C.M., B.J.S., A.A., F.B., E.F., S.H., S.M., N.I.N.P., A.P., E.S., M.A.; writing—review and editing, B.J.S., C.M., E.S., M.A.; supervision, M.A. All authors have read and agreed to the published version of the manuscript.

Funding: All authors were supported by the EU H2020 project PANDORA, grant number 671881.

Institutional Review Board Statement: Not applicable.

Informed Consent Statement: Not applicable.

Acknowledgments: The authors warmly acknowledge the project coordinator Diana Boraschi for her strong support during the whole project period, and all the PIs (L. Canesi, D. Drobne, A. Duschl, M.A. Ewart, J. Horejs-Hoeck, P. Italiani, B. Kemmerling, P. Kille, A. Pinsino, P. Procházková, V.F. Puntes, D.J. Spurgeon, C. Svendsen, C.J. Wilde) for the offered opportunity. The authors wish also to acknowledge Paola Cesaroni for her immense organizational help. Special thanks to our Project Officer Giuliana Donini for making PANDORA a successful story.

Conflicts of Interest: The authors declare no conflict of interest.

References

1. Casals, E.; Gonzalez, E.; Puntes, V.F. Reactivity of Inorganic Nanoparticles in Biological Environments: Insights into Nanotoxicity Mechanisms. *J. Phys. D Appl. Phys.* **2012**, *45*, 443001. [CrossRef]
2. Aitken, R.J.; Chaudhry, M.Q.; Boxall, A.B.A.; Hull, M. Manufacture and Use of Nanomaterials: Current Status in the UK and Global Trends. *Occup. Med.* **2006**, *56*, 300–306. [CrossRef] [PubMed]
3. Maynard, A.D.; Aitken, R.J.; Butz, T.; Colvin, V.; Donaldson, K.; Oberdorster, G.; Philbert, M.A.; Ryan, J.; Seaton, A.; Stone, V. Safe Handling of Nanotechnology. *Nature* **2006**, *444*, 267–269. [CrossRef] [PubMed]
4. Schmid, K.; Riediker, M. Use of Nanoparticles in Swiss Industry: A Targeted Survey. *Environ. Sci. Technol.* **2008**, *42*, 2253–2260. [CrossRef]
5. Bogart, L.K.; Pourroy, G.; Murphy, C.J.; Puntes, V.; Pellegrino, T.; Rosenblum, D.; Peer, D. Nanoparticles for Imaging, Sensing, and Therapeutic Intervention. *ACS Nano* **2014**, *8*, 16. [CrossRef] [PubMed]
6. Pulit-Prociak, J.; Banach, M. Silver Nanoparticles—A Material of the Future . . . ? *Open Chem.* **2016**, *14*. [CrossRef]
7. Boraschi, D. From Antigen Delivery System to Adjuvanticy: The Board Application of Nanoparticles in Vaccinology. *Vaccines* **2015**, *10*, 930–939. [CrossRef]
8. Lehner, R. Intelligent Nanomaterials for Medicine: Carrier Platforms and Targeting Strategies in the Context of Clinical Application. *Nanomedicine* **2013**, *16*, 742–757. [CrossRef]
9. Boraschi, D. Interaction of Engineered Nanomaterials with the Immune System: Health-Related Safety and Possible Benefits. *Curr. Opin. Toxicol.* **2018**, *10*, 74–83. [CrossRef]
10. Moghimi, S.M.; Hunter, A.C.; Murray, J.C. Nanomedicine: Current Status and Future Prospects. *FASEB J.* **2005**, *19*, 311–330. [CrossRef]
11. Nel, A.; Xia, T. Toxic Potential of Materials at the Nanolevel. *Science* **2006**, *311*, 622–627. [CrossRef]
12. Dobrovolskaia, M.; McNeil, S. Immunological Properties of Engineered Nanomaterials. *Nat. Nanotechnol.* **2007**, *2*, 10. [CrossRef]
13. Fadeel, B.; Garcia-Bennett, A.E. Better Safe than Sorry: Understanding the Toxicological Properties of Inorganic Nanoparticles Manufactured for Biomedical Applications. *Adv. Drug Deliv. Rev.* **2010**, *13*, 362–374. [CrossRef]
14. Jiang, Z.; Jacob, J.A.; Li, J.; Wu, X.; Wei, G.; Vimalanathan, A.; Mani, R.; Nainangu, P.; Rajadurai, U.M.; Chen, B. Influence of Diet and Dietary Nanoparticles on Gut Dysbiosis. *Microb. Pathog.* **2018**, *118*, 61–65. [CrossRef]
15. Spurgeon, D.J.; Lahive, E.; Schultz, C.L. Nanomaterial Transformations in the Environment: Effects of Changing Exposure Forms on Bioaccumulation and Toxicity. *Small* **2020**, *16*. [CrossRef]
16. Mittal, D.; Kaur, G.; Singh, P.; Yadav, K.; Ali, S.A. Nanoparticle-Based Sustainable Agriculture and Food Science: Recent Advances and Future Outlook. *Front. Nanotechnol.* **2020**, *2*, 579954. [CrossRef]
17. Bundschuh, M. Nanoparticles in the Environment: Where Do We Come from, Where Do We Go To? *Environ. Sci. Eur.* **2018**, *30*, 6. [CrossRef]

18. Graca, B.; Zgrundo, A.; Zakrzewska, D.; Rzodkiewicz, M.; Karczewski, J. Origin and Fate of Nanoparticles in Marine Water-Preliminary Results. *Chemosphere* **2018**, *206*, 359–368. [CrossRef]
19. Gottschalk, F.; Lassen, C.; Kjoelholt, J.; Christensen, F.; Nowack, B. Modeling Flows and Concentrations of Nine Engineered Nanomaterials in the Danish Environment. *Int. J. Environ. Res. Public Health* **2015**, *12*, 5581–5602. [CrossRef]
20. Rocha, T.L.; Gomes, T.; Sousa, V.S.; Mestre, N.C.; Bebianno, M.J. Ecotoxicological Impact of Engineered Nanomaterials in Bivalve Molluscs: An Overview. *Mar. Environ. Res.* **2015**, *111*, 74–88. [CrossRef]
21. Boraschi, D.; Alijagic, A.; Auguste, M.; Barbero, F.; Ferrari, E.; Hernadi, S.; Mayall, C.; Michelini, S.; Pacheco, N.I.N.; Prinelli, A.; et al. Addressing Nanomaterial Immunosafety by Evaluating Innate Immunity across Living Species. *Small* **2020**, *16*. [CrossRef] [PubMed]
22. Swartzwelter, B.J.; Fux, A.C.; Johnson, L.; Swart, E.; Hofer, S.; Hofstätter, N.; Geppert, M.; Italiani, P.; Boraschi, D.; Duschl, A.; et al. The Impact of Nanoparticles on Innate Immune Activation by Live Bacteria. *Int. J. Mol. Sci.* **2020**, *23*, 9695. [CrossRef] [PubMed]
23. Boraschi, D.; Duschl, A. *Nanoparticles and the Immune System: Safety and Effects*; Elsevier/AP: Amsterdam, The Netherlands, 2014; ISBN 978-0-12-408005-0.
24. Mitchell-Olds, T. Arabidopsis Thaliana and Its Wild Relatives: A Model System for Ecology and Evolution. *Trends Ecol. Evol.* **2001**, *16*. [CrossRef]
25. Bevan, M.; Walsh, S. The Arabidopsis Genome: A Foundation for Plant Research. *Genome Res.* **2005**, *15*, 1632–1642. [CrossRef] [PubMed]
26. The Arabidopsis Genome Iniative. Analysis of the Genome Sequence of the Flowering Plant Arabidopsis Thaliana. *Nature* **2000**, *408*, 796–815. [CrossRef]
27. OECD. *Test No 222. Earthworm Reproduction Test (Eisenia Fetida/Eisenia Andrei)*; OECD: Paris, France, 2016.
28. Edwards, C.A.; Bohlen, P.J. *Biology and Ecology of Earthworms*; Chapman&Hall: London, UK, 1996.
29. Van Gestel, C.A.M.; Loureiro, S.; Zidar, P. Terrestrial Isopods as Model Organisms in Soil Ecotoxicology: A Review. *Zookeys* **2018**, *801*, 127–162. [CrossRef]
30. Malev, O. Effects of CeO$_2$ Nanoparticles on Terrestrial Isopod Porcellio Scaber: Comparison of CeO$_2$ Biological Potential with Other Nanoparticles. *Arch. Environ. Contam. Toxicol.* **2017**, *72*, 303–311. [CrossRef]
31. Novak, S.; Romih, T.; Dra, B.; Ferraris, P.; Sorieul, S.; Zieba, M.; Sebastian, V.; Arruebo, M.; Ho, S.B. The in Vivo Effects of Silver Nanoparticles on Terrestrial Isopods, Porcellio Scaber, Depend on a Dynamic Interplay between Shape, Size and Nanoparticle Dissolution Properties. *Analyst* **2019**, *2*. [CrossRef]
32. Beyer, J.; Green, N.W.; Brooks, S.; Allan, I.J.; Ruus, A.; Gomes, T.; Bråte, I.L.N.; Schøyen, M. Blue Mussels (*Mytilus Edulis* spp.) as Sentinel Organisms in Coastal Pollution Monitoring: A Review. *Mar. Environ. Res.* **2017**, *130*, 338–365. [CrossRef]
33. Fernández Robledo, J.A.; Yadavalli, R.; Allam, B.; Pales Espinosa, E.; Gerdol, M.; Greco, S.; Stevick, R.J.; Gómez-Chiarri, M.; Zhang, Y.; Heil, C.A.; et al. From the Raw Bar to the Bench: Bivalves as Models for Human Health. *Dev. Comp. Immunol.* **2019**, *92*, 260–282. [CrossRef]
34. Chou, H.-Y.; Lun, C.M.; Smith, L.C. SpTransformer Proteins from the Purple Sea Urchin Opsonize Bacteria, Augment Phagocytosis, and Retard Bacterial Growth. *PLoS ONE* **2018**, *13*, e0196890. [CrossRef]
35. Pandora-H2020. Available online: https://www.Pandora-H2020.Eu/ (accessed on 16 February 2021).
36. Pinsino, A.; Bastús, N.G.; Busquets-Fité, M.; Canesi, L.; Cesaroni, P.; Drobne, D.; Duschl, A.; Ewart, M.-A.; Gispert, I.; Horejs-Hoeck, J.; et al. Probing the Immune Responses to Nanoparticles across Environmental Species. A Perspective of the EU Horizon 2020 Project PANDORA. *Environ. Sci. Nano* **2020**, *7*, 3216–3232. [CrossRef]
37. Soderhall, K. *Invertebrate Immunity*. *Advances in Experimental Medicine and Biology*; Landes Bioscience and Springer Science+Business Media, LLC: New York, NY, USA, 2010; ISBN 978-1-4419-8058-8.
38. Canesi, L.; Procházková, P. The Invertebrate Immune System as a Model for Investigating the Environmental Impact of Nanoparticles. In *Nanoparticles and the Immune System Safety and Effects*; Boraschi, D., Duschl, A., Eds.; Academic Press: Cambridge, MA, USA, 2014; pp. 91–112.
39. Jones, J.D.G.; Dangl, J.L. The Plant Immune System. *Nature* **2006**, *444*, 323–329. [CrossRef]
40. Takeuchi, O.; Akira, S. Pattern Recognition Receptors and Inflammation. *Cell* **2010**, *140*, 805–820. [CrossRef]
41. Sarma, J.V.; Ward, P.E. The Complement System. *Cell Tissue Res.* **2011**, *343*, 227–235. [CrossRef]
42. Bilej, M.; Baetselier, P.D.; Dijck, E.V.; Stijlemans, B.; Colige, A.; Beschin, A. Distinct Carbohydrate Recognition Domains of an Invertebrate Defense Molecule Recognize Gram-Negative and Gram-Positive Bacteria. *J. Biol. Chem.* **2001**, *276*, 45840–45847. [CrossRef]
43. Soderhall, K.; Cerenius, L. Role of the Prophenoloxidase-Activating System in Invertebrate Immunity. *Curr. Opin. Immunol.* **1998**, *10*, 23–28. [CrossRef]
44. Jaenicke, E.; Fraune, S.; May, S.; Irmak, P.; Augustin, R.; Meesters, C.; Decker, H.; Zimmer, M. Is Activated Hemocyanin Instead of Phenoloxidase Involved in Immune Response in Woodlice? *Dev. Comp. Immunol.* **2009**, *33*, 1055–1063. [CrossRef]
45. Motion, G.B.; Huitema, E. Nuclear Processes Associated with Plant Immunity and Pathogen Susceptibility. *Brief Funct. Genom.* **2015**, *14*, 243–252. [CrossRef]
46. Coll, N.; Epple, P.; Dangl, J. Programmed Cell Death in the Plant Immune System. *Cell Death Differ.* **2011**, *18*, 1247–1256. [CrossRef]
47. Newman, M.-A. MAMP (Microbe-Associated Molecular Pattern) Triggered Immunity in Plants. *Front. Plant Sci.* **2013**, *4*, 139. [CrossRef] [PubMed]

48. Miescher-Institut, F.; Box, P.O. FLS2: An LRR Receptor–like Kinase Involved in the Perception of the Bacterial Elicitor Flagellin in Arabidopsis. *Mol. Cell* **2000**, *5*, 1003–1011.
49. Boutrot, F.; Zipfel, C. Function, Discovery, and Exploitation of Plant Pattern Recognition Receptors for Broad-Spectrum Disease Resistance. *Annu. Rev. Phytopathol.* **2017**, *55*, 257–286. [CrossRef] [PubMed]
50. Dangl, J.L.; Horvath, D.M.; Staskawicz, B.J. Pivoting the Plant Immune System from Dissection to Deployment. *Science* **2013**, *14*. [CrossRef] [PubMed]
51. Gust, A.A.; Pruitt, R.; Nürnberger, T. Sensing Danger: Key to Activating Plant Immunity. *Trends Plant Sci.* **2017**, *22*, 779–791. [CrossRef] [PubMed]
52. Sukarta, O.C.A. Structure-Informed Insights for NLR Functioning in Plant Immunity. *Semin. Cell Dev. Biol.* **2016**, *56*, 134–149. [CrossRef]
53. Thomma, B.P.H.J.; Nürnberger, T.; Joosten, M.H.A.J. Of PAMPs and Effectors: The Blurred PTI-ETI Dichotomy. *Plant. Cell* **2011**, *23*, 4–15. [CrossRef]
54. Tao, Y.; Xie, Z.; Chen, W.; Glazebrook, J.; Chang, H.-S.; Han, B.; Zhu, T.; Zou, G.; Katagiri, F. Quantitative Nature of Arabidopsis Responses during Compatible and Incompatible Interactions with the Bacterial Pathogen Pseudomonas Syringae. *Plant Cell* **2003**, *15*, 317–330. [CrossRef]
55. Bigeard, J. Signaling Mechanisms in Pattern-Triggered Immunity (PTI). *Mol. Plant* **2015**, *8*, 521–539. [CrossRef]
56. Chagas, F.O.; Pessotti, R.D.C.; Caraballo-Rodrıguez, A.M.; Pupo, M.T. Chemical Signaling Involved in Plant–Microbe Interactions. *Chem. Soc. Rev.* **2018**, *47*, 1652–1704. [CrossRef]
57. Halim, V.A.; Vess, A.; Scheel, D.; Rosahl, S. The Role of Salicylic Acid and Jasmonic Acid in Pathogen Defence. *Plant Biol.* **2006**, *8*, 307–313. [CrossRef]
58. Kachroo, P.; Kachroo, A. The Roles of Salicylic Acid and Jasmonic Acid in Plant Immunity. In *Molecular Plant Immunity*; Sessa, G., Ed.; Wiley-Blackwell: Oxford, UK, 2012; pp. 55–79, ISBN 978-1-118-48143-1.
59. Bilej, M.; Procházková, P.; Silerova, M.; Joskova, R. Earthworm immunity. In *Invertebrate Immunity*; Landes Bioscience and Springer Science: New York, NY, USA, 2010; pp. 66–79.
60. Cooper, E.L.; Kauschke, E.; Cossarizza, A. Digging for Innate Immunity since Darwin and Metchnikoff. *BioEssays* **2002**, *24*, 319–333. [CrossRef]
61. Molnár, L. Cold-Stress Induced Formation of Calcium and Phosphorous Rich Chloragocyte Granules (Chloragosomes) in the Earthworm Eisenia Fetida. *Comp. Biochem. Physiol.* **2012**, *11*, 199–209. [CrossRef]
62. Beschin, A.; Bilej, M.; Hanssens, F.; Raymakers, J.; Dyck, E.V.; Revets, H.; Brys, L.; Gomez, J.; Baetselier, P.D.; Timmermans, M. Identification and Cloning of a Glucan- and Lipopolysaccharide- Binding Protein from Eisenia Foetida Earthworm Involved in the Activation of Prophenoloxidase Cascade. *J. Biol. Chem.* **1998**, *273*, 24948–24954. [CrossRef]
63. Škanta, F.; Roubalová, R.; Dvořák, J.; Procházková, P.; Bilej, M. Molecular Cloning and Expression of TLR in the Eisenia Andrei Earthworm. *Dev. Comp. Immunol.* **2013**, *41*, 694–702. [CrossRef]
64. Škanta, F. LBP/BPI Homologue in Eisenia Andrei Earthworms. *Dev. Comp. Immunol.* **2016**, *54*, 1–6. [CrossRef]
65. Silerova, M.; Prochazkova, P.; Joskova, R.; Josens, G.; Beschin, A.; De Baetselier, P.; Bilej, M. Comparative Study of the CCF-like Pattern Recognition Protein in Different Lumbricid Species. *Dev. Comp. Immunol.* **2006**, *30*, 765–771. [CrossRef]
66. Cotuk, A.; Dales, R.P. Lyzomyme Activity in the Coelomic Fluid and Coelomocytes of the Earthworm Eisenia Foetida Sav. in Relation to Bacterial Infection. *Comp. Biochem. Physiol.* **1984**, *78A*, 469–474. [CrossRef]
67. Joskova, R.; Šilerová, M. Identification and Cloning of an Invertebrate-Type Lysozyme from Eisenia Andrei. *Dev. Comp. Immunol.* **2009**, *33*, 932–938. [CrossRef]
68. Lassegues, M.; Milochau', A.; Doignon, F.; Pasquier, L.D.; Valembois, P. Sequence and Expression of an Eisenia-Fetida-Derived CDNA Clone That Encodes the 40-KDa Fetidin Antibacterial Protein. *JBIC J. Biol. Inorg. Chem.* **1997**, *246*, 756–762.
69. Sekizawa, Y.; Hagiwara, K.; Nakajima, T.; Kobayashi, H. A Novel Protein, Lysenin, That Causes Contraction of the Isolated Rat Aorta: Its Purification from the Coelomic Fluid of the Earthworm Eisenia Foetida. *Biomed. Res.* **1996**, *17*, 197–203. [CrossRef]
70. Chevalier, F.; Herbinière-Gaboreau, J.; Bertaux, J.; Raimond, M.; Morel, F.; Bouchon, D.; Grève, P.; Braquart-Varnier, C. The Immune Cellular Effectors of Terrestrial Isopod Armadillidium Vulgare: Meeting with Their Invaders, Wolbachia. *PLoS ONE* **2011**, *6*, e18531. [CrossRef] [PubMed]
71. Kostanjšek, R. Pathogenesis, Tissue Distribution and Host Response to Rhabdochlamydia Porcellionis Infection in Rough Woodlouse Porcellio Scaber. *J. Invertebr. Pathol.* **2015**, *125*, 56–67. [CrossRef]
72. Liu, H. Phenoloxidase Is an Important Component of the Defense against Aeromonas Hydrophila Infection in a Crustacean, Pacifastacus Leniusculus. *J. Biol. Chem.* **2007**, *282*, 33593–33598. [CrossRef] [PubMed]
73. Zhou, Y. Ginger Extract Extends the Lifespan of Drosophila Melanogaster through Antioxidation and Ameliorating Metabolic Dysfunction. *J. Funct. Foods* **2018**, *49*, 295–305. [CrossRef]
74. Jiravanichpaisal, P.; Lee, B.L.; Söderhäll, K. Cell-Mediated Immunity in Arthropods: Hematopoiesis, Coagulation, Melanization and Opsonization. *Immunobiology* **2006**, *211*, 213–236. [CrossRef] [PubMed]
75. Yeh, F.-C.; Wu, S.-H.; Lai, C.-Y.; Lee, C.-Y. Demonstration of Nitric Oxide Synthase Activity in Crustacean Hemocytes and Anti-Microbial Activity of Hemocyte-Derived Nitric Oxide. *Comp. Biochem. Physiol. Part B Biochem. Mol. Biol.* **2006**, *144*, 11–17. [CrossRef]
76. Rosa, R.; Barracco, M. Antimicrobial Peptides in Crustaceans. *Invert. Surviv. J.* **2010**, *7*, 262–284.

77. Chevalier, F.; Herbinière-Gaboreau, J.; Charif, D.; Mitta, G.; Gavory, F.; Wincker, P.; Grève, P.; Braquart-Varnier, C.; Bouchon, D. Feminizing Wolbachia: A Transcriptomics Approach with Insights on the Immune Response Genes in Armadillidium Vulgare. *BMC Microbiol.* **2012**, *12*, S1. [CrossRef]
78. Canesi, L.; Pruzzo, C. Specificity of Innate Immunity in bivalves: A Lesson From Bacteria. In *Lessons in Immunity: From Single-Cell Organisms to Mammals*; Ballarin, L., Cammarata, M., Eds.; Academic Press: Cambridge, MA, USA, 2016; pp. 79–92.
79. Gerdol., M.; Gomez-Chiari, M.; Castillo, M.G.; Figueras, A.; Fiorito, G.; Moreira, R.; Novoa, B.; Pallavicini, A.; Ponte, G.; Roumbedakis, K.; et al. Immunity in Molluscs: Recognition and Effector Mechanisms, with a Focus on Bivalvia. In *Advances in Comparative Immunology*; Cooper, E., Ed.; Springer: Berlin/Heidelberg, Germany, 2018; pp. 225–342.
80. Pezzati, E.; Canesi, L.; Damonte, G.; Salis, A.; Marsano, F.; Grande, C.; Vezzulli, L.; Pruzzo, C. Susceptibility of *V Ibrio Aestuarianu* s 01/032 to the Antibacterial Activity of *M Ytilus* Haemolymph: Identification of a Serum Opsonin Involved in Mannose-Sensitive Interactions: *Vibrio Aestuarianus* and Bivalve Haemocytes. *Environ. Microbiol.* **2015**, *17*, 4271–4279. [CrossRef]
81. Song, L.; Wang, L.; Qiu, L.; Zhang, H. Bivalve immunity. In *Invertebrate Immunity*; Landes Bioscience and Springer Science: New York, NY, USA, 2010.
82. Allam, B.; Raftos, D. Immune Responses to Infectious Diseases in Bivalves. *J. Invertebr. Pathol.* **2015**, *131*, 121–136. [CrossRef]
83. Luna-Acosta, A.; Breitwieser, M.; Renault, T.; Thomas-Guyon, H. Recent Findings on Phenoloxidases in Bivalves. *Mar. Pollut. Bull.* **2017**, *122*, 5–16. [CrossRef]
84. Pinsino, A. Sea Urchin Immune Cells as Sentinels of Environmental Stress. *Dev. Comp. Immunol.* **2015**, *49*, 198–205. [CrossRef]
85. Smith, L.C.; Arizza, V.; Hudgell, M.A.B.; Barone, G.; Bodnar, A.G.; Buckley, K.M.; Cunsolo, V.; Dheilly, N.M.; Franchi, N.; Fugmann, S.D.; et al. Echinodermata: The complex immune system in echinoderms. In *Advances in Comparative Immunology*; Cooper, E.L., Ed.; Springer International Publishing AG: New York, NY, USA, 2018; pp. 409–501.
86. Sea Urchin Genome Sequencing Consortium. The Genome of the Sea Urchin Strongylocentrotus Purpuratus. *Science* **2006**, *10*, 941–952. [CrossRef]
87. Rast, J.P.; Smith, L.C.; Loza-Coll, M.; Hibino, T.; Litman, G.W. Genomic Insights into the Immune System of the Sea Urchin. *Science* **2006**, *314*, 952–956. [CrossRef]
88. Echinoderm Antimicrobial peptides: The ancient arms of the Deuterostome inna immune system. In *Lessons in Immunity: From Single Cell Organisms to Mammals*; Academic Press: Cambridge, MA, USA; Elsevier Inc.: Amsterdam, The Netherlands, 2016; pp. 145–153.
89. Schillaci, D.; Arizza, V.; Parrinello, N.; Di Stefano, V.; Fanara, S.; Muccilli, V.; Cunsolo, V.; Haagensen, J.J.A.; Molin, S. Antimicrobial and Antistaphylococcal Biofilm Activity from the Sea Urchin Paracentrotus Lividus: Antimicrobial and Antistaphylococcal Biofilm Activity. *J. Appl. Microbiol.* **2010**, *108*, 17–24. [CrossRef]
90. Alijagic, A. Gold Nanoparticles Coated with Polyvinylpyrrolidone and Sea Urchin Extracellular Molecules Induce Transient Immune Activation. *J. Hazard. Mater.* **2021**, *402*, 123793. [CrossRef]
91. Liu, M.-C.; Liao, W.-Y.; Buckley, K.M.; Yang, S.Y.; Rast, J.P.; Fugmann, S.D. AID/APOBEC-like Cytidine Deaminases Are Ancient Innate Immune Mediators in Invertebrates. *Nat. Commun.* **2018**, *9*, 1948. [CrossRef]
92. Chernecky, C.C.; Berger, B.J. *Laboratory Tests and Diagnostic Procedures-E-Book*; Elsevier Health Science: St. Louis, MO, USA, 2012.
93. Tsou, C.-L.; Peters, W.; Si, Y.; Slaymaker, S.; Aslanian, A.M.; Weisberg, S.P.; Mack, M.; Charo, I.F. Critical Roles for CCR2 and MCP-3 in Monocyte Mobilization from Bone Marrow and Recruitment to Inflammatory Sites. *J. Clin. Investig.* **2007**, *117*, 902–909. [CrossRef]
94. Italiani, P. From Monocytes to M1/M2 Macrophages: Phenotypical vs. Functional Differentiation. *Front. Immunol.* **2014**, *5*, 514. [CrossRef]
95. Bain, C.C.; Bravo-Blas, A.; Scott, C.L.; Perdiguero, E.G.; Geissmann, F.; Henri, S.; Malissen, B.; Osborne, L.C.; Mowat, A.M. Constant Replenishment from Circulating Monocytes Maintains the Macrophage Pool in Adult Intestine. *Nat. Immunol.* **2014**, *15*, 929–937. [CrossRef] [PubMed]
96. Mills, C.D.; Kincaid, K.; Alt, J.M.; Heilman, M.J.; Hill, A.M. M-1/M-2 Macrophages and the Th1/Th2 Paradigm. *J. Immunol.* **2000**, *164*, 6166–6173. [CrossRef] [PubMed]
97. Mosser, D.M.; Edwards, J.P. Exploring the Full Spectrum of Macrophage Activation. *Nat. Rev. Immunol.* **2008**, *8*, 958–969. [CrossRef] [PubMed]
98. Hoppstädter, J.; Seif, M.; Dembek, A.; Cavelius, C.; Huwer, H.; Kraegeloh, A.; Kiemer, A.K. M2 Polarization Enhances Silica Nanoparticle Uptake by Macrophages. *Front. Pharmacol.* **2015**, *6*. [CrossRef]
99. Medzhitov, R.; Preston-Hurlburt, P.; Janewayr, C.A. A Human Homologue of the Drosophila Toll Protein Signals Activation of Adaptive Immunity. *Nat. Cell Biol.* **1997**, *388*, 4. [CrossRef]
100. Diebold, S.S.; Kaisho, T.; Hemmi, H.; Akira, S. Innate Antiviral Responses by Means of TLR7-Mediated Recognition of Single-Stranded RNA. *Science* **2004**, *303*, 4. [CrossRef]
101. Peiser, L.; Mukhopadhyay, S.; Gordon, S. Scavenger Receptors in Innate Immunity. *Curr. Opin. Immunol.* **2002**, *14*, 123–128. [CrossRef]
102. Brown, G.D.; Taylor, P.R.; Reid, D.M.; Willment, J.A.; Williams, D.L.; Martinez-Pomares, L.; Wong, S.Y.C.; Gordon, S. Dectin-1 Is A Major β-Glucan Receptor On Macrophages. *J. Exp. Med.* **2002**, *196*, 407–412. [CrossRef]
103. Davis, B.K.; Wen, H.; Ting, J.P.-Y. The Inflammasome NLRs in Immunity, Inflammation, and Associated Diseases. *Annu. Rev. Immunol.* **2011**, *29*, 707–735. [CrossRef]

104. Kato, H.; Takeuchi, O.; Sato, S.; Yoneyama, M.; Yamamoto, M.; Matsui, K.; Uematsu, S.; Jung, A.; Kawai, T.; Ishii, K.J.; et al. Differential Roles of MDA5 and RIG-I Helicases in the Recognition of RNA Viruses. *Nat. Cell Biol.* **2006**, *441*, 101–105. [CrossRef]
105. Martinon, F. NLRs Join TLRs as Innate Sensors of Pathogens. *Trends Immunol.* **2005**, *26*, 447–454. [CrossRef]
106. Connor, E.E.; Mwamuka, J.; Gole, A.; Murphy, C.J.; Wyatt, M.D. Gold Nanoparticles Are Taken Up by Human Cells but Do Not Cause Acute Cytotoxicity. *Small* **2005**, *1*, 325–327. [CrossRef]
107. Barbero, F.; Moriones, O.H.; Bastús, N.G.; Puntes, V. Dynamic Equilibrium in the Cetyltrimethylammonium Bromide–Au Nanoparticle Bilayer, and the Consequent Impact on the Formation of the Nanoparticle Protein Corona. *Bioconjugate Chem.* **2019**, *30*, 2917–2930. [CrossRef]
108. Li, Y.; Boraschi, D. Endotoxin Contamination: A Key Element in the Interpretation of Nanosafety Studies. *Nanomedicine* **2016**, *11*, 269–287. [CrossRef]
109. Treuel, L.; Docter, D.; Maskos, M.; Stauber, R.H. Protein Corona-from Molecular Adsorption to Physiological Complexity. *Beilstein J. Nanotechnol.* **2015**, *6*, 857–873. [CrossRef]
110. Fleischer, C.C.; Payne, C.K. Nanoparticle–Cell Interactions: Molecular Structure of the Protein Corona and Cellular Outcomes. *Acc. Chem. Res.* **2014**, *47*, 2651–2659. [CrossRef]
111. Lundqvist, M.; Stigler, J.; Elia, G.; Lynch, I.; Cedervall, T.; Dawson, K.A. Nanoparticle Size and Surface Properties Determine the Protein Corona with Possible Implications for Biological Impacts. *Proc. Natl. Acad. Sci. USA* **2008**, *105*, 14265–14270. [CrossRef]
112. Casals, E.; Pfaller, T.; Duschl, A.; Oostingh, G.J.; Puntes, V. Time Evolution of the Nanoparticle Protein Corona. *ACS Nano* **2010**, *4*, 3623–3632. [CrossRef]
113. Monopoli, M.P.; Walczyk, D.; Campbell, A.; Elia, G.; Lynch, I.; Baldelli Bombelli, F.; Dawson, K.A. Physical−Chemical Aspects of Protein Corona: Relevance to in Vitro and in Vivo Biological Impacts of Nanoparticles. *J. Am. Chem. Soc.* **2011**, *133*, 2525–2534. [CrossRef]
114. Tenzer, S.; Docter, D.; Kuharev, J.; Musyanovych, A.; Fetz, V.; Hecht, R.; Schlenk, F.; Fischer, D.; Kiouptsi, K.; Reinhardt, C.; et al. Rapid Formation of Plasma Protein Corona Critically Affects Nanoparticle Pathophysiology. *Nat. Nanotech.* **2013**, *8*, 772–781. [CrossRef]
115. Silvio, D.D. Effect of Protein Corona Magnetite Nanoparticles Derived from Bread in Vitro Digestion on Caco-2 Cells Morphology and Uptake. *Int. J. Biochem.* **2016**, *75*, 212–222. [CrossRef] [PubMed]
116. Piella, J.; Bastús, N.G.; Puntes, V. Size-Dependent Protein–Nanoparticle Interactions in Citrate-Stabilized Gold Nanoparticles: The Emergence of the Protein Corona. *Bioconjugate Chem.* **2017**, *28*, 88–97. [CrossRef] [PubMed]
117. Barbero, F.; Russo, L.; Vitali, M.; Piella, J.; Salvo, I.; Borrajo, M.L.; Busquets-Fité, M.; Grandori, R.; Bastús, N.G.; Casals, E.; et al. Formation of the Protein Corona: The Interface between Nanoparticles and the Immune System. *Semin. Immunol.* **2017**, *34*, 52–60. [CrossRef] [PubMed]
118. Saha, K.; Rahimi, M.; Yazdani, M.; Kim, S.T.; Moyano, D.F.; Hou, S.; Das, R.; Mout, R.; Rezaee, F.; Mahmoudi, M.; et al. Regulation of Macrophage Recognition through the Interplay of Nanoparticle Surface Functionality and Protein Corona. *ACS Nano* **2016**, *10*, 4421–4430. [CrossRef] [PubMed]
119. Hayashi, Y.; Miclaus, T.; Scavenius, C.; Kwiatkowska, K.; Sobota, A. Species Differences Take Shape at Nanoparticles: Protein Corona Made of the Native Repertoire Assists Cellular Interaction. *Environ. Sci. Technol.* **2013**, *47*, 14367–14375. [CrossRef]
120. Canesi, L.; Balbi, T.; Fabbri, R.; Salis, A.; Damonte, G.; Volland, M.; Blasco, J. Biomolecular Coronas in Invertebrate Species: Implications in the Environmental Impact of Nanoparticles. *NanoImpact* **2017**, *8*, 89–98. [CrossRef]
121. Marques-Santos, L.F.; Grassi, G.; Bergami, E.; Faleri, C.; Balbi, T.; Salis, A.; Damonte, G.; Canesi, L.; Corsi, I. Cationic Polystyrene Nanoparticle and the Sea Urchin Immune System: Biocorona Formation, Cell Toxicity, and Multixenobiotic Resistance Phenotype. *Nanotoxicology* **2018**, *12*, 847–867. [CrossRef]
122. Grassi, G.; Landi, C.; Della Torre, C.; Bergami, E.; Bini, L.; Corsi, I. Proteomic Profile of the Hard Corona of Charged Polystyrene Nanoparticles Exposed to Sea Urchin *Paracentrotus Lividus* Coelomic Fluid Highlights Potential Drivers of Toxicity. *Environ. Sci. Nano* **2019**, *6*, 2937–2947. [CrossRef]
123. Mueller, N.C.; Nowack, B. Exposure Modeling of Engineered Nanoparticles in the Environment. *Environ. Sci. Technol.* **2008**, *42*, 4447–4453. [CrossRef]
124. Nowack, B. Nanosilver Revisited Downstream. *Science* **2010**, *330*, 1054–1055. [CrossRef]
125. Nowack, B.; Krug, H.F.; Height, M. 120 Years of Nanosilver History: Implications for Policy Makers. *Policy Anal.* **2011**, *45*, 1177–1183.
126. Dale, A.L.; Casman, E.A.; Lowry, G.V.; Lead, J.R.; Viparelli, E.; Baalousha, M. Modeling Nanomaterial Environmental Fate in Aquatic Systems. *Environ. Sci. Technol.* **2015**, *49*, 2587–2593. [CrossRef]
127. Nasser, F.; Constantinou, J.; Lynch, I. Nanomaterials in the Environment Acquire an "Eco-Corona" Impacting Their Toxicity to *Daphnia Magna*—A Call for Updating Toxicity Testing Policies. *Proteomics* **2020**, *20*, 1800412. [CrossRef]
128. Saavedra, J.; Stoll, S.; Slaveykova, V.I. Influence of Nanoplastic Surface Charge on Eco-Corona Formation, Aggregation and Toxicity to Freshwater Zooplankton. *Environ. Pollut.* **2019**, *252*, 715–722. [CrossRef]
129. Barbero, F.; Mayall, C.; Drobne, D.; Saiz-Poseu, J.; Bastús, N.G.; Puntes, V. Formation and Evolution of the Nanoparticle Environmental Corona: The Case of Au and Humic Acid. *Sci. Total Environ.* **2021**, *768*, 144890. [CrossRef]
130. Batley, G.E.; Kirby, J.K.; Mclaughlin, M.J. Fate and Risks of Nanomaterials in Aquatic and Terrestrial Environments. *Accounts Chem. Res.* **2013**, *46*, 854–862. [CrossRef]

131. Nowack, B.; Rose, J. Potential Scenarios for Nanomaterial Release and Subsequent Alteration in the Environment. *Environ. Toxicol. Chem.* **2011**, *31*, 50–59. [CrossRef]
132. Peijnenburg, W.J.G.M.; Baalousha, M.; Chen, J.; Chaudry, Q.; Von der kammer, F.; Kuhlbusch, T.A.J.; Lead, J.; Nickel, C.; Quik, J.T.K.; Renker, M.; et al. A Review of the Properties and Processes Determining the Fate of Engineered Nanomaterials in the Aquatic Environment. *Crit. Rev. Environ. Sci. Technol.* **2015**, *45*, 2084–2134. [CrossRef]
133. Svendsen, C.; Spurgeon, D.J.; Hankard, P.K.; Weeks, J.M. A Review of Lysosomal Membrane Stability Measured by Neutral Red Retention: Is It a Workable Earthworm Biomarker? *Ecotoxicol. Environ. Saf.* **2004**, *57*, 20–29. [CrossRef]
134. Eyambe, G.S.; Goven, A.J.; Fitzpatrick, L.C.; Venables, B.J.; Cooper, E.L. A Non-Invasive Technique for Sequential Collection of Earthworm (*Lumbricus Terrestris*) Leukocytes during Subchronic Immunotoxicity Studies. *Lab. Anim.* **1991**, *25*, 61–67. [CrossRef]
135. Garcia-Velasco, N. Selection of an Optimal Culture Medium and the Most Responsive Viability Assay to Assess AgNPs Toxicity with Primary Cultures of Eisenia Fetida Coelomocytes. *Ecotoxicol. Environ. Saf.* **2019**, *183*, 109545. [CrossRef] [PubMed]
136. Yang, Y.; Xiao, Y.; Li, M.; Ji, F.; Hu, C.; Cui, Y. Evaluation of Complex Toxicity of Canbon Nanotubes and Sodium Pentachlorophenol Based on Earthworm Coelomocytes Test. *PLoS ONE* **2017**, *12*, e0170092. [CrossRef] [PubMed]
137. Hayashi, Y. Time-Course Profiling of Molecular Stress Responses to Silver Nanoparticles in the Earthworm Eisenia Fetida. *Ecotoxicol. Environ. Saf.* **2013**, *98*, 219–226. [CrossRef] [PubMed]
138. Semerad, J.; Pacheco, N.I.N.; Grasserova, A.; Prochazkova, P.; Pivokonsky, M.; Pivokonska, L.; Cajthaml, T. In Vitro Study of the Toxicity Mechanisms of Nanoscale Zero-Valent Iron (NZVI) and Released Iron Ions Using Earthworm Cells. *Nanomaterials* **2020**, *10*, 2189. [CrossRef]
139. Pacheco, N.I.N.; Roubalova, R.; Semerad, J.; Grasserova, A.; Benada, O.; Kofronova, O.; Cajthaml, T.; Dvorak, J.; Bilej, M.; Prochazkova, P. In Vitro Interactions of TiO_2 Nanoparticles with Earthworm Coelomocytes: Immunotoxicity Assessment. *Nanomaterials* **2021**, *11*, 250. [CrossRef]
140. Swart, E.; Dvorak, J.; Hernádi, S.; Goodall, T.; Kille, P.; Spurgeon, D.; Svendsen, C.; Prochazkova, P. The Effects of In Vivo Exposure to Copper Oxide Nanoparticles on the Gut Microbiome, Host Immunity, and Susceptibility to a Bacterial Infection in Earthworms. *Nanomaterials* **2020**, *10*, 1337. [CrossRef]
141. Dolar, A. Modulations of Immune Parameters Caused by Bacterial and Viral Infections in the Terrestrial Crustacean Porcellio Scaber: Implications for Potential Markers in Environmental Research. *Dev. Comp. Immunol.* **2020**, *113*, 103789. [CrossRef]
142. Canesi, L.; Ciacci, C.; Balbi, T. Invertebrate Models for Investigating the Impact of Nanomaterials on Innate Immunity: The Example of the Marine Mussel Mytilus spp. *CBNT* **2017**, *2*, 77–83. [CrossRef]
143. Barrick, A.; Guillet, C.; Mouneyrac, C.; Châtel, A. Investigating the Establishment of Primary Cultures of Hemocytes from Mytilus Edulis. *Cytotechnology* **2018**, *70*, 1205–1220. [CrossRef]
144. Katsumiti, A.; Tomovska, R.; Cajaraville, M.P. Intracellular Localization and Toxicity of Graphene Oxide and Reduced Graphene Oxide Nanoplatelets to Mussel Hemocytes in Vitro. *Aquat. Toxicol.* **2017**, *188*, 138–147. [CrossRef]
145. Sendra, M.; Volland, M.; Balbi, T.; Fabbri, R.; Yeste, M.P.; Gatica, J.M.; Canesi, L.; Blasco, J. Cytotoxicity of CeO_2 Nanoparticles Using in Vitro Assay with Mytilus Galloprovincialis Hemocytes: Relevance of Zeta Potential, Shape and Biocorona Formation. *Aquat. Toxicol.* **2018**, *200*, 13–20. [CrossRef]
146. Balbi, T.; Fabbri, R.; Montagna, M.; Camisassi, G.; Canesi, L. Seasonal Variability of Different Biomarkers in Mussels (*Mytilus Galloprovincialis*) Farmed at Different Sites of the Gulf of La Spezia, Ligurian Sea, Italy. *Mar. Pollut. Bull.* **2017**, *116*, 348–356. [CrossRef]
147. Katsumiti, A.; Gilliland, D.; Arostegui, I.; Cajaraville, M.P. Cytotoxicity and Cellular Mechanisms Involved in the Toxicity of CdS Quantum Dots in Hemocytes and Gill Cells of the Mussel Mytilus Galloprovincialis. *Aquat. Toxicol.* **2014**, *153*, 39–52. [CrossRef]
148. Canesi, L.; Auguste, M.; Bebianno, M.J. Sublethal Effects of Nanoparticles on Aquatic Invertebrates, from Molecular to Organism Level. In *Ecotoxicology of Nanoparticles in Aquatic Systems*; Blasco, J., Corsi, I., Eds.; CRC Press: Boca Raton, FL, USA, 2019; pp. 38–61.
149. Kádár, E.; Lowe, D.M.; Solé, M.; Fisher, A.S.; Jha, A.N.; Readman, J.W.; Hutchinson, T.H. Uptake and Biological Responses to Nano-Fe versus Soluble FeCl3 in Excised Mussel Gills. *Anal. Bioanal. Chem.* **2010**, *396*, 657–666. [CrossRef]
150. Pinsino, A.; Alijagic, A. Sea Urchin Paracentrotus Lividus Immune Cells in Culture: Formulation of the Appropriate Harvesting and Culture Media and Maintenance Conditions. *Biol. Open* **2019**, *8*, 7. [CrossRef]
151. Alijagic, A.; Gaglio, D.; Napodano, E.; Russo, R.; Costa, C.; Benada, O.; Kofronova, O.; Pinsino, A. Titanium Dioxide Nanoparticles Temporarily Influence the Sea Urchin Immunological State Suppressing Inflammatory-Relate Gene Transcription and Boosting Antioxidant Metabolic Activity. *J. Hazard. Mater.* **2020**, *11*. [CrossRef]
152. Nurnberger, T.; Brunner, F.; Kemmerling, B.; Piater, L. Innate Immunity in Plants and Animals: Striking Similarities and Obvious Differences. *Immunol. Rev.* **2004**, *198*, 249–266. [CrossRef]
153. Michelini, S.; Barbero, F.; Prinelli, A.; Steiner, P.; Weiss, R.; Verwanger, T.; Andosch, A.; Lütz-Meindl, U.; Puntes, V.F.; Drobne, D.; et al. Gold Nanoparticles (AuNPs) Impair LPS-Driven Immune Responses by Promoting a Tolerogenic-like Dendritic Cell Phenotype with Altered Endosomal Structures. *Nanoscale* **2021**. [CrossRef]
154. Koeffler, H.P. Human Myeloid Leukemia Cell Lines: A Review. *Blood* **1980**, *56*, 344–350. [CrossRef]
155. Kroll, A.; Pillukat, M.H.; Hahn, D.; Schnekenburger, J. Current in Vitro Methods in Nanoparticle Risk Assessment: Limitations and Challenges. *Eur. J. Pharm. Biopharm.* **2009**, *72*, 370–377. [CrossRef]

156. Pott, G.; Chan, E.; Dinarello, C.A.; Shapiro, L. A-1-Antitrypsin Is an Endogenous Inhibitor of Proinflammatory Cytokine Production in Whole Blood. *J. Leukoc. Biol.* **2009**, *85*, 11. [CrossRef] [PubMed]
157. Beguin, Y.; Noizat-Pirenne, F.; Pirenne, J.; Gathy, R.; Dehart, I.; Igot, D.; Baudrihaye, M.; Delacroix, D.; Franchimontl, P. Direct stimulation of cytokines (il-lp, tnf-a, il-6, il-2, ifn-y and gm-csf) in whole blood. I. Comparison with isolated pbmc stimulation. *Cytokine* **1992**, *4*, 239–248.
158. Kiertscher, S.M.; Roth, M.D. Human CD14 [+] Leukocytes Acquire the Phenotype and Function of Antigen-Presenting Dendritic Cells When Cultured in GM-CSF and IL-4. *J. Leukoc. Biol.* **1996**, *59*, 208–218. [CrossRef] [PubMed]
159. Pfeiffer, I.A. Leukoreduction System Chambers Are an Efficient, Valid, and Economic Source of Functional Monocyte-Derived Dendritic Cells and Lymphocytes. *Immunobiology* **2013**, *218*, 1392–1401. [CrossRef]
160. Arts, R.J.W. BCG Vaccination Protects against Experimental Viral Infection in Humans through the Induction of Cytokines Associated with Trained Immunity. *Cell Host Microbe* **2018**, *23*, 89–100.e5. [CrossRef]
161. Pfaller, T.; Colognato, R.; Nelissen, I.; Favilli, F.; Casals, E.; Ooms, D.; Leppens, H.; Ponti, J.; Stritzinger, R.; Puntes, V.; et al. The Suitability of Different Cellular in Vitro Immunotoxicity and Genotoxicity Methods for the Analy. *Nanotoxicology* **2010**, *4*, 52–72. [CrossRef]
162. Irvine, D.J.; Hanson, M.C.; Rakhra, K.; Tokatlian, T. Synthetic Nanoparticles for Vaccines and Immunotherapy. *Chem. Rev.* **2015**, *115*, 11109–11146. [CrossRef]
163. Siddiqui, D.M.H.; Al-Whaibi, M.H.; Mohammad, F. *Nanotechnology and Plant. Sciences: Nanoparticles and Their Impact on Plants*; Springer: New York, NY, USA; Berlin/Heidelberg, Germany, 2015; ISBN 978-3-319-14501-3.
164. Ma, X.; Geiser-Lee, J.; Deng, Y.; Kolmakov, A. Interactions between Engineered Nanoparticles (ENPs) and Plants: Phytotoxicity, Uptake and Accumulation. *Sci. Total Environ.* **2010**, *408*, 3053–3061. [CrossRef]
165. Koelmel, J.; Leland, T.; Wang, H.; Amarasiriwardena, D.; Xing, B. Investigation of Gold Nanoparticles Uptake and Their Tissue Level Distribution in Rice Plants by Laser Ablation-Inductively Coupled-Mass Spectrometry. *Environ. Pollut.* **2013**, *174*, 222–228. [CrossRef]
166. Avellan, A.; Schwab, F.; Masion, A.; Chaurand, P.; Borschneck, D.; Vidal, V.; Rose, J.; Santaella, C.; Levard, C. Nanoparticle Uptake in Plants: Gold Nanomaterial Localized in Roots of Arabidopsis Thaliana by X-Ray Computed Nanotomography and Hyperspectral Imaging. *Environ. Sci. Technol.* **2017**, *51*, 8682–8691. [CrossRef]
167. Kolenčík, M.; Ernst, D.; Komár, M.; Urík, M.; Šebesta, M.; Dobročka, E.; Černý, I.; Illa, R.; Kanike, R.; Qian, Y.; et al. Effect of Foliar Spray Application of Zinc Oxide Nanoparticles on Quantitative, Nutritional, and Physiological Parameters of Foxtail Millet (Setaria Italica L.) under Field Conditions. *Nanomaterials* **2019**, *9*, 1559. [CrossRef]
168. Al-Khaishany, M.Y. Role of Nanoparticles in Plants. In *Nanotechnology and Plant Sciences*; Siddiqui, M.H., Al-Whaibi, M.H., Mohammad, F., Eds.; Springer International Publishing: Cham, Swizterland, 2015; pp. 19–35, ISBN 978-3-319-14501-3.
169. Hayashi, Y.; Miclaus, T.; Engelmann, P.; Autrup, H.; Sutherland, D.S.; Scott-Fordsmand, J.J. Nanosilver Pathophysiology in Earthworms: Transcriptional Profiling of Secretory Proteins and the Implication for the Protein Corona. *Nanotoxicology* **2016**, *10*, 303–331. [CrossRef]
170. Waalewijn-Kool, P.L.; Ortiz, M.D. Effect of Different Spiking Procedures on the Distribution and Toxicity of ZnO Nanoparticles in Soil. *Ecotoxicol.* **2012**, *21*, 1797–1804. [CrossRef]
171. Boraschi, D.; Oostingh, G.J.; Casals, E.; Italiani, P.; Nelissen, I.; Puntes, V.F.; Duschl, A. Nano-Immunosafety: Issues in Assay Validation. *J. Phys. Conf. Ser.* **2011**, *304*, 9. [CrossRef]
172. Moret, Y.; Moreau, J. The Immune Role of the Arthropod Exoskeleton. *Invert. Surviv. J.* **2012**, *9*, 200–206.
173. Mayall, C.; Dolar, A.; Jemec Kokalj, A.; Novak, S.; Razinger, J.; Barbero, F.; Puntes, V.; Drobne, D. Stressor-Dependant Changes in Immune Parameters in the Terrestrial Isopod Crustacean, Porcellio Scaber: A Focus on Nanomaterials. *Nanomaterials* **2021**, *11*, 934. [CrossRef]
174. Duroudier, N.; Katsumiti, A.; Mikolaczyk, M.; Schäfer, J.; Bilbao, E.; Cajaraville, M.P. Dietary Exposure of Mussels to PVP/PEI Coated Ag Nanoparticles Causes Ag Accumulation in Adults and Abnormal Embryo Development in Their Offspring. *Sci. Total Environ.* **2019**, *655*, 48–60. [CrossRef]
175. Ward, J.E.; Kach, D.J. Marine Aggregates Facilitate Ingestion of Nanoparticles by Suspension-Feeding Bivalves. *Mar. Environ. Res.* **2009**, *68*, 137–142. [CrossRef]
176. Barmo, C.; Ciacci, C.; Canonico, B.; Fabbri, R.; Cortese, K.; Balbi, T.; Marcomini, A.; Pojana, G.; Gallo, G.; Canesi, L. In Vivo Effects of N-TiO_2 on Digestive Gland and Immune Function of the Marine Bivalve Mytilus Galloprovincialis. *Aquat. Toxicol.* **2013**, *132–133*, 9–18. [CrossRef]
177. Auguste, M. In Vivo Immunomodulatory and Antioxidant Properties of Nanoceria ($NCeO_2$) in the Marine Mussel Mytilus Galloprovincialis. *Comp. Biochem. Physiol. Part C Toxicol. Pharmacol.* **2019**, *219*, 95–102. [CrossRef]
178. Falugi, C. Toxicity of Metal Oxide Nanoparticles in Immune Cells of the Sea Urchin. *Mar. Environ. Res.* **2012**, *76*, 114–121. [CrossRef] [PubMed]
179. Pinsino, V.; Russo, P.; Bonaventura, R.; Brunelli, A.; Marcomini, A.; Matranga, V. Titanium Dioxide Nanoparticles Stimulate Sea Urchin Immune Cell Phagocytic Activity Involving TLR/P38 MAPK-Mediated Signalling Pathway. *Sci. Rep.* **2015**, *5*, 14492. [CrossRef] [PubMed]
180. Chivasa, S.; Ndimba, B.K.; Simon, W.J.; Lindsey, K.; Slabas, A.R. Extracellular ATP Functions as an Endogenous External Metabolite Regulating Plant Cell Viability. *Plant Cell* **2005**, *17*, 3019–3034. [CrossRef] [PubMed]

181. Bigorgne, E.; Foucaud, L.; Caillet, C.; Giamberini, L.; Nahmani, J.; Thomas, F.; Rodius, F. Cellular and Molecular Responses of E. Fetida Cœlomocytes Exposed to TiO$_2$ Nanoparticles. *J. Nanopart. Res.* **2012**, *14*, 1–17. [CrossRef]
182. Oostingh, G.J.; Casals, E.; Italiani, P.; Colognato, R.; Stritzinger, R.; Ponti, J.; Pfaller, T.; Kohl, Y.; Ooms, D.; Favilli, F.; et al. Problems and Challenges in the Development and Validation of Human Cell-Based Assays to Determine Nanoparticle-Induced Immunomodulatory Effects. *Part. Fibre Toxicol.* **2011**, *8*, 8. [CrossRef]
183. Jones, K.; Kim, D.W.; Park, J.S.; Khang, C.H. Live-Cell Fluorescence Imaging to Investigate the Dynamics of Plant Cell Death during Infection by the Rice Blast Fungus Magnaporthe Oryzae. *BMC Plant Biol.* **2016**, *16*, 69. [CrossRef]
184. Huang, C.-N.; Cornejo, M.J.; Bush, D.S.; Jones, R.L. Estimating Viability of Plant Protoplasts Using Double and Single Staining. *Protoplasma* **1986**, *135*, 80–87. [CrossRef]
185. Ciacci, C.; Canonico, B.; Bilaničová, D.; Fabbri, R.; Cortese, K.; Gallo, G.; Marcomini, A.; Pojana, G.; Canesi, L. Immunomodulation by Different Types of N-Oxides in the Hemocytes of the Marine Bivalve Mytilus Galloprovincialis. *PLoS ONE* **2012**, *7*, e36937. [CrossRef]
186. Moyen, N.E.; Bump, P.A.; Somero, G.N.; Denny, M.W. Establishing Typical Values for Hemocyte Mortality in Individual California Mussels, Mytilus Californianus. *Fish Shellfish Immunol.* **2020**, *100*, 70–79. [CrossRef]
187. de Araújo, R.F., Jr.; de Araújo, A.A.; Pessoa, J.B.; Freire Neto, F.P.; da Silva, G.R.; Leitão Oliveira, A.L.; de Carvalho, T.G.; Silva, H.F.; Eugênio, M.; Sant'Anna, C.; et al. Anti-Inflammatory, Analgesic and Anti-Tumor Properties of Gold Nanoparticles. *Pharmacol. Rep.* **2017**, *69*, 12. [CrossRef]
188. Ikegawa, H.; Yamamoto, Y.; Matsumoto, H. Cell Death Caused by a Combination of Aluminum and Iron in Cultured Tobacco Cells. *Physiol. Plant.* **1998**, *104*, 474–478. [CrossRef]
189. Katsumiti, A.; Gilliland, D.; Arostegui, I.; Cajaraville, M.P. Mechanisms of Toxicity of Ag Nanoparticles in Comparison to Bulk and Ionic Ag on Mussel Hemocytes and Gill Cells. *PLoS ONE* **2015**, *10*, e0129039. [CrossRef]
190. Fernández-Bautista, N.; Domínguez-Núñez, J.; Moreno, M.M.; Berrocal-Lobo, M. Plant Tissue Trypan Blue Staining During Phytopathogen Infection. *Bio-Protocol* **2016**, *6*. [CrossRef]
191. Gupta, S.; Kushwah, T.; Yadav, S. Earthworm Coelomocytes as Nanoscavenger of ZnO NPs. *Nanoscale Res. Lett* **2014**, *9*, 259. [CrossRef]
192. Parisi, M.G. Effects of Organic Mercury on Mytilus Galloprovincialis Hemocyte Function and Morphology. *J. Comp. Physiol. B* **2021**, *191*, 143–158. [CrossRef]
193. Murano, C.; Bergami, E.; Liberatori, G.; Palumbo, A.; Corsi, I. Interplay Between Nanoplastics and the Immune System of the Mediterranean Sea Urchin Paracentrotus Lividus. *Front. Mar. Sci.* **2021**, *8*, 647394. [CrossRef]
194. Karlsson, H.L.; Cronholm, P.; Gustafsson, J.; Moller, L. Copper Oxide Nanoparticles Are Highly Toxic: A Comparison between Metal Oxide Nanoparticles and Carbon Nanotubes. *Chem. Res. Toxicol.* **2008**, *21*, 1726–1732. [CrossRef]
195. Watanabe, M.; Setoguchi, D.; Uehara, K.; Ohtsuka, W.; Watanabe, Y. Apoptosis-like Cell Death of *Brassica Napus* Leaf Protoplasts. *New Phytol.* **2002**, *156*, 417–426. [CrossRef]
196. Wang, H.; Zhu, X.; Li, H.; Cui, J.; Liu, C.; Chen, X.; Zhang, W. Induction of Caspase-3-like Activity in Rice Following Release of Cytochrome-f from the Chloroplast and Subsequent Interaction with the Ubiquitin-Proteasome System. *Sci. Rep.* **2015**, *4*, 5989. [CrossRef]
197. Canesi, L.; Ciacci, C.; Bergami, E.; Monopoli, M.P.; Dawson, K.A.; Papa, S.; Canonico, B.; Corsi, I. Evidence for Immunomodulation and Apoptotic Processes Induced by Cationic Polystyrene Nanoparticles in the Hemocytes of the Marine Bivalve Mytilus. *Mar. Environ. Res.* **2015**, *111*, 34–40. [CrossRef]
198. Kumar, G.; Degheidy, H.; Casey, B.J.; Goering, P.L. Flow Cytometry Evaluation of in Vitro Cellular Necrosis and Apoptosis Induced by Silver Nanoparticles. *Food Chem. Toxicol.* **2015**, *85*, 45–51. [CrossRef]
199. Irizar, A. Establishment of Toxicity Thresholds in Subpopulations of Coelomocytes (Amoebocytes vs. Eleocytes) of Eisenia Fetida Exposed in Vitro to a Variety of Metals: Implications for Biomarker Measurements. *Ecotoxicology* **2015**, *24*, 1004–1013. [CrossRef] [PubMed]
200. Auguste, M.; Canesi, L. Shift in Immune Parameters After Repeated Exposure to Nanoplastics in the Marine Bivalve Mytilus. *Front. Immunol.* **2020**, *11*, 11. [CrossRef] [PubMed]
201. Rocha, T.L.; Gomes, T.; Cardoso, C.; Letendre, J.; Pinheiro, J.P.; Sousa, V.S.; Teixeira, M.R.; Bebianno, M.J. Immunocytotoxicity, Cytogenotoxicity and Genotoxicity of Cadmium-Based Quantum Dots in the Marine Mussel Mytilus Galloprovincialis. *Mar. Environ. Res.* **2014**, *101*, 29–37. [CrossRef] [PubMed]
202. Tomic, S.; Đokic, J.; Vasilijic, S.; Ogrinc, N.; Rudolf, R.; Pelicon, P.; Vučević, D.; Milosavljevic, P.; Rupnik, M.S.; Friedrich, B. Size-Dependent Effects of Gold Nanoparticles Uptake on Maturation and Antitumor Functions of Human Dendritic Cells In Vitro. *PLoS ONE* **2014**, *9*, e96584. [CrossRef]
203. Yan, A.; Chen, Z. Impacts of Silver Nanoparticles on Plants: A Focus on the Phytotoxicity and Underlying Mechanism. *IJMS* **2019**, *20*, 1003. [CrossRef]
204. Taylor, A.F.; Rylott, E.L.; Anderson, C.W.N.; Bruce, N.C. Investigating the Toxicity, Uptake, Nanoparticle Formation and Genetic Response of Plants to Gold. *PLoS ONE* **2014**, *9*, e93793. [CrossRef]
205. Hayashi, Y. Earthworms and Humans in Vitro: Characterizing Evolutionarily Conserved Stress and Immune Responses to Silver Nanoparticles. *Environ. Sci. Technol.* **2012**, *46*, 4166–4173. [CrossRef]

206. Auguste, M.; Mayall, C.; Barbero, F.; Hočevar, M.; Alberti, S.; Grassi, G.; Puntes, V.F.; Drobne, D.; Canesi, L. Functional and Morphological Changes Induced in Mytilus Hemocytes by Selected Nanoparticles. *Nanomaterials* **2021**, *11*, 470. [CrossRef]
207. Canesi, L.; Ciacci, C.; Fabbri, R.; Balbi, T.; Salis, A.; Damonte, G.; Cortese, K.; Caratto, V.; Monopoli, M.P.; Dawson, K.; et al. Interactions of Cationic Polystyrene Nanoparticles with Marine Bivalve Hemocytes in a Physiological Environment: Role of Soluble Hemolymph Proteins. *Environ. Res.* **2016**, *150*, 73–81. [CrossRef]
208. Katsumiti, A.; Arostegui, I.; Oron, M.; Gilliland, D.; Valsami-Jones, E.; Cajaraville, M.P. Cytotoxicity of Au, ZnO and SiO$_2$ NPs Using in Vitro Assays with Mussel Hemocytes and Gill Cells: Relevance of Size, Shape and Additives. *Nanotoxicology* **2015**, *10*, 185–193. [CrossRef]
209. Swartzwelter, B.J.; Barbero, F.; Verde, A.; Mangini, M.; Pirozzi, M.; Luca, A.C.D.; Puntes, V.F.; Leite, L.C.C.; Italiani, P.; Boraschi, D. Gold Nanoparticles Modulate BCG-Induced Innate Immune Memory in Human Monocytes by Shifting the Memory Response towards Tolerance. *Nanomaterials* **2019**, *9*, 1354. [CrossRef]
210. Kurepa, J.; Paunesku, T.; Vogt, S.; Arora, H.; Rabatic, B.M.; Lu, J.; Wanzer, M.B.; Woloschak, G.E.; Smalle, J.A. Uptake and Distribution of Ultrasmall Anatase TiO$_2$ Alizarin Red S Nanoconjugates in *Arabidopsis thaliana*. *Nano Lett.* **2010**, *10*, 2296–2302. [CrossRef]
211. Timmers, A.C.J.; Tirlapur, U.K.; Schel, J.H.N. Vacuolar Accumulation of Acridine Orange and Neutral Red in Zygotic and Somatic Embryos of Carrot (*Daucus Carota* L.). *Protoplasma* **1995**, *188*, 236–244. [CrossRef]
212. Weeks, J.M.; Svendsen, C. Neutral Red Retention by Lysosomes from Earthworm (*Lumbricus rubellus*) Coelomocytes: A Simple Biomarker of Exposure to Soil Copper. *Environ. Toxicol. Chem.* **1996**, *15*, 1801–1805. [CrossRef]
213. Long, J. Internalization, Cytotoxicity, Oxidative Stress and Inflammation of Multi-Walled Carbon Nanotubes in Human Endothelial Cells: Influence of Pre-Incubation with Bovine Serum Albumin. *RSC Adv.* **2018**, *8*, 9253–9260. [CrossRef]
214. Liu, Y.; Schiff, M.; Czymmek, K.; Tallóczy, Z.; Levine, B.; Dinesh-Kumar, S.P. Autophagy Regulates Programmed Cell Death during the Plant Innate Immune Response. *Cell* **2005**, *121*, 567–577. [CrossRef]
215. Patel, S.; Dinesh-Kumar, S.P. Arabidopsis ATG6 Is Required to Limit the Pathogen-Associated Cell Death Response. *Autophagy* **2008**, *4*, 20–27. [CrossRef]
216. Auguste, M. Effects of Nanosilver on Mytilus Galloprovincialis Hemocytes and Early Embryo Development. *Aquat. Toxicol.* **2018**, *203*, 107–116. [CrossRef]
217. Borges, J.; Porto-Neto, L.; Mangiaterra, M.; Jensch-Junior, B.; da Silva, J. Phagocytosis in Vitro and in Vivo in the Antarctic Sea Urchin Sterechinus Neumayeri at 0 °C. *Polar Biol.* **2002**, *25*, 891–897. [CrossRef]
218. Gustafson, H.H.; Holt-Casper, D.; Grainger, D.W.; Ghandehari, H. Nanoparticle Uptake: The Phagocyte Problem. *Nano Today* **2015**, *10*, 487–510. [CrossRef] [PubMed]
219. Thwala, M.; Musee, N.; Sikhwivhilu, L.; Wepener, V. The Oxidative Toxicity of Ag and ZnO Nanoparticles towards the Aquatic Plant Spirodela Punctuta and the Role of Testing Media Parameters. *Environ. Sci. Processes Impacts* **2013**, *15*, 1830. [CrossRef] [PubMed]
220. Sharma, P.; Bhatt, D.; Zaidi, M.G.H.; Saradhi, P.P.; Khanna, P.K.; Arora, S. Silver Nanoparticle-Mediated Enhancement in Growth and Antioxidant Status of Brassica Juncea. *Appl. Biochem. Biotechnol.* **2012**, *167*, 2225–2233. [CrossRef] [PubMed]
221. Moreira, R.; Romero, A.; Rey-Campos, M.; Pereiro, P.; Rosani, U.; Novoa, B.; Figueras, A. Stimulation of Mytilus Galloprovincialis Hemocytes With Different Immune Challenges Induces Differential Transcriptomic, MiRNomic, and Functional Responses. *Front. Immunol.* **2020**, *11*, 606102. [CrossRef]
222. Magesky, A.; de Oliveira Ribeiro, C.A.; Beaulieu, L.; Pelletier, É. Silver Nanoparticles and Dissolved Silver Activate Contrasting Immune Responses and Stress-Induced Heat Shock Protein Expression in Sea Urchin: Nanosilver and Dissolved Ag Effects in Sea Urchins. *Environ. Toxicol. Chem.* **2017**, *36*, 1872–1886. [CrossRef]
223. Minai, L.; Yeheskely-Hayon, D.; Yelin, D. High Levels of Reactive Oxygen Species in Gold Nanoparticle-Targeted Cancer Cells Following Femtosecond Pulse Irradiation. *Sci. Rep.* **2013**, *3*, srep02146. [CrossRef]
224. Shi, J. Inflammatory Caspases Are Innate Immune Receptors for Intracellular LPS. *Nat. Cell Biol.* **2014**, *514*, 187–192. [CrossRef]
225. Reddy Pullagurala, V.L.; Adisa, I.O.; Rawat, S.; Kalagara, S.; Hernandez-Viezcas, J.A.; Peralta-Videa, J.R.; Gardea-Torresdey, J.L. ZnO Nanoparticles Increase Photosynthetic Pigments and Decrease Lipid Peroxidation in Soil Grown Cilantro (Coriandrum Sativum). *Plant Physiol. Biochem.* **2018**, *132*, 120–127. [CrossRef]
226. Capolupo, M.; Valbonesi, P.; Fabbri, E. A Comparative Assessment of the Chronic Effects of Micro- and Nano-Plastics on the Physiology of the Mediterranean Mussel Mytilus Galloprovincialis. *Nanomaterials* **2021**, *11*, 649. [CrossRef]
227. Paciorek, P. Products of Lipid Peroxidation as a Factor in the Toxic Effect of Silver Nanoparticles. *Materials* **2020**, *13*, 2460. [CrossRef]
228. Chen, W.; Provart, N.J.; Glazebrook, J.; Katagiri, F.; Chang, H.-S.; Eulgem, T.; Mauch, F.; Luan, S.; Zou, G.; Whitham, S.A.; et al. Expression Profile Matrix of Arabidopsis Transcription Factor Genes Suggests Their Putative Functions in Response to Environmental Stresses. *Plant Cell* **2002**, *14*, 559–574. [CrossRef]
229. Tripathi, D.K.; Singh, S.; Singh, S.; Srivastava, P.K.; Singh, V.P.; Singh, S.; Prasad, S.M.; Singh, P.K.; Dubey, N.K.; Pandey, A.C.; et al. Nitric oxide alleviates silver nanoparticles (AgNps)-induced phytotoxicity in Pisum sativum seedlings. *Plant Physiol. Biochem.* **2017**, *110*, 167–177. [CrossRef]
230. Homa, J.; Zorska, A.; Wesolowski, D.; Chadzinska, M. Dermal Exposure to Immunostimulants Induces Changes in Activity and Proliferation of Coelomocytes of Eisenia Andrei. *J. Comp. Physiol. B* **2013**, *183*, 313–322. [CrossRef]

231. Ma, J.S.; Kim, W.J.; Kim, J.J.; Kim, T.J.; Ye, S.K.; Song, M.D.; Kang, H.; Kim, D.W.; Moon, W.K.; Lee, K.H. Gold Nanoparticles Attenuate LPS-Induced NO Production through the Inhibition of NF-κB and IFN-β/STAT1 Pathways in RAW264.7 Cells. *Nitric Oxide* **2010**, *23*, 214–219. [CrossRef]
232. Sakthivel, M.; Karthikeyan, N.; Palani, P. Detection and analysis of lysozyme activity in some tuberous plants and calotropis procera's latex. *J. Phytol.* **2010**, *2*, 65–72.
233. Fiołka, M.J.; Zagaja, M.P.; Hułas-Stasiak, M.; Wielbo, J. Activity and Immunodetection of Lysozyme in Earthworm Dendrobaena Veneta (Annelida). *J. Invertebr. Pathol.* **2012**, *109*, 83–90. [CrossRef]
234. Auguste, M.; Lasa, A.; Balbi, T.; Pallavicini, A.; Vezzulli, L.; Canesi, L. Impact of Nanoplastics on Hemolymph Immune Parameters and Microbiota Composition in Mytilus Galloprovincialis. *Mar. Environ. Res.* **2020**, *159*, 105017. [CrossRef]
235. Shimizu, M.; Kohno, S.; Kagawa, H.; Ichise, N. Lytic Activity and Biochemical Properties of Lysozyme in the Coelomic Fluid of the Sea UrchinStrongylocentrotus Intermedius. *J. Invertebr. Pathol.* **1999**, *73*, 214–222. [CrossRef]
236. Pagliara, P.; Stabili, L. Zinc Effect on the Sea Urchin Paracentrotus Lividus Immunological Competence. *Chemosphere* **2012**, *89*, 563–568. [CrossRef]
237. Ragland, S.A.; Criss, A.K. From Bacterial Killing to Immune Modulation: Recent Insights into the Functions of Lysozyme. *PLoS Pathog.* **2017**, *13*, e1006512. [CrossRef]
238. Dinarello, C.A. Historical Insights into Cytokines. *Eur. J. Immunol.* **2007**, *37*, S34–S45. [CrossRef] [PubMed]
239. Smith-Garvin, J.E.; Koretzky, G.A.; Jordan, M.S. T Cell Activation. *Annu. Rev. Immunol.* **2009**, *27*, 591–619. [CrossRef] [PubMed]
240. Procházková, P.; Silerova, M.; Stijlemans, B.; Dieu, M.; Halada, P.; Joskova, R.; Beschin, A.; De Baetselier, P.; Bilej, M. Evidence for Proteins Involved in Prophenoloxidase Cascade Eisenia Fetida Earthworms. *J. Comp. Physiol. B* **2006**, *176*, 581–587. [CrossRef] [PubMed]
241. Cheng, Y. Identification and Characterization of Proteins with Phenoloxidase-like Activities in the Sea Urchin Strongylocentrotus Nudus. *Fish Shellfish. Immunol.* **2015**, *47*, 117–121. [CrossRef] [PubMed]
242. Kumar, V.; Guleria, P.; Kumar, V.; Yadav, S.K. Gold Nanoparticle Exposure Induces Growth and Yield Enhancement in Arabidopsis Thaliana. *Sci. Total Environ.* **2013**, *462–468*. [CrossRef]
243. Bergami, E.; Krupinski Emerenciano, A.; González-Aravena, M.; Cárdenas, C.A.; Hernández, P.; Silva, J.R.M.C.; Corsi, I. Polystyrene Nanoparticles Affect the Innate Immune System of the Antarctic Sea Urchin Sterechinus Neumayeri. *Polar Biol.* **2019**, *42*, 743–757. [CrossRef]
244. Mincarelli, L. Evaluation of Gene Expression of Different Molecular Biomarkers of Stress Response as an Effect of Copper Exposure on the Earthworm EIsenia Andrei. *Ecotoxicology* **2019**, *28*, 938–948. [CrossRef]
245. Chan, S.L.; Mukasa, T.; Santelli, E.; Low, L.Y.; Pascual, J. The Crystal Structure of a TIR Domain from Arabidopsis Thaliana Reveals a Conserved Helical Region Unique to Plants. *Protein Sci.* **2009**. [CrossRef]
246. Vasilichin, V.A.; Tsymbal, S.A.; Fakhardo, A.F.; Anastasova, E.I.; Marchenko, A.S.; Shtil, A.A.; Vinogradov, V.V.; Koshel, E.I. Effects of Metal Oxide Nanoparticles on Toll-Like Receptor MRNAs in Human Monocytes. *Nanomaterials* **2020**, *10*, 127. [CrossRef]
247. Iizasa, S.; Iizasa, E.; Matsuzaki, S.; Tanaka, H.; Kodama, Y.; Watanabe, K.; Nagano, Y. Arabidopsis LBP/BPI Related-1 and -2 Bind to LPS Directly and Regulate PR1 Expression. *Sci. Rep.* **2016**, *6*, 27527. [CrossRef]
248. OSPAR. Background Document and Technical Annexes for Biological Effects Monitoring. 2013. Available online: https://mcc.jrc.ec.europa.eu/documents/OSPAR/OSPAR_CoordinatedEnvironmentalMonitoringProgramme_CEMP.pdf (accessed on 8 June 2021).
249. Conte, C.; Dal Poggetto, G.; Swartzwelter, B.; Esposito, D.; Ungaro, F.; Laurienzo, P.; Boraschi, D.; Quaglia, F. Surface Exposure of PEG and Amines on Biodegradable Nanoparticles as a Strategy to Tune Their Interaction with Protein-Rich Biological Media. *Nanomaterials* **2019**, *9*, 1354. [CrossRef]
250. Gautam, A. Immunotoxicity of Copper Nanoparticle and Copper Sulfate in a Common Indian Earthworm. *Ecotoxicol. Environ. Saf.* **2018**, *148*, 620–631. [CrossRef]
251. Dvořák, J.; Mančíková, V.; Pižl, V.; Elhottová, D.; Šilerová, M.; Roubalová, R.; Škanta, F.; Procházková, P.; Bilej, M. Microbial Environment Affects Innate Immunity in Two Closely Related Earthworm Species Eisenia Andrei and Eisenia Fetida. *PLoS ONE* **2013**, *8*, e79157.
252. Dvořák, J. Sensing Microorganisms in the Gut Triggers the Immune Response in Eisenia Andrei Earthworms. *Dev. Comp. Immunol.* **2016**, *57*, 67–74. [CrossRef]
253. Bhattacharya, K. *Fundamentals of Qualitative Research A Practical Guide*; Routledge: London, UK, 2017.
254. Banchereau, J.; Steinman, R.M. Dendritic Cells and the Control of Immunity. *Nature* **1998**, *392*, 245–252. [CrossRef]
255. Buffet, P.-E.; Richard, M.; Caupos, F.; Vergnoux, A.; Perrein-Ettajani, H.; Luna-Acosta, A.; Akcha, F.; Amiard, J.-C.; Amiard-Triquet, C.; Guibbolini, M.; et al. A Mesocosm Study of Fate and Effects of CuO Nanoparticles on Endobenthic Species (Scrobicularia Plana, Hediste Diversicolor). *Environ. Sci. Technol.* **2013**, 130110104824003. [CrossRef]
256. van Straalen, N.M.; Feder, M.E. Ecological and Evolutionary Functional Genomics—How Can It Contribute to the Risk Assessment of Chemicals? *Environ. Sci. Technol.* **2012**, *46*, 3–9. [CrossRef]
257. Maleck, K.; Levine, A.; Eulgem, T.; Morgan, A.; Schmid, J.; Lawton, K.A.; Dietrich, R.A. The Transcriptome of Arabidopsis Thaliana during Systemic Acquired Resistance. *Nat. Genet.* **2000**, *26*, 8. [CrossRef]
258. Détrée, C.; Gallardo-Escárate, C. Single and Repetitive Microplastics Exposures Induce Immune System Modulation and Homeostasis Alteration in the Edible Mussel Mytilus Galloprovincialis. *Fish Shellfish Immunol.* **2018**, *83*, 52–60. [CrossRef]

259. Felice, B.D.; Parolini, M. Can Proteomics Be Considered as a Valuable Tool to Assess the Toxicity of Nanoparticles in Marine Bivalves? *J. Mar. Sci. Eng.* **2020**, *8*, 1033. [CrossRef]
260. Duroudier, N. Changes in Protein Expression in Mussels Mytilus Galloprovincialis Dietarily Exposed to PVP/PEI Coated Silver Nanoparticles at Different Seasons. *Aquat. Toxicol.* **2019**, *210*, 56–68. [CrossRef] [PubMed]
261. Syu, Y. Impacts of Size and Shape of Silver Nanoparticles on Arabidopsis Plant Growth and Gene Expression. *Plant Physiol. Biochem.* **2014**, *83*, 57–64. [CrossRef] [PubMed]

MDPI
St. Alban-Anlage 66
4052 Basel
Switzerland
Tel. +41 61 683 77 34
Fax +41 61 302 89 18
www.mdpi.com

Nanomaterials Editorial Office
E-mail: nanomaterials@mdpi.com
www.mdpi.com/journal/nanomaterials

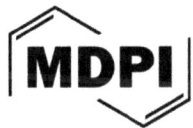